ADVANCED MEDICAL LIFE SUPPORT: ADULT MEDICAL EMERGENCIES

Mikel A. Rothenberg, M.D.
Emergency Care Educator
Department of Emergency Medicine
Lutheran Medical Center
Fairview General Hospital
Cleveland, Ohio

The C.V. Mosby Company
St. Louis ■ Toronto ■ Washington, D.C. ■ 1987

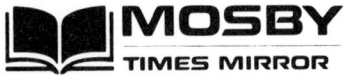

Executive Editor: David T. Culverwell
Senior Editor: Richard A. Weimer
Editorial Project Manager: Lisa G. Cunninghis
Project Manager: Janis K. Oppelt
Indexer: A. Tony Melendez

Library of Congress Cataloging-in-Publication Data

Rothenberg, Mikel A.
  Advanced medical life support.

  Bibiliography: p.
  Includes index.
  1. Emergency medicine. I. Title.
RC86.7.R685 1987   616′.025   87-24715
ISBN 0-8016-4284-1

Printed in the United States of America

The C.V. Mosby Company
11830 Westline Industrial Drive, St. Louis, Missouri 63146

BI/DC/DC 9 8 7 6 5 4 3

01/A/026

NOTICE
The indications and dosages of all drugs, procedures, and protocols in this text have been recommended in the medical literature and conform to the practices of the general medical community. The medications described do not necessarily have specific approval by the Food and Drug Administration (FDA) for use in the diseases and dosages for which they are recommended. The package insert for each drug should be consulted for use and dosage as approved by the FDA. Because standards for usage change, keep advised of revised recommendations.

To Diane, Kara, and Marc

About the Author

Dr. Rothenberg is a board certified internal medicine specialist with a special interest in critical care and emergency medicine. He has served as an ICU/CCU director as well as physician advisor for both air and ground ambulance services. While in private practice for four years in Montana, Dr. Rothenberg was active in several state wide emergency medicine related committees. Dr. Rothenberg is well-known for his work with the advanced cardiac life support course and the ACLS affiliate faculty of both the Montana and Washington Heart Association. He is also the executive editor of an advanced cardiac life support update newsletter entitled ''ACLS Alert,'' the author of ''Life Disc,'' a computerized ACLS review program, and ''Emergency Department Standards of Care: A Lawyer's Guide,'' a textbook on Emergency Department negligence for attorneys. In addition to working as an emergency physician and medicolegal expert in Cleveland, Ohio, Dr. Rothenberg travels nationally presenting courses on ACLS, adult medical emergencies, and medical negligence to both health care professionals and attorneys.

Preface

Advanced Medical Life Support: Adult Medical Emergencies (AMLS) is designed to bridge a large gap in the currently available literature covering Advanced Life Support. The focus of this text is to teach and review the rapid diagnosis and treatment of adult medical emergencies. Trauma is not discussed specifically, though there are certain areas where an overlap is unavoidable.

The scope of this text ranges from initial field care to initial Intensive Care Unit (ICU) procedures. Sophisticated critical care is not dealt with here. Though this work is specifically intended for Emergency Department/ICU nurses and physicians, the advanced Paramedic or Emergency Medical Technician may find selected sections of particular benefit. Many of the situations discussed occur commonly on the hospital ward as well. Prehospital procedures and recommendations are discussed because it is critically important that nurses and physicians understand the care given their patients before arrival at the hospital.

The organization of the didactic chapters follows a standardized format. Any necessary introductory material is presented first. Common problems are then discussed in order of significance and occurrence. Each entity is defined and causes listed. Diagnosis of the problem according to history (Hx), physical (Px), lab and other studies is then presented.

Emergency treatment, starting in the field, is listed and discussed next and, by necessity, presented in a "cookbook" format. Any protocol must be modified according to local regulation and patient necessity. The Appendices have a slightly different format.

The final section on each disease entity is entitled "Pearls to Remember." This is an attempt to share "words of wisdom" gleaned from the literature as well as from my personal experience in the field, Emergency Department, and ICU/CCU. These may be the most worthwhile suggestions in the text in terms of practical applicability. The Appendices should serve as reference material to delve further into areas not detailed in the format text.

Much of the information in this text is taken from current medical literature. Due to its timeliness, it is unlikely to be found in any but the most recent reference books. For this reason, I have included relevant journal references in the textual material as necessary, rather than group them all together in the Bibliography.

As this is a pilot effort, I welcome feedback and suggestions. I eventually hope to see a standardized course on adult medical emergencies presented from this material, including pre- and posttests and patient evaluation stations. I sincerely hope the reader finds this an educational and pleasant endeavor.

Mikel A. Rothenberg, M.D.

Acknowledgments

There are so many people to thank in preparing a work such as this that I am hard-pressed on where to begin. I honestly believe that the feedback I have received over the last four years from thousands of students in my Advanced Adult Medical Life Support classes throughout the country has been the single most helpful tool in preparing this final manuscript. Without their openness and honesty, this book could not have been.

Thanks to Drs. Timothy O'Dea and Jay Winship for reviewing the original Table of Contents and suggesting revisions. The time taken away from these physicians' busy practices is most appreciated.

Jim Brower of the St. Mary Medical Center Print Shop in Walla Walla, Washington is a special friend and expert. Without his assistance, the preliminary versions of this text, as well as my teaching materials, would not have been.

To Rick Weimer, Senior Editor of this project, I owe a special "thank you." Rick encouraged the continuation of this project when I was ready to stop. His honesty and efforts are sincerely appreciated.

To my wife, Diane, and my children, Kara and Marc: thank you for providing love and support. Your understanding of my need for frequent travel and many long hours locked in my office behind the computer mean everything to me. I love you.

Finally, thanks to modern technology. Without my computer and its word processing abilities, I could not have written this text. I am convinced that any individual's personal productivity can at least triple with the proper use of a computer.

Mikel A. Rothenberg, M.D.
July 17, 1989

General Principles

Certain general principles must be adhered to in the care of any emergency patient. The A, B, C,'s of Basic Life Support should always remain foremost in one's mind. Airway and oxygenation problems must be corrected before proceeding to other matters. If airway obstruction or poor oxygenation are ignored, the outcome will be poor regardless of how appropriate other Basic and Advanced Life Support measures have been.

It is essential that medical personnel be able to *recognize* and *respond* promptly to emergent difficulties. Attention to the A, B, C's as mentioned above is, of course, the first step in this response. Based on a brief history and physical, the patient's problem should be classified into a basic category of disease (i.e., respiratory, GI, etc.). Appropriate treatment can then be undertaken.

Shock must be recognized and managed according to the type. Ongoing monitoring of patient status is essential in all situations. The patient should be positioned for comfort unless their medical condition would dictate otherwise. This includes elevation of the legs for hypovolemic and neurogenic shock as well as elevation of the head and chest for respiratory distress.

Communication—beginning with the first patient contact—is essential. The exchange from patient to rescuer, rescuer to base station, base station to ED/ICU requires clear and concise transmission of information. This is the responsibility of all personnel. It is, finally, very important that all individuals involved in emergency care be able to anticipate and recognize unstable conditions requiring immediate treatment and/or transport.

Contents

Patient Assessment

Patient assessment is the key to identification and treatment of any medical problem. The components of an emergency patient assessment include:

- Environmental survey
- Primary survey
- Resuscitation phase
- Secondary survey
- Definitive care
- History.

As will be seen, there is often some overlap between various phases as life-threatening problems are treated. Protocols should NEVER replace sound judgment!

ENVIRONMENTAL SURVEY

The environmental survey is done as the patient is first approached, whether it be in the field or in the Emergency Department. Obvious environmental hazards, which may threaten the well-being of the rescuer, must be promptly identified. Once assured of their own safety, medical personnel should identify themselves, rapidly ascertain the patient's chief complaint, and note the position of the patient. This is the time to call for back-up if necessary (police if in the field, additional personnel if in the hospital).

PRIMARY SURVEY

The primary survey should take 30 seconds or less. It is easily remembered by the mnemonic "ABCDE":

- A—Airway
- B—Breathing
- C—Circulation
- D—Disability (neurological status)
- E—Expose (as necessary).

The **airway** is at least partially open if the patient is able to speak. Otherwise, utilize the chin lift or jaw thrust to open it. Debris should be cleared and potential airway problems such as dentures and a thick neck noted.

Breathing is checked by observation and by rapidly auscultating the anterior chest bilaterally for breath sounds. Respiratory noises and unusual efforts (wheezes, retractions) should be listened for. Skin color is noted as well as the patient's behavior. Remember, hypoxia can cause unusual behavior.

Adequacy of the **circulation** is best checked by the patient's pulse and capillary refill. Blood pressure measurement at this time is not an optimal use of resources. The quality, rate, and regularity of the pulse are easily discerned. A "ballpark" estimate of the blood pressure can be rapidly made by the location of palpable pulses. Presence of a radial pulse suggests a systolic blood pressure (BP) of at least 80 mm Hg, femoral pulse at least 70 mm Hg, and carotid pulse at least 60 mm Hg.

Capillary refill is checked by compressing the hypothenar eminence (fleshy part of palm across from the thumb). The color normally returns within two seconds (about the time it takes to say "capillary return"). Poor capillary refill suggests low cardiac output. This test is unreliable in a hypothermic patient or a cold environment.

Disability is evaluated and prevented by a brief neurological exam. Pupillary size and reaction is rapidly determined. The level of consciousness (LOC) is then evaluated based on the "AVPU" scale:

- A—Alert
- V—responds to *verbal* stimuli
- P—responds to *painful* stimuli
- U—unresponsive.

It may be necessary to **expose** (undress) the patient (preserving modesty) to evaluate their condition.

The 30 second primary survey is summarized in Table 1-1.

Table 1-1. Primary Survey (30 Seconds)

A—Airway

Open
Clear
Note problems (dentures, thick neck)

B—Breathing

Auscultate rapidly
Skin color
Behavior

C—Circulation

Pulse:
- Quality
- Rate, regularity
- Site obtained (radial = 80, femoral = 70, carotid = 60)

Capillary refill (normal = < 2 seconds)

D—Disability

Pupils
Level of consciousness:
- A—alert
- V—responds to verbal stimuli
- P—responds to painful stimuli
- U—Unresponsive

E—Expose

RESUSCITATION PHASE

The resuscitation phase should take place concomitantly with the primary survey. Airway maintenance, CPR, and other lifesaving modalities should be initiated when the problem is identified. DO NOT wait until the end of the primary survey just to be systematic.

Resuscitation, as a general rule, always involves placing the patient on oxygen. For most situations, 3–4 liters per minute (LPM) by nasal prongs (NP) will suffice. Higher or lower concentrations may be necessary, depending on the circumstances. A brief review of oxygen delivery systems is outlined below:

1. *Nasal prongs*—depend on respiratory frequency and depth of respiration. The fraction of inspired oxygen (FIO_2) is roughly $20 + (4 \times O_2$ flow in LPM). This system is ideal when a precise O_2 concentration is unimportant.

2. *Standard mask*—FIO_2 35%–55%, depending on O_2 flow and patient's ventilation; delivers an intermediate FIO_2 when the precise concentration, again, is unimportant.

3. *Partial rebreathing reservoir mask*—FIO_2 40%–90%.

4. *Nonrebreathing reservoir mask*—FIO_2 90%.

5. *Venturi mask*—delivers a specific low FIO_2 to the oxygen-sensitive patient; several masks are available. Uncomfortable for prolonged use; do not provide proper humidification.

An intravenous (IV) line is necessary to treat emergent situations. It is helpful if blood is drawn when the IV is inserted for glucose, electrolytes, and anything else deemed necessary. Many ambulance services have a standard "pack" of colored-top tubes they routinely fill when starting IVs—a procedure that is easily applied in an ED as well. The type of solution and rate of infusion depend upon the circumstances. D_5W or Ringer's Lactate (RL) at "to keep open" (TKO) will suffice for most clinical circumstances.

Military anti-shock trousers (MAST) can be applied if there is a possibility of shock, especially if the IV is difficult to start. They are inflated as necessary. Monitoring of the heart rhythm is necessary in almost all cases. Depending on the situation, a urinary catheter and/or nasogastric (NG) tube can be inserted; these are not routinely considered field procedures. The resuscitation phase is summarized in Table 1-2.

Table 1-2. Resuscitation Phase

- Supplemental oxygen—3–4 LPM via NP
- Draw blood
- IV—D$_5$W, RL TKO or as directed
- MAST suit—inflate if indicated
- EKG monitor
- Urinary catheter—if indicated
- NG tube—if indicated

SECONDARY SURVEY

The secondary survey is then performed. This outline is designed for examination of the patient with a purely *medical* problem. Certain vital steps in the treatment of a trauma patient are deliberately omitted.

The **head and face** are examined for deformities. Can the patient wrinkle their forehead? The mouth is then observed for patency of the airway, loose teeth, and tongue and jaw movements. Ears and nose are examined for discharge and bleeding. Eyes are checked for contact lenses, foreign bodies, pupillary responses, and extraocular movements. The fundi should also be visualized.

The **neck** is observed for venous distention and tracheal deviation. Is the patient using his accessory muscles of respiration? Be sure to check for a tracheostomy stoma and Medi-Alert tags.

The **chest** is observed for symmetry and the pattern of breathing—shallow, rapid, deep? Are retractions present? The lung fields are now more extensively auscultated for symmetry of breath sounds as well as extraneous noises. Abnormal respiratory sounds should be noted. Those experienced in cardiac auscultation should listen for dysrhythmias, gallops, clicks, and murmurs.

The **back** is briefly checked for tenderness, deformity, and edema, especially over the sacral area. The **abdomen** is auscultated for the presence of bowel sounds, palpated for tenderness and for rigidity. This examination will be further detailed on pages 113 to 115 where the acute abdomen is discussed.

The **extremities** are checked for the presence of pulses, color, Medi-Alert tags, and edema. **Neurological** function is assessed by determining strength, sensation, and the presence of reflexes. A **rectal** exam assesses sphincter tone, masses, and any blood in the stool. This is not considered to be a field procedure.

The **level of consciousness (LOC)** is assessed using the Glasgow Coma Scale as illustrated in Table 1-3. The mnemonic ''motor vehicle exam'' may be helpful in remembering the components of motor, verbal, and eye opening.

Table 1-3. Glasgow Coma Scale

Eye Opening
Never	1
Pain (responds to painful stimuli)	2
Speech (responds to verbal stimuli)	3
Spontaneous	4

Best Verbal
None	1
Garbled	2
Inappropriate	3
Confused	4
Oriented	5

Best Motor
None	1
Extension	2
Flexion	3
Withdrawal	4
Localizes pain	5
Obeys commands	6
Total	15

The secondary survey should take 3–5 minutes to complete. It should be systematic, though the exact order may vary from patient to patient. DO NOT interrupt this part of the evaluation for treatment unless deterioration in the A, B, C's is noted. Quantitative vital signs should be obtained AFTER the secondary survey unless the patient shows signs of shock, in which case they may be obtained earlier. The secondary survey is summarized in Table 1-4.

Definitive care depends on the particular situation. Lab and X-ray workup will be discussed under each individual entity.

The **history** can usually be obtained while doing the physical. Initially (often during the primary survey), an abbreviated "AMPLE" history can be taken:

A—Allergies
M—Medications (including over-the-counter, birth control)
P—Past illnesses
L—Last meal
E—Events surrounding problem.

With the above patient assessment, it should be relatively easy to embark on a course of further workup and initial treatment. In summary, the components of patient assessment are again:

- Environmental survey
- Primary survey
- Resuscitation phase
- Secondary survey
- Definitive care
- History.

Table 1-4. Secondary Survey

Head and Face
Deformity
Mouth—airway, loose teeth, tongue/jaw movements
Ears/Nose—discharge, bleeding
Eyes—pupils, foreign body, contacts, extraocular movements, fundi

Neck
Venous distension
Tracheal deviation
Accessory muscles of respiration
Stoma? Medi-Alert tag?

Chest
Inspection—symmetry, retractions, paradoxical movements
Breathing—shallow, rapid, deep
Breath sounds—symmetry, extraneous/abnormal sounds
Heart—rhythm, gallops, clicks, murmurs

Back
Tenderness, deformity
Edema

Abdomen
Bowel sounds
Tenderness, rigidity

Extremities/Neurological
Pulses, color
Medi-Alert tag
Strength, sensation, reflexes
Edema

Rectal
Tone, masses
Blood

Level of Consciousness
Glasgow Coma Scale—eyes (4), verbal (5), motor (6)

Cardiovascular Emergencies

The majority of true medical emergencies encompass those of a cardiovascular nature. Of these, cardiac arrest, dysrhythmias, and chest pain are the most common. The American Heart Association's Advanced Cardiac Life Support course covers much of this information. This section will cover:

- Acute pulmonary edema
- Hypertensive crisis
- Syncope
- Chest pain.

The final chapter, "Synthesis," beginning on page 159, will review the general approach to the "shocky" patient.

ACUTE PULMONARY EDEMA

Acute pulmonary edema can be defined as the filling of the pulmonary interstitial spaces, and then the alveoli, with fluid from the capillary bed. Although many mechanisms play a role, the two most common causes will be presented here.

Fluid can extravasate due to either increased capillary pressure or from increased capillary permeability. The former mechanism is responsible for pulmonary edema in myocardial infarction, congestive heart failure, and fluid overload. Elevated pulmonary and cardiac pressures may be responsible for the formation of pulmonary edema during acute epiglottitis as well [Ann Emerg Med, January 1985, Vol. 14, pp. 60-63]. Ischemic pulmonary edema

without concurrent myocardial infarction is associated with a two-year mortality of 70% in patients over 70 years of age. Coronary artery bypass in this group can result in marked improvement of symptoms [NEJM, 1985, Vol. 313, p. 1207].

Increased permeability is responsible for edema formation in hypoxia (Adult Respiratory Distress Syndrome—ARDS), chemical irritation, sepsis, and heroin overdose—so-called noncardiogenic pulmonary edema. Ethylene glycol ingestion has also been reported to cause permeability pulmonary edema [Ann Emerg Med, June 1985, Vol. 14, pp. 594-596]. Anaphylactic shock is felt to occasionally result in pulmonary edema via the same mechanism.

An interesting syndrome of unilateral pulmonary edema occurs following rapid suction expansion of a spontaneous pneumothorax that is over three days old. Thus, a simple underwater seal or frequent small aspirations of air should be used, rather than suction, on these patients [J. Em Med, 1983, Vol. 1, pp. 29-36].

Numerous other causes of noncardiogenic pulmonary edema have been reported including trauma [J. Trauma, 1986, Vol. 26, p. 409], airway obstruction [Ped Emerg Care, 1986, Vol. 2, p. 235], intravenous ethclorvynol [Am J Emerg Med, 1986, Vol. 4, p. 549], and intrabiliary infusion of agents for gallstone dissolution [Crit Care Med, 1986, Vol. 14, p. 659].

The increase in capillary permeability occurs due to damage of the tight junctions which hold endothelial cells together. Thus, fluid and proteins are able to leak out with relatively little (if any) change in transmural pressures. It is felt that oxygen-derived free radicals generated from complement-activated granulocytes are possibly involved in the vascular damage that leads to permeability changes [*Ann Emerg Med,* August 1985, Vol. 14, pp. 724—728]. Irrespective of the mechanism, the end point in pulmonary edema is a shunt effect where nonfunctional alveoli are unable to reoxygenate venous blood. This shunt effect as well as the differences between hydrostatic and permeability pulmonary edema are illustrated in Figures 2.1 and 2.2.

NORMAL ALVEOLUS WHICH COMPLETELY OXYGENATES THE BLOOD PASSING IT

DEOXYGENATED BLOOD FROM THE RIGHT-SIDED CIRCULATION (RIGHT HEART)

PARTICALY OXYGENATED BLOOD DUE TO SHUNT FROM "FLOODED" ALVEOLUS

Deoxygenated Blood

Oxygenated Blood

Alveolus filled with edema fluid cannot oxygenate blood

Figure 2.1. Shunt effect of pulmonary edema.

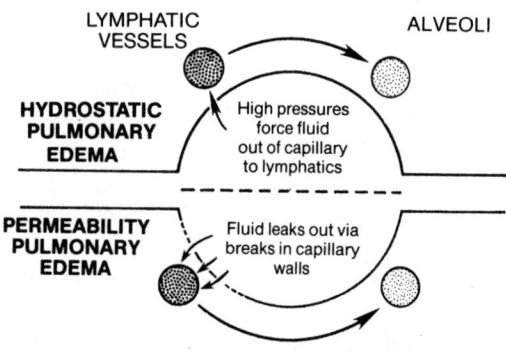

LYMPHATIC VESSELS

ALVEOLI

HYDROSTATIC PULMONARY EDEMA

High pressures force fluid out of capillary to lymphatics

PERMEABILITY PULMONARY EDEMA

Fluid leaks out via breaks in capillary walls

Figure 2.2. Differences in hydrostatis versus permeability pulmonary edema.

Neurogenic pulmonary edema has always been classified as being of the "permeability" type. It should be noted that several workers have proposed that, initially, there is a period of increased hydrostatic pressure which leads to endothelial cell damage. It is felt these secondary effects lead to increased permeability [*J Aeromedical Health Care,* September/October 1985, p. 14]. This hypothesis is not uniformly accepted.

Diagnosis

History

A patient in acute pulmonary edema may give a history of acute or chronic symptoms with sudden exacerbation. They are dyspneic (short of breath) and may be terrified with a sensation of "impending doom." Often, there is a history of orthopnea (increased shortness of breath with reclining). The patient may actually have awakened at night with difficulty breathing—paroxysmal nocturnal dyspnea (PND). Cough and/or chest pain may be prominent complaints.

Physical examination

The physical exam reveals a patient who is usually sitting upright. They appear tachypneic with rapid, labored respirations. Wheezes and rales may be prominent. The neck veins are distended, and the measured jugular venous pressure is elevated (greater than 10 cm). Gallop rhythms, edema, and cyanosis may be present. Pink, frothy sputum is seen late in the course of the disease but is highly suggestive of the diagnosis. Interestingly, in one large study, jugular venous distention was noted in only 45.7%, an S_3 (gallop) in 25.5%, and peripheral edema in 34% of patients [*Arch Intern Med,* 1986, Vol. 146, pp. 489—493].

Laboratory tests

Lab tests are optional in making the diagnosis. If obtained, arterial blood gases will most commonly show a respiratory alkalosis or a combined metabolic acidosis-respiratory alkalosis.

The **chest X-ray** may not reflect the severity of the disease but often shows increased heart size. Haziness in the peripheral fields, so-called perivascular cuffing, may be noted. As pulmonary edema progresses, homogeneous radiopacities radiating symmetrically from the hila in the well-known "butterfly" configuration may be seen. In late stages, bilateral "white-outs" of both lung fields are present. It has also been established that although the chest X-ray may show pulmonary edema-type changes, findings do not necessarily correlate with extravascular lung water in critically ill patients [*Chest,* 1985, Vol. 88, pp. 649–652]. A typical chest film of florid pulmonary edema is shown in Figure 2.3.

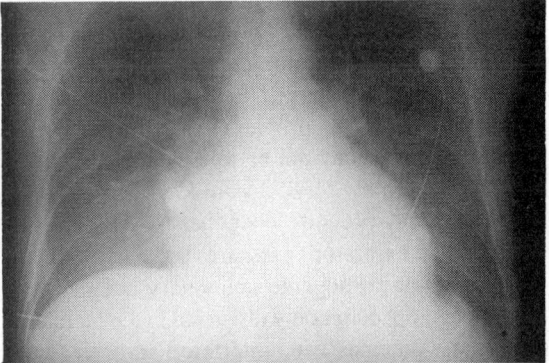

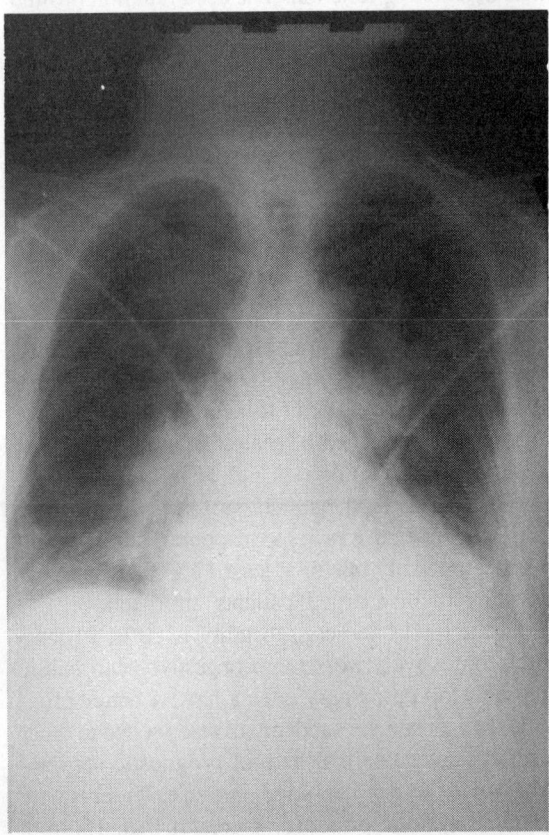

Figure 2.3. Typical chest X-rays of pulmonary edema.

Treatment

Treatment for acute hydrostatic pulmonary edema is initiated by placing the patient in an upright, sitting position and administering 4–6 LPM of oxygen, preferably by nasal prongs. Many believe it is an error to place an oxygen mask over the mouth and nose of a patient who is already markedly short of breath and feeling "smothered."

An IV line of D_5W is started. Once established, medications can be given as follows:

1. MORPHINE SULFATE—This is the single most important drug due to its vasodilating and antianxiety effects. The dose is 2–4 mg IV every 3–5 minutes as needed.
2. FUROSEMIDE (LASIX)—40 mg IV— may be repeated at double this dose in 10–15 minutes if necessary. This drug has three important actions in pulmonary edema (see Table 2-1). These may be different from its action in chronic congestive heart failure without pulmonary edema where furosemide has been shown to transiently increase the left ventricular filling pressure and decrease the cardiac index [*Ann Int Med,* 1985, Vol. 103, pp. 1–6].
3. AMINOPHYLLINE—This decreases pulmonary venous pressure, increases cardiac contractility, and produces a bronchodilatory effect. The loading dose is 6 mg/kg over 15–20 minutes IV (mix in D_5W, 100 cc). Depending on the response, a drip may then be given at .6–.9 mg/kg/hr.
4. DIGOXIN—This is optional, in acute pulmonary edema, since its acute effects are probably limited to the treatment of supraventricular dysrhythmias. If these are present, digoxin is definitely indicated.
    Severely compromised patients who fail to respond to diuretics, morphine, and vasodilators may also benefit from digitalization [*Jrnl Am Coll Card,* 1987, Vol. 9, pp. 849–857].
5. NITROGLYCERIN—Use either the sublingual or intravenous form of this drug.

Table 2-1. The Actions of Furosemide

Diuretic

Causes diuresis within 5–15 minutes when given intravenously

Venodilatory

- Causes rapid venodilation with decreased preload in acute pulmonary edema
- In chronic congestive failure, may cause an initial increase in systemic vascular resistance

Lymphatic

Increases efferent lymphatic flow from the lungs, resulting in a net flow of fluid from the pulmonary interstitium and avleoli into the circulatory system

Thus, the administration of furosemide causes an eflux of fluid from the lungs to the central vascular space, a decrease in ventricular preload, and diuresis. These actions work synergistically to decrease pulmonary edema.

See Appendix B on page 180 for further guidelines.

6. NITROPRUSSIDE—Some feel that, due to its mixed vasodilator effect, this agent may be the drug of choice in acute pulmonary edema; the literature on this is very limited at this point, but this drug should be considered in difficult patients [*Emergency Medical Services,* May 1986, pp. 22-B–22-L].

7. AMRINONE—This newer positive inotropic agent can dramatically increase the cardiac output. Again, its use should be considered in difficult patients.

8. CHLORPROMAZINE—This drug, given 5 mg IV every few hours, has been reported to treat neurogenic pulmonary edema via an alpha-receptor blockade (a central effect) [*Crit Care Med,* 1985, Vol. 13, pp. 210–211].

In either type of pulmonary edema, continuous positive airway pressure (CPAP) may be given via a face mask. The only problem is that the mask must fit tightly, and it may not be tolerated by the ill patient [*Am J Cardio,* 1985, Vol. 55, pp. 296–300]. Positive airway pressure via either CPAP or PEEP (positive end expiratory pressure) is the treatment of choice for noncardiogenic pulmonary edema.

Though not commonly discussed in the literature, pulmonary edema can interfere severely with mechanical lung function. The accumulation of fluid leads to decreased lung volumes and compliance with an increase in airway resistance. Large transpulmonary gradients and negative pleural pressures are required to maintain adequate alveolar ventilation. This great work of breathing can easily lead to a decrease in ventricular performance. Thus, consideration of intubation and mechanical ventilation may be necessary in the patient who does not respond to the above therapies [*Int Crit Care Dig,* 1985, Vol. 4, pp. 29–31].

MAST garments are absolutely contraindicated in acute pulmonary edema. Rotating tourniquets have been used but are difficult to manage and may have no true clinical or hemodynamic affect [*Annals Em Med,* July, 1987, Vol. 16, pp. 764–767].

The survival in patients suffering cardiogenic pulmonary edema appears to be poor. There is an in-hospital mortality rate of at least 17%. The one-year mortality of discharged patients approaches 40%. Thus, the total one-year mortality is 50%. Patients with progressively worsening congestive heart failure who develop pulmonary edema have a better prognosis than those who suddenly develop it due to other cardiac causes. A final helpful prognostic sign appears to be the systolic blood pressure. Patients with an initial systolic pressure of greater than 160 mm Hg seem to do better [*Arch Intern Med,* 1986, Vol. 146, pp. 489–493]. The approach to acute pulmonary edema is summarized in Table 2-2.

Table 2-2. Acute Pulmonary Edema

Mechanisms
Increased capillary pressure (MI, CHF, fluid overload)
Increased capillary permeability (ARDS, sepsis, heroin)

History
Dyspnea, sense of "impending doom"
Orthopnea, paroxysmal nocturnal dyspnea
Cough, chest pain

Physical
Sitting, upright position
Tachypnea, rapid and labored respirations
Wheezes, rales
Jugular venous distension
Cardiac gallop rhythm
Edema, cyanosis, pink frothy sputum

Lab
ABG—respiratory alkalosis or metabolic acidosis/respiratory alkalosis
CXR—cardiomegaly, haziness, "butterfly," white-out

Treatment, General
Sitting, upright position
4–6 LPM NP
IV D$_5$W
Cardiac monitoring
Rotating tourniquets
(Note: MAST garment contraindicated)

Treatment, Drug
Morphine sulfate
Furosemide
Aminophylline
Digoxin
Nitroglycerin

HYPERTENSIVE CRISIS

A hypertensive crisis (hypertensive emergency) is a true life-threatening emergency. It is extremely important to distinguish between a **hypertensive emergency** (crisis) and a **hypertensive urgency.**

Emergencies are those conditions in which severe end-organ damage is present, the diastolic blood pressure is usually > 120, and a delay in appropriate therapy might result in progression of end-organ damage with major complications, a poorer overall prognosis, or death (intracranial hemorrhage/thrombotic stroke, subarachnoid hemorrhage, hypertensive encephalopathy, acute aortic dissection, acute pulmonary edema, eclampsia, pheochromocytoma, severe eye changes, acute renal insufficiency, myocardial insufficiency syndromes).

Of these, hypertensive encephalopathy is of particular concern. There appears to be a loss of the cerebral autoregulatory mechanism, which normally maintains normal cerebral blood flow despite wide fluctuations in systemic arterial pressure. Thus, there is diffuse cerebral dysfunction. Headaches, lethargy, confusion, gastrointestinal symptoms, disturbed vision, and neurological signs may be noted.

Urgencies include those conditions with minimal or no end-organ damage and a diastolic blood pressure usually > 120 mm Hg in which the risk of immediate complications is less likely to occur, and the immediate prognosis is better if appropriate therapy is instituted. Progression to a hypertensive emergency is likely if treatment is not rapidly undertaken (early eye changes, postoperative HBP, preoperative uncontrolled hypertension). The differences between hypertensive urgencies and emergencies are summarized in Table 2-3.

The cause of hypertensive crisis is usually an acute exacerbation of idiopathic hypertension, but other conditions may less commonly be associated. Acute left ventricular failure or coronary insufficiency may significantly elevate the blood pressure, though the effect is usually the opposite. Eclampsia of pregnancy, acute glomerulonephritis, dissecting aortic aneurysm, and pheochromocytoma (epinephrine-producing tumor) can cause crises. Finally, some postoperative patients, and often individuals with head injury or intracranial hemorrhage, can have hypertensive crises.

Table 2-3. Hypertensive Urgencies Versus Emergencies

Emergencies
Severe end-organ damage present
- Intracranial hemorrhage
- Thrombotic stroke
- Hypertensive encephalopathy
- Acute aortic dissection
- Acute pulmonary edema
- Severe eye-ground (fundus) changes
- Acute renal insufficiency

Diastolic blood pressure is usually over 120 mm Hg; delay may result in:
- Progression of organ damage
- Poorer prognosis
- Death

Urgencies
Minimal or no end-organ damage;
Progression to an emergency likely if not treated
- Early eye changes
- Postoperative hypertension
- Myocardial infarction
- Uncontrolled essential hypertension

The acute withdrawal of many antihypertensive agents (especially clonidine) has led to massive blood pressure elevations. In rare cases, clonidine withdrawal leads to such significant rebound catecholamine release that the blood pressure may actually be unobtainable without intra-arterial monitoring. This is due to an extremely high systemic vascular resistance. Doses of > 1.0 mg/day are often required. Most patients are on considerably less. Interestingly, rebound hypertension has been associated with the clonidine transdermal administration system when an area of local dermatitis develops at the patch placement site [*West J Med,* July 1986, p. 102].

Diagnosis

History
There is often a history of inadequately treated hypertension. The patient may complain of a severe, generalized headache. Blurring of vision, vomiting, confusion, or a comatose state may be present.

Physical examination
On physical exam, the blood pressure is usually noted to be > 250/150 mm Hg unless the crisis is hyperacute (i.e., head injury, intracranial bleeding, eclampsia). It should be noted that hypertensive crisis can present with signs of cerebral insufficiency with a relatively modest elevation in the blood pressure if the patient has a low baseline reading (such as 100/70, where 160/100 is potentially a "crisis" level).

Possibly, there may be evidence of trauma. On funduscopic exam, hemorrhage, exudates, spasm, or papilledema may be present. Nuchal rigidity (stiff neck) suggests subarachnoid hemorrhage.

Laboratory tests
Lab findings are nonspecific. One should order a complete blood count (CBC), urinalysis (UA), electrolytes, BUN/creatinine, and electrocardiogram (EKG).

A **chest X-ray** may be helpful if aortic dissection or heart failure is a strong consideration.

Treatment

The initial treatment consists of providing oxygen (4–6 LPM NP) and starting an IV line. It is important to remember NOT to use D_5W alone if increased intracranial pressure is suspected, as this will further elevate it. Normal saline is preferable. Remember, isolated intracranial problems rarely cause *hypotension* except in their very late stages; if your patient is deteriorating and hypotensive, be sure to look for another cause.

Numerous drug regimens are published for the treatment of hypertensive crises of different etiologies. The goal, generally, is to safely reduce the blood pressure within one hour. Listed below is a regimen that may be used for hypertensive emergencies under ALL circumstances, is safe, and will usually work:

1. NITROPRUSSIDE—50 mg in 250 cc D_5W IV and titrate. NO other diluent other than D_5W should be used with nitroprusside. This is the BEST drug choice as it is not contraindicated in any form of emergently elevated blood pressure. Many recommend the use of an intra-arterial line for ongoing assessment, though, several experts feel this to be optional, as long as the patient's blood is monitored frequently using standard methods. The average dose is 3 mg/Kg/min with a range of 0.5–10 mg/Kg/min. Though cyanide toxicity can occur with prolonged infusions this is not a realistic consideration in the emergent situation. This agent has been shown to be safe in pregnancy-associated hypertension as well [*Obstet Gynecol,* 1982, Vol. 60, p. 533].

2. NITROGLYCERIN—The IV form of this (50–100 mg in 250 cc D_5W and titrated) is generally a good second choice EXCEPT in dissecting aortic aneurysm and in cases where increased intracranial pressure is present—venodilation caused by this agent will further elevate it.

3. PROPRANOLOL should be added to nitroprusside in suspected dissecting aortic aneurysm. Alternatively, use TRIMETHA-PHAN (Arfonad) 500 mg in 500 cc D_5W at 3–4 micrograms per minute IV.

4. FUROSEMIDE—Given 40 mg IV along with other drugs to offset fluid retention that may be caused by vasodilators and ganglionic blockers.

Other agents, especially diazoxide (Hyperstat) and hydralazine (Apresoline) have too many side effects and contraindications to make their inclusion in standard protocols worthwhile. A new agent, labetolol, has been recently released in an IV form that is indicated for acute hypertensive crises. Its beta-blocking properties prevent use in patients with asthma, congestive heart failure, and heart block. The data is inconclusive at this time though it may be especially helpful in a hypertensive crisis resulting from ingestion of a mixed alpha/beta-stimulatory agent such as cocaine or pseudoephedrine. In this case, treatment of the beta effects alone (such as with propranolol) may lead to a paradoxical elevation of the blood due to unopposed alpha stimulation [*Am J Emerg Med,* 1985, Vol. 4, pp. 141–142].

Several studies suggest that sublingual nifedipine is safe and effective in both hypertensive crises and urgencies. It has a rapid onset of action (buccal, 5–15 minutes; oral, 30–45 minutes) and peak effect (buccal, 30 minutes; oral, 60 minutes). The duration of action is 4–6 hours with mean BP drop of 21.6% [*Am J Emerg Med,* 1985, Vol. 3, pp. 524–530]. Either 10 or 20 mg of sublingual nifedipine initiated a smooth and predictable decline in blood pressure within 5 minutes and produced a peak effect between 30 and 60 minutes. One report has suggested that chewing the capsule and swallowing the contents may lead to more rapid absorption [*Am J Med,* 1986, Vol. 81 (suppl 6A), p. 2], though the majority of experts favor the sublingual route [*J Clin Hypertens,* 1986, Vol. 3, p. 55S].

The most attractive feature of this method of treatment is the fact that the acute hypotensive effect of sublingual nifedipine can predict the efficacy of subsequent oral nifedipine used on a chronic basis [*Am J Med,* 1986, Vol. 81 (suppl 6A), p. 35]. One case of syncope and conduction disturbance following sublingual nifedipine for a hypertensive crisis has been reported [*Ann Emerg Med,* October 1985, Vol. 14, pp. 1005–1006].

One study has noted efficacy using sublingual captopril (25 mg) in hypertensive crisis [*Lancet,* July 6, 1986, p. 34]. It appears that the decrease in blood pressure using this agent is not associated with reflex tachycardia so often seen with nifedipine. This agent should still be considered highly experimental for hypertensive crisis at the present time.

Clonidine has been used via a rapid-loading oral regimen in both hypertensive emergencies and urgencies. The oral regimen is now generally recommended only for **urgencies.** The initial dose is .1–.2 mg followed by hourly oral doses of .1 mg to a total loading dose of .7 mg or until blood pressure control is achieved. A significant reduction occurs in 91% of patients. This method is smooth, quick, and predictable with a low incidence of clinical side effects (sedation, dizziness, and dry mouth are the most common—hypotension or orthostasis was rare—0–5%) [*Cardiovascular Reviews & Reports,* November 1985, p. 1249]. Naloxone may be used to reverse clonidine-induced hypotension if this complication occurs. Doses of 2 mg every hour as needed have been used [*Ann Emerg Med,* October 1986, Vol. 15, p. 1229]. Hypertensive crisis is summarized in Table 2-4.

A final note should be made regarding an unusual, though potentially fatal, cause of hypertensive crisis which does not nicely fit into the above scheme—**autonomic dysreflexia** in the patient whose spinal cord is injured. This syndrome occurs in quadriplegics and paraplegics whose lesion is at or above the T6 (sixth thoracic) vertebral level. Due to an imbalance between ingoing and outgoing autonomic nervous signals, certain visceral stimuli (particularly from the bladder, colon, rectum, uterus, and skin) can lead to reflex vasoconstriction below the level of the spinal cord lesion, leading to severe hypertension.

The more common **cause** of this problem is bladder distension. Others include: rectal distension (occurring from procedures such as sigmoidoscopy and colonoscopy), acute abdominal conditions (appendicitis, perforated ulcer), childbirth, garments that are too tight, and decubitus ulcers.

The **history** is that of spinal cord damage. Often the patient is aware of the diagnosis and will provide it by name. Anxiety, headache, blurred vision, nausea, and flushing may be noted.

Physical findings include hypertension and the expected concomitants of any hypertensive crisis discussed above. Additionally, bradycardia and piloerection may be noted. Examination of the bladder may reveal distension. Rectal examination may show the presence of a fecal impaction. Particular attention should be paid to the presence of abdominal signs suggesting peritoneal irritation.

Table 2-4. Hypertensive Crisis

Causes (Diastolic Blood Pressure > 140 mm Hg)
Acute exacerbation of hypertension
Left ventricular failure
Acute coronary insufficiency
Pregnancy
Acute glomerulonephritis
Dissecting aortic aneurysm
Acute withdrawal of antihypertensive agents
Surgery
Head injury, intracranial hemorrhage

History
Inadequately controlled hypertension, abrupt discontinuation of antihypertensive medications
Severe generalized headache
Blurred vision, vomiting, confusion

Physical
Blood pressure usually > 250/150 mm Hg
? Evidence of trauma
Fundi—hemorrhage, exudates, spasm, papilledema
Nuchal rigidity

Lab
CBC, UA, lytes, BUN/creatinine—nonspecific
EKG, chest X-ray

Treatment
Oxygen, 4–6 LPM NP
IV, normal saline, TKO
Drugs:
- Nitroprusside
- Nitroglycerin
- Propranolol/trimethaphan (dissecting aneurysm only)
- Furosemide

The **treatment** of autonomic dysreflexia is basically removal of the causative stimulus. The patient is seated upright, and all tight clothing is removed. The bladder is checked first. If a Foley catheter is in place, it is immediately replaced if there is any suggestion of blockage. If a distended bladder is decompressed, it should be irrigated with 30 cc of 2% lidocaine to inhibit further sensory stimulation. Similar principles apply to the rectal exam (though lidocaine jelly should be used instead). Standard drug therapy (as discussed above) should be used if these methods do not result in prompt decreases in blood pressure.

Autonomic dysreflexia may be prevented in spinal cord-injured patients by administering ganglionic-blocking drugs 20–30 minutes prior to performing any urological or gastrointestinal procedures. If a patient has previously experienced this problem, either general, spinal, or epidural anesthesia may be required [*Rehab Nursing,* 1983, Vol. 16, p. 9].

SYNCOPE

Syncope is defined as a transient state of unconsciousness caused by inadequate perfusion of the brain *from which the patient has recovered.* If the victim is still unconscious, they should be treated according to the "coma" protocol. Syncope can be caused by any factor that leads to a sudden decrease in cardiac output or venous return. Categories of syncope include: neurogenic, vascular, cardiac, metabolic, and psychiatric.

The commonest neurogenic cause of syncope is the vasovagal or simple "faint." Consciousness returns quickly once the patient is recumbent. Cerebral ischemia, either from intracerebral disease (seizure) or vascular problems (subclavian steal, cough/micturition syncope) can also lead to syncope. Disorders of the carotid sinus can cause bradycardia and vasodepressor reactions.

Vascular causes of syncope include blood or fluid loss, especially from occult gastrointestinal bleeding. Impairment of vascular tone due to peripheral neurologic impairment (autonomic neuropathy), poor muscle tone, and venous insufficiency can also lead

to syncope. The medicines associated commonly with vascular syncope are: chlorpromazine (Thorazine), guanethidine, nitroglycerin, isosorbide dinitrate (Sorbitrate), quinidine, and captopril.

The most common cardiac disorders associated with syncope are, of course, the dysrhythmias. Both tachydysrhythmias (ventricular fibrillation, ventricular tachycardia, atrial fibrillation with rapid ventricular response) or bradydysrhythmias (complete heart block, sinus arrest, sick sinus syndrome) may play a role. When attributing syncope to a dysrhythmia, a heart rate of > 150 BPM or < 40 BPM is usually required but not absolutely necessary.

Structural cardiac lesions such as aortic stenosis, hypertrophic cardiomyopathy, or atrial myxoma may cause life-threatening syncopal spells. Syncope in aortic stenosis is an ominous sign. It is caused by peripheral vasodilation in face of a fixed cardiac output due to valvular obstruction which leads to decreased forward flow. Obstruction of left ventricular output by the hypertrophied intraventricular septum or of left atrial output by a myxomatous tumor will also lead to decreased cardiac output.

Functional causes of cardiac syncope include myocardial infarction and acute pulmonary hypertension, such as that caused by a pulmonary embolism (blood clot in the lung). In fact, syncope is the commonest presenting sign of a massive pulmonary embolus.

Metabolic causes of syncope include intoxications (drugs, alcohol) and hypoglycemia. The blood sugar is usually extremely low and the victim elderly. Psychiatric problems can also lead to syncope. "Hyperventilation" is a true entity with numbness and tingling in the feet and hands and even loss of consciousness. It is important to also remember that this same pattern can occur secondary to anoxia, encephalopathy, and salicylate toxicity. Hysteria may be present in a syncopal patient, who appears otherwise normal, yet remains recumbent with normal vital signs. The causes of syncope are summarized in Table 2-5.

Diagnosis

History
Essential history to be obtained in patients who have had a syncopal spell include the onset and du-

ration of the episode and the presence/absence of seizure activity. This is especially important because transient cerebral hypoperfusion often accompanies a vasovagal faint, leading to short-lived myoclonic jerks. These are often perceived by lay individuals as seizures and reported as such.

It is important to discern the position of the patient before the event occurred. Was the patient getting up from a chair (suggests orthostatic hypotension), walking (perhaps arrhythmia or IHSS), or lying down (suggests a cardiac cause)? Could the patient be pregnant (ruptured ectopic pregnancy, venous compression from uterine mass)?

Physical examination

During the physical exam, vital signs are especially important. Orthostatic blood pressure and pulse measurements may be very helpful. The level of consciousness, neurological status, and any signs of head trauma are noted. Cardiac dysrhythmias MUST be sought as they are a common cause of syncope, especially in older individuals.

Laboratory tests

Lab tests may or may not be helpful. Electrolytes, glucose (most importantly), CBC, arterial blood gas (ABG), and drug screens should be obtained. An EKG is crucial; constant cardiac monitoring may also be especially helpful if symptoms correlate with noted dysrhythmias. An electroencephalogram (EEG) may be indicated if seizure activity is suspected.

The diagnostic yield of various tests in the initial workup of syncope has been explored. Diagnosis was provided as follows: history—25%, physical—10%, EKG—5%, lab (BS, K+, Ca++)—< 5%, and 24–48 hour Holter monitoring—15%. The investigators felt that because there is a 50–70% likelihood that syncope will not recur, if the above types of investigations are negative, there is no need to proceed further. Of course, if syncope recurs, further testing—such as EEGs and electrophysiological studies—are warranted [*Mod Con CV Dis,* May 1985]. If electrophysiological studies are done, a high diagnostic yield (up to 70%) may be expected [*Am Heart J,* 1986, Vol. 110, pp. 469–479].

Table 2-5. Causes of Syncope

Neurogenic
  Vasovagal faint
  Cerebral ischemia
  Intracerebral disease (seizure)
  Vascular (subclavian steal, micturition/cough)
  Carotid sinus disorders

Vascular
  Blood/fluid loss
  Impairment of vascular tone
  • Poor muscle tone
  • Venous insufficiency
  Drugs
  • Chlorpromazine
  • Guanethidine
  • Nitroglycerin
  • Isosorbide dinitrate
  • Quinidine
  • Captopril

Cardiac
  Dysrhythmias (tachycardia, bradycardia)
  Structural lesions
  • Aortic stenosis
  • Hypertrophic cardiomyopathy (IHSS)
  • Left atrial myxoma
  Functional
  • Myocardial infarction
  • Acute pulmonary hypertension (pulmonary embolus)

Metabolic
  Intoxication (drugs, alcohol)
  Hypoglycemia

Psychiatric
  Hyperventilation
  Hysteria

Treatment

The general treatment plan for any patient who

has recovered from a syncopal episode is as follows:

1. Position of comfort—do not sit the patient up prematurely.

2. If vital signs are unstable or if the patient is greater than 30 years old:

   ■ O_2, 4–6 LPM, NP
   ■ IV D_5W TKO
   ■ Cardiac monitor
   ■ EKG.

Pearls to Remember

Most syncope is vasovagal not cardiac. The recumbent position should be sufficient to restore vital signs and level of consciousness to normal in the majority of patients. Despite this, syncope of recent onset in a middle-aged or elderly patient is often cardiac and deserves special consideration. Patients greater than 30 years old, even though apparently normal, should be transported to and observed in the Emergency Department. If indicated, they should be admitted to the hospital. The approach to syncope is summarized in Table 2-6.

CHEST PAIN

Chest pain is always a worrisome symptom. This subject is dealt with extensively in the American Heart Association's (AHA) Advanced Cardiac Life Support course along with myocardial infarction and dysrhythmias. Due to its overwhelming importance, though, it will be briefly reviewed in this chapter as well.

There has been a recent decrease in the incidence of coronary artery disease (CAD) over the last decade. Reasons for this are uncertain. It is hypothesized that better attention to health habits (stopping smoking, controlling hypertension, losing weight, etc.) has played the strongest role. Improved prehospital, Emergency Department, and ICU care for myocardial infarction and cardiac arrest victims are likely also responsible. Nonetheless, if one examines the statistics, coronary artery disease is still present

in epidemic proportions and accounts for the highest percentage of sudden death cases.

Table 2-6. Syncope

Causes
  (See Table 2-4)

History
  Onset, duration
  Presence of seizure activity
  Position of patient before event
  Pregnant

Physical
  Orthostatic BP changes
  Level of consciousness
  Neurological status
  Signs of head trauma
  Dysrhythmias

Lab
  Lytes, glucose, CBC, ABG
  ? Drug screens
  EKG
  EEG if indicated

Treatment
  Position of comfort—don't sit prematurely.
  For patients who are unstable or > 30 years old:
  • Oxygen, 4–6 LPM NP
  • IV D_5W TKO
  • Cardiac monitor
  • EKG

Myocardial ischemia (lack of oxygen to the heart muscle) is potentially the most lethal and the most treatable cause of acute chest pain, especially in the prehospital setting. For this reason, *every* patient with chest pain should be approached as having a possible coronary event. This is even more important when one considers the fact that patients suffering chest pains tend to experience much denial—they minimize their symptoms and often fail to report them accurately. This is so common that most consider it a major diagnostic point when dealing with coronary artery disease. Thus, patients tend to wait hours to seek medical attention.

This long lag-time before seeking help can be very dangerous. The incidence of serious life-threatening dysrhythmias is greatest in the first two hours following onset of symptoms. Thus, 50–60% of the deaths from myocardial infarction (MI) occur prior to hospital admission. The majority of these are secondary to ventricular fibrillation, and many are NOT preceded by so-called "warning dys-rhythmias."

There are numerous entities that can cause chest pain. Myocardial ischemia, of course, is the most worrisome and dangerous. Pericarditis is commonly caused by a viral infection but may follow a my-ocardial infarction or open heart surgery as well. Dis-section of the aorta, pulmonary embolism, and costochondritis (viral inflammation of the rib car-tilage) can cause chest pain that is sometimes difficult to differentiate from that of myocardial infarction. At times, patients with mitral valve prolapse have vague chest pains that can be very bothersome. Reflux esophagitis may lead to spasm of the esophageal mus-culature. This pain mimics that of myocardial infarc-tion almost exactly. The major **causes** of chest pain are summarized in Table 2-7.

Table 2-7. Major Causes of Chest Pain

- Myocardial ischemia
- Pericarditis
- Mitral valve prolapse
- Aortic dissection
- Pulmonary embolus
- Reflux esophagitis
- Costochondritis

Diagnosis

There are several **principles of emergency care** that should be adhered to when treating a patient who complains of chest pains. Most importantly, emer-gency care should err on the side of overtreating a number of relatively low-risk suspects rather than un-dertreating a potential myocardial infarction. In other words, if there is a possibility that one's pain may be due to myocardial ischemia, they should be treated that way. The risks of this form of treatment are rela-tively low.

Chest pain patients need monitoring of their cardiac rhythm. Prophylactic lidocaine should be strongly considered in a patient under 70 years of age. With some of the newer methods of reperfusion (such as intravenous or intracoronary streptokinase) avail-able, time becomes of the essence. Thus, patients should be transported to a properly staffed and equipped Emergency Department as soon as possi-ble BUT with allowance for performing essential functions in the field.

History

The history is the most important item. The "classical presentation" of myocardial infarction consists of pain located beneath the sternum. It is described as crushing, pressing, squeezing, or burn-ing in nature. It may radiate to one or both arms, the neck, jaw, or back. A patient often holds their "clenched fist" over the sternum—this is felt by many to be a classic sign of myocardial pain. This discomfort generally builds up gradually to a maxi-mum lasting minutes to hours. The patient's subjec-tive impression of the pain intensity varies greatly from person to person. It is sometimes helpful to have the patient use a "rating scale" where "0" is pain-free and "10" represents the worst pain they could imagine.

Associated symptoms may include diaphoresis, shortness of breath, nausea, and vomiting. Appre-hension, a sense of impending doom ("Doctor, I think I'm going to die!"), and denial are very common.

At times, more atypical presentations appear. The most common of these is pain either to the left of the breastbone or in the epigastric region. Epigas-tric discomfort is usually more of a gnawing nature, and left upper chest pain is sharper than typical sub-sternal pain. Myocardial ischemia may present with other types of symptoms (such as toothache, elbow-ache, or neckache), but these are far more difficult to recognize. A high index of suspicion is always necessary. Table 2-8 summarizes the historical features of chest pain.

Table 2-8. Historical Features of Chest Pain

Classical Presentation
  Crushing, pressing, squeezing, burning
  Substernal or epigastric (clenched fist)
  Radiation to one or both arms, back,
    neck, jaw

Course
  Builds up gradually to a maximum
  Lasts minutes to hours
  Subjective ''intensity'' varies

Associated Symptoms
  Diaphoresis
  Shortness of breath
  Nausea, vomiting
  Apprehension, impending doom
  Denial

Atypical
  Left upper chest—sharp
  Epigastric—gnawing
  Toothache
  Neckache
  Elbow ache

Physical examination

On physical exam, attention must first be paid to the A, B, C's. Vital signs (especially pulse rate and regularity) are particularly important. Hypotension is a sign of cardiogenic shock. Auscultation of the lung fields will reveal the presence of rales if the patient is in left ventricular failure. Additional diagnostic clues include the presence/absence of jugular venous pressure elevation and peripheral edema.

Laboratory tests

Laboratory evaluation should include a CBC, electrolytes, and cardiac enzymes. These are important in the early care of the chest pain patient. Cardiac enzymes are obtained to detect the presence/absence of damage to the heart, i.e., myocardial infarction. Although important to obtain, one must remember that the initial EKG in myocardial infarction is *normal* greater than 50% of the time. Thus, it is poor practice to send someone home from the hospital who gives a good history for possible myocardial ischemia because ''their EKG was normal.'' Baseline **chest x-ray** should also be obtained, looking for cardiac enlargement and signs of left ventricular failure.

Treatment

Therapeutic modalities include, first, oxygen. Low-grade hypoxemia is common in myocardial infarction, and supplemental oxygen is helpful. A reasonable choice is 3 LPM via nasal prongs. An IV line—through which one may give medications and manage shock—comes next. Normally, this is D_5W TKO, but may be NS, RL, or Plasmanate if the patient is hypotensive. EKG monitoring is applied as soon as possible. The heart rhythm is monitored throughout the patient's first few days of observation.

Drug treatment should be directed towards prevention of serious cardiac dysrhythmias and pain control. Often, these go hand in hand. Unless the patient is over 70 years old or a high-grade AV block is present, the current recommendation of the AHA in a patient with suspected acute myocardial infarction is to start a prophylactic lidocaine infusion to prevent the occurrence of ventricular fibrillation.

The recommended dose of lidocaine is 1 mg/kg intravenous bolus, repeated at one-half the original dose in 5 minutes. A 4:1 drip (2 grams in 500 cc D_5W) is then run at 2 mg/minute. In the field, 300–400 mg intramuscularly has also been used effectively.

Effective analgesics include nitroglycerin (NTG) and morphine sulfate (MS). Nitroglycerin acts to relax vascular smooth muscle, thus decreasing spasm and ischemic injury. It is felt by many to actually decrease the size of a myocardial infarction. This is a distinct change from the philosophy several years ago that nitroglycerin causes a ''coronary steal'' by selectively overdilating the ''good'' vessels, thus further drawing life-giving blood from the infarcted area. The ''coronary steal'' philosophy simply has not held up to scrutiny.

Nitroglycerin is generally used in its sublingual form (dissolves under the tongue). The weakest strength (1/200) seems to result in fewer untoward hypotensive reactions with equal antianginal efficacy. If should be given every 3–4 minutes or so to a total of 3 pills in 10 minutes. An intravenous form is available which can be titrated to control chest pain in an easy fashion. Though popular, the intravenous form of nitroglycerin is not currently recommended by the AHA as first drug of choice. A lingual spray which releases 0.4 mg/spray has been released and looks promising as well. If nitroglycerin does not completely relieve pain, morphine sulfate (MS) should be used.

It is the opinion of many experts that MS is the single *best* cardiac drug currently available. It acts as a sedative and is an excellent pain reliever. It also causes vasodilation, thus decreasing the amount of blood the damaged heart has to pump (i.e., the preload). This leads to decreased myocardial oxygen consumption. There is no other analgesic that has these combined effects. Rarely, it may cause hypotension, nausea, and bradycardia. But, used in the dose of 2 mg IV every 5 minutes as needed to relieve pain, the data shows this to be an extremely safe drug.

It is also important to remember that MS can cause the release of histamine (leading to redness and hives) along the course of a vein or throughout the body. This is a DIRECT effect of this agent as well as several others (particularly Demerol). It **DOES NOT** imply that the patient is allergic to morphine. Antihistamines can be given and morphine sulfate still safely used if necessary.

Table 2-9 summarizes a general protocol for the approach to the patient with chest pains.

Table 2-9. General Chest Pain Protocol

- Supplemental oxygen
- Cardiac monitor
- IV D_5W
- Nitroglycerin, then morphine sulphate
- Prophylactic lidocaine (patient < 70 years old)

A final aspect of drug treatment should be mentioned—reperfusion therapy (RPT). RPT consists of giving a drug, either intravenously or directly into the coronary arteries, which is designed to reopen the ''clogged'' vessel. It is a well-known fact that early in myocardial infarction the involved coronary artery is often blocked by a thrombus, which totally occludes a lumen already narrowed by atherosclerotic plaque. In the late seventies, it was established that 90% of patients have a thrombus in the affected coronary artery in the first four hours. This frequency decreases to 50% in the next 12–24 hours and further hence.

Studies also showed that intracoronary nitroglycerin (NTG) or calcium antagonists *rarely* (< 3% of cases) ''reopened'' occluded arteries, suggesting that spasm is not often a final cause of acute MI. It is most likely that some type of ''dynamic interaction'' of defects in the coronary vessel wall, spasm, and platelet activation lead to the formation of a thrombus—this is indeed the final common pathway to infarction. Therefore, over 90% of acute transmural myocardial infarctions ARE caused by thrombi in the coronary arteries. The percentage is much lower in subendocardial infarctions—these events are thought to result from acute, severe imbalances between the O_2 supply and demand.

Three agents are available (two commercially) that will lyse these clots and may decrease the amount of myocardial damage. The most widely studied is STREPTOKINASE. This is an enzyme originally made by the bacterial genus *Streptococcus*. It is now commercially prepared in a much purer form. This agent, like UROKINASE (which is also currently available), acts to stimulate the fibrinolytic system of the body. This is the mechanism by which excessive blood clotting is controlled. Thus, the clot in the coronary artery is dissolved. Unfortunately, any other significant clots in the rest of the body may also be affected, leading to significant bleeding.

Nonetheless, both intravenous and intracoronary streptokinase have been shown to lyse clots in coronary arteries if given within 4–6 hours of the onset of chest pain. Most literature at the time of this writing suggests that either form is efficacious in decreasing infarction size and, perhaps, in reducing mortality. Less vast is the literature on urokinase.

A new compound, **tissue plasminogen activat-**

ing factor, has been used as well. This has the advantage of relatively local thrombolysis in the vicinity of the intracoronary clot itself, rather than activation of the entire body fibrinolytic system. Early data is highly promising.

Though thrombolytic therapy appears to work well, it is worth keeping in mind that many, including the AHA, at the time of this writing, have not recognized it as standard therapy in the treatment of acute myocardial infarction. Hopefully, this will change in the near future.

Pearls to Remember

Patients with chest pain tend to deny either the existence and/or the significance of their symptoms. Thus, there is often a crucial delay in seeking medical help. With the advent of new reperfusion techniques, greatest efficacy is achieved if these agents are used in the first few hours of pain onset. Therefore, it is very important that patients be brought to medical attention as soon as possible. It is also mandatory to recognize the fact that the initial EKG in a myocardial infarction may be normal in > 50% of patients. The *history* should be the deciding factor in admission NOT the EKG.

[Author's note: Three excellent references on chest pain and myocardial infarction are:

Textbook of Advanced Cardiac Life Support, American Heart Association, 1981 (the definitive text—should be replaced by a newer edition shortly).

Journal of the American Medical Association, June 6, 1986 (contains the new recommendations of the American Heart Association for both Advanced Cardiac and Basic Life Support).

Circulation, Part 2, Volume 74, December 1986 (contains the formal Proceedings of the 1985 National Conference on Standards and Guidelines for Cardiopulmonary Resuscitation and Emergency Cardiac Care during which the standards published in the second reference were decided upon).

Respiratory Emergencies

Emergencies involving the respiratory system are quite common. They are intertwined with cardiovascular problems. Respiratory arrest and airway obstruction are covered in the ACLS and BLS courses. Though they will be alluded to, specific coverage is omitted here. Nonetheless, there remain several significant respiratory emergencies all medical care providers should be familiar with:

- Anaphylaxis
- Asthma
- Chronic obstructive pulmonary disease (COPD) exacerbation
- Near-drowning
- Spontaneous pneumothorax
- Pulmonary embolism
- Toxic gas inhalation.

ANAPHYLAXIS

Anaphylaxis, or anaphylactic shock, is defined as an acute, life-threatening systemic allergic reaction resulting from released chemical mediators in a sensitized person exposed to a foreign substance (antigens). Basically, three distinct events must take place for anaphylaxis to occur. First of all, an antigen-antibody reaction must occur. Pharmacologically active mediators must then be released. Finally, the host must demonstrate a response to these compounds.

The majority of life-threatening anaphylactic reactions are mediated by the antibody IgE. These are referred to as Type I reactions and involve the coupling of a specific IgE molecule with the antigen on mast cells. The mast cells then release various chemical mediators in a process known as **degranulation.** These include histamine, slow-reacting substance of anaphylaxis, and eosinophilic chemotactic factor of anaphylaxis. There may also be activation of the complement and kallikrein systems, as well as involvement of prostaglandins. All of these compounds are likely interrelated in a complex fashion beyond the scope of this discussion [*J Emerg Med,* 1986, Vol. 4, p. 227].

Causes of anaphylaxis are usually injected substances. Most common are drugs. The list includes penicillin, cephalosporins, sulfonamides, iron, heparin, and thiamine. Anaphylaxis occurs in 1–2% of all patients treated with penicillin (PCN). The frequency of anaphylactic reactions to oral penicillin range from .3% to 2.5%, depending on the study. For the parenteral preparations, the figures are similar: .3%–1%. Small amounts of the drug are actually absorbed in the oropharynx. IgE-coated mast cells have been noted to be present in the epithelium of the tonsils and adenoids. These may be responsible for the rapid anaphylactic response that occurs in some patients with oral ingestion of penicillins [*Am J Emerg Med,* 1986, Vol. 4, pp. 241–246].

Positive skin tests are found in 10% of the general population. Interestingly, 75% of individuals suffering fatal anaphylactic reactions report NO history of prior allergy. It appears that people who have an atopic (highly allergic) tendency are at increased risk [*J Emerg Med,* 1983, Vol. 1, pp. 83–95]. It behooves one to observe a patient for 20–30 minutes following a PCN injection.

Iodinated contrast media causes what is referred to as an anaphylactoid reaction, which is somewhat different, but the problems and treatment are the same. Interestingly, the ionic or nonionic nature of the contrast media used may determine the compound's reactivity [*Am J Med,* 1986, Vol. 80, p. 382].

The local anesthetics, procaine (Novacaine) and xylocaine (Lidocaine), are responsible for several anaphylactic reactions each year. It is important to note that these two drugs DO NOT cross-react. Because of differences in their chemical structures, a person may be allergic to one and not to the other.

Exercise-induced anaphylaxis is fairly common. In distinction to other types, wheezing and gastrointestinal symptoms are uncommon. A familial susceptibility has been reported and the syndrome is more common in the atopic individual [*West J Med,* March 1986, Vol. 144, pp. 329–337]. Several variant forms of exercise-induced anaphylaxis have been reported involving concomitant food sensitivity. Patients seem to develop anaphylaxis only if a particular foodstuff was ingested in close relation to exercise. Various foods have been implicated, including celery [*J Emerg Med,* 1986, Vol. 4, p. 195].

Some people are highly allergic to various types of antisera and vaccines (especially horse serum). Insect stings are responsible for a significant proportion of anaphylactic deaths each year. In fact, more people die from allergic reactions to bee stings than snake bites. Interestingly, many insect bites other than those of the Class Hymenoptera (bees, wasps, etc.) can cause anaphylaxis. These include deer flies, gnats, horse flies, mosquitoes, fire ants, cockroaches, miller moths, and exposure to butterfly larvae [*Internal Medicine News,* 1985, Vol. 18, p. 53].

Anaphylaxis has been reported following intravenous corticosteroid administration [*J Emerg Med,* 1986, Vol. 4, p. 213] and in gila monster bites [*Ann Emerg Med,* 1986, Vol. 15, p. 959]. Several food items are particularly likely to cause problems—shellfish, egg albumin, nuts, and chocolate. Food additives, especially preservatives often used in restaurants, have been commonly implicated as well [*Arch Intern Med,* 1986, Vol. 149, p. 2129]. Idiopathic anaphylaxis, for which no inciting agent is ever determined, is well-described in the literature. Table 3-1 summarizes the causes of anaphylaxis.

Table 3-1. Causes of Anaphylaxis

Drugs (Usually Injected)
Penicillin
Cephalosporins
Sulfonamides
Iron
Heparin
Thiamine
Procaine/Xylocaine

IV Contrast Media (Anaphylactoid Reaction)
Antisera and Vaccines (Especially Horse)
Insect Stings
Foods
- Shellfish
- Egg albumin
- Nuts
- Chocolate

Diagnosis

History

Most reactions occur within 30 minutes following exposure, though the onset of symptoms can vary from several seconds to hours. The patient often gives a history of known allergy but not always. They will note the onset of sudden anxiety, restlessness, and a feeling of doom. Intense itching, especially of the feet and hands may be present along with a pounding headache. There may be coughing and difficulty with breathing. Nausea and abdominal cramps are common. Seizures may occur but are relatively unusual.

The principal manifestations of anaphylaxis occur where the concentrations of mast cells are the highest: the skin, the lungs, and the gastrointestinal tract. Thus, urticaria, erythema, and angioedema are common. In fact, the cause of death in greater than one-half of cases is angioedema in the epiglottis, larynx, or hypopharynx.

Physical examination

The patient will be noted to have often dramatic hypotension. Urinary incontinence, wheezing, stridor, chest retractions, hoarseness, and loud upper airway noises may be present. Hives and/or flushed skin can be seen. Edema, either generalized or local (lips, tongue, uvula, face), may be obvious.

Laboratory tests

No immediate lab work is indicated due to the urgent need for rapid treatment. Cardiac rhythm monitoring is appropriate, though. Numerous arrhythmias have been reported including ST-T changes. These are present prior to treatment and NOT thought to be secondary to epinephrine. Myocardial infarction has been reported to complicate anaphylactic shock [*Am Heart J,* 1976, Vol. 91, p. 365]. Table 3-2 summarizes the diagnostic features of anaphylactic shock.

Table 3-2. Diagnosis of Anaphylaxis

History
Often known allergy
Sudden onset of anxiety, restlessness, doom
Intense itching (especially of feet and hands)
Headache
Cough
Difficulty with breathing
Nausea, abdominal cramps
Seizures (rare)

Physical
Dramatic hypotension
Urinary incontinence
Wheezing, stridor, chest retraction
Hoarseness, loud upper airway noises
Hives, flushed skin
Edema (generalized or local—lips, tongue, face)

Treatment

Anaphylaxis is an acutely life-threatening problem. Immediate treatment is necessary. The following steps should be rapidly taken:

1. Protect the airway—suction or intubate if needed.

2. Remove the injection mechanism if still present (i.e., the stinger), BUT don't waste time if you encounter any difficulty.

3. Oxygen—10–15 LPM by mask (high-flows are preferred here because of the acute life-threatening nature of this problem).

4. Place patient supine with legs elevated unless severe respiratory distress is present (then patient should be seated).

5. IV-large bore (#14–16)—NS or RL; run wide open if systolic BP < 85; 200 cc/h if between 85–110, and TKO if > 110 mm Hg.

6. Cardiac monitor.

Specific **drug therapy** of anaphylaxis should proceed as rapidly as possible as follows:

1. EPINEPHRINE—the drug of choice— give as soon as possible. This agent vasoconstricts, bronchodilates, and counteracts the effects of histamine and has an inotropic effect—all of these actions are indeed helpful in anaphylaxis. For life-threatening problems, give .5 mg IV (5 cc of a 1:10,000 solution) and repeat every 5–10 minutes as needed. This may also be given as a sublingual injection (.3–.5 cc of 1:1000 solution) or into an endotracheal (ET) tube as well. Realistically, use of the sublingual injection route may be the easiest. Despite the unpleasant sound of this choice, there is usually so much edema as to render the injection totally painless to the patient!

For less-threatening situations, give .3–.5 mg subcutaneously (SQ) (.3–.5 cc of a 1:1000 solution); this may be repeated every 20–30 minutes for a total of three doses. This is likely appropriate when symptoms such as shortness of breath, rash, and anxiety occur without significant hypotension.

Due to a few reports of complications from bolus IV epinephrine administration, some recommend the use of a 1:100,000 dilution [*JAMA,* 1984, Vol. 251, p. 2118]. The data on this is inconclusive at this time.

2. AMINOPHYLLINE—for bronchospasm—bolus with 6 mg/kg IV over 20–30 minutes; a maintenance infusion should be run at .5–1 mg/kg/hr (see page 31 on COPD exacerbation for exceptions). In addition to bronchodilation, aminophylline may have a direct positive inotropic effect on the heart via the intracellular translocation of calcium ions. It is recommended that this drug only be used if bronchospasm is present though, due to the possibility of side effects, including hypotension [*JAMA,* 1974, Vol. 227, p. 1431].

3. HYDROCORTISONE—500 mg IV every 6 hours. Generally, steroids take from 4–6 hours to achieve their maximum therapeutic benefit.

4. DIPHENHYDRAMINE (Benadryl)— 25–50 mg IV every 6 hours.

5. At the site of an injected antigen, place a tourniquet proximal to the site to occlude lymphatic and venous drainage (but NOT arterial flow). Inject .3 cc of 1:100 EPINEPHRINE SQ into the site.

6. A few reports have documented the efficacy of cimetidine infusion (300 mg IV over 15 minutes) in treating acute allergic urticaria in response to insect stings refractory to other measures [*Ann Emerg Med,* November 1986, Vol. 15, p. 1363].

Table 3-3 summarizes the treatment of anaphylactic shock.

Table 3-3. Treatment of Anaphylaxis

General Therapy
  Protect airway
  Remove injection mechanism (don't waste time)
  Oxygen (10–15 LPM, mask)
  Patient seated with legs elevated unless too short of breath
  IV NS or RL
  Cardiac monitor

Drug Therapy
  Epinephrine—3–5 cc of a 1:10,000 SLN IV, ET, or SL (use 1:1,000 strength)
  Aminophylline—6 mg/kg IV bolus then .5–1 mg/kg/hr drip
  Hydrocortisone—500 mg IV every 6 hours
  Diphenhydramine—25–50 mg IV every 6 hours

  Note: Place tourniquet above site of an injected antigen and inject .3 cc of 1:1000 epinephrine)

Pearls to Remember

Patients who have suffered an anaphylactic reaction should be observed at least 6, and preferably 12 hours, for delayed problems.

1. Be SURE you are using the proper dilution and dose of epinephrine.

2. Anxiety, tremor, palpitations, tachycardia, and headache are *common* with the administration of epinephrine. Vomiting may occur in children.

3. Epinephrine should NOT be given without

signs *and* symptoms of anaphylaxis. Don't rely on the history alone. Hyperventilators may *think* they are having an anaphylactic reaction.

4. Lethal edema may be localized to the tongue, uvula, or other parts of the upper airway. Be prepared for cricothyroidotomy if necessary.

5. DO NOT let treatment of the injection site distract you from the IV treatment of life-threatening anaphylaxis.

6. Epinephrine and other injected adrenergic stimulants have been reported to cause hypokalemia (decreased potassium). This value should be watched carefully, especially in a patient who has been on a diuretic and is, therefore, more likely to have a low total serum potassium to begin with.

7. Patients with a history of anaphylactic reactions should not be on beta-blockers (Inderal, Tenormin, Corgard, Lo-Pressor, etc.). The severity of the respiratory component to bee-sting allergy anaphylaxis is increased, and the entire syndrome is much more difficult to treat [*Emerg Med,* March 1985, p. 94].

8. A new self-injector, the "Epi-Pen," is available by prescription. It is carried by the anaphylaxis-prone patient, similar to the currently used epinephrine kits. A spring-loaded syringe gives .5 cc of epinephrine intramuscularly into the anterior thigh when applied by the patient.

9. Venom immunotherapy is available to densitize patients allergic to bee and wasp stings. It appears to be highly efficacious. It has been shown that if urticaria is the sole manifestation of insect-sting anaphylaxis, severe reactions on retesting are unlikely; these patients are NOT candidates for immunotherapy [*J Allergy Clin Immunol,* 1975, Vol. 76, pp. 735–740]. Patients having large local reactions are likely to have the same type again and have a small, but not significantly increased, risk of anaphylaxis.

ASTHMA

Asthma is defined as a reversible respiratory condition of airflow obstruction that usually results from hypersensitivity in the lower airways to various stimuli. The **pathophysiology** of asthma is not always clear. However, exaggerated responsiveness to stimuli, some identifiable and some not, does exist.

During an asthmatic attack, bronchospasm and constriction of the smaller airways occur. By definition, these are totally reversible in pure asthma. There is also swelling of the mucous membranes of the bronchial walls and plugging of the bronchi with thick mucus. This results in normally perfused alveoli being hypoventilated. Thus, an abnormality in the ventilation/perfusion ratio occurs, leading to hypoxemia. Carbon dioxide elimination generally increases with increasing ventilatory efforts until a point when expiratory airflow is severely reduced (forced expiratory volume, FEV_1, < 25% of predicted normal) and retention begins.

Asthma may be classified according to the severity of the attack. A slight attack involves wheezing and sputum production. A moderate attack consists of dyspnea on exertion and more pronounced wheezing. A patient with a severe attack will have dyspnea at rest, cough, wheezing, and distant breath sounds. **Status asthmaticus** is a severe attack that doesn't respond to conventional therapy.

The **causes** or trigger factors of an asthmatic condition are not always readily identifiable. Commonly identified conditions include:

1. Allergic reactions—smoking, medicines, pollen, dust. Of particular note are asthmatic reactions provoked by sulfite preservatives used in commercial foods [*Am J Med,* 1986, Vol. 81, p. 816].

2. Respiratory infection—usually viral, with later bacterial invasion or overgrowth.

3. Changes in environmental conditions—humidity or temperature.

4. Emotional response to stress. One study has reported that 80% of patients with the hyperventilation syndrome have concomitant asthma [*Am J Med,* 1986, Vol. 81, p. 989].

5. Exercise—the motion of air over the posterior oropharynx area may stimulate bronchospasm in sensitive individuals. Interestingly, this may be more common than previously thought, especially in highly trained athletes [*Chest,* 1986, Vol. 90, p. 23].

6. Medications—aspirin sensitivity may be present in up to 20% of asthmatic patients (see page 30). Ingestion of aspirin or similar non-steroidal anti-inflammatory agents can lead to severe consequences. The ophthalmic preparation of timolol is a strong beta-blocker and has been shown to be systemically absorbed, potentially leading to worsening of airway obstruction in both asthmatics and those with chronic obstructive lung disease [*Am Rev Respir Dis,* 1986, Vol. 133, p. 264].

Diagnosis

History

The asthmatic patient will often give a history of previous attacks. They may have had a recent respiratory infection with sputum production. This is especially common, and one must ask about *changes* in the color, amount, and character of the sputum. The patient will often relate a story of acute or gradual onset of shortness of breath and wheezing from a previously healthy state. Most worrisome is the patient's statement of getting "too tired to breathe anymore."

Physical examination

The patient is usually seated and in obvious respiratory distress. Expiratory (and sometimes inspiratory) wheezes may be heard. A quiet-sounding chest in an asthmatic in obvious respiratory distress is a bad sign—they are too "tight" to wheeze. Thus, the presence of wheezing suggests that there is at least enough airflow to cause turbulence. Tachycardia,

tachypnea, cough, and the use of accessory muscles of respiration (intercostal and supraclavicular retractions) may be noted. In a severe attack, pulsus paradoxus may be present (a difference in the auscultated systolic BP of 10 mm Hg or greater between the expiratory and inspiratory phases of respiration). Somnolence or agitation are also signs of a worsening condition. Table 3-4 summarizes the clinical signs of a severe asthma attack.

Table 3-4. Clinical Signs of Severe Asthma

- Diaphoresis
- Seated posture
- Somnolence, agitation
- Pulsus paradoxus
- Heart rate > 130
- Retractions—supraclavicular, intercostal
- Quiet chest to auscultation

Laboratory tests

Lab work should include arterial blood gases and, possibly, a CBC. Between attacks, the ABGs of a pure asthmatic should be normal. With an acute attack, they show mild hypoxemia and respiratory alkalosis with an average pH = 7.5 and pCO_2 = 25. If the patient is tachypneic and ABGs are "normal," be ever alert to the strong possibility of CO_2 retention in a tiring patient, as these results are clearly NOT compatible with the dyspneic, hyperventilating asthmatic. If epinephrine has been used, the CBC will show an increase in the white blood cell count (due to catecholamine-induced demargination of WBCs, making this determination less helpful in the management of an acute attack.

Muscle-specific creatine phosphokinase (MM-CPK) elevations are commonly noted in asthmatics. The source may be from skeletal muscle that is stressed from the work of breathing. It does not have any prognostic significance and no further workup is necessary unless there is a clinical suggestion of myocardial, central nervous system, or skeletal muscle injury or disease [*West J Med,* March 1986, Vol. 144, pp. 321-323].

Chest X-ray may show an acute pneumonia. More often, mild hyperexpansion is noted. A chest X-ray is not indicated in every acute asthmatic attack. Though it may certainly be needed later (especially if the patient is to be admitted), other items have greater value.

Bedside spirometry is helpful if available. The volume of air expired in the first second of a forced expiration (FEV_1) is measured. If it is initially less than 800 ml or fails to increase by greater than 400 ml after 3–4 hours of outpatient treatment, the patient should be admitted to the hospital. An easier, though less accurate, test is the Peak Expiratory Flow Rate (PEFR). If < 100 LPM initially or if treatment fails to improve PEFR to > 300 LPM, a severe attack is usually present. PEFR is helpful as a "trend" to monitor rather than as an absolute determinant.

Numerous papers have appeared in the Emergency Medicine literature trying to establish a "gold standard" for determination of when an asthmatic should be admitted. Though appealing conceptually, there is no widely proven and accepted standard. It would be helpful to have an objective means of judging the severity of an asthmatic attack in the Emergency Department. As of the this writing, though, there is no clear-cut consensus [*Ann Emerg Med,* January 1987, Vol. 16, p. 79].

Treatment

Treatment of mild to moderately severe asthma first involves placing the patient on low-flow oxygen (2–3 LPM, NP). This may be later adjusted according to ABGs (if they are drawn). As these patients are often dehydrated, an IV of D_5W 1/2 NS at 125 cc/hr may be necessary. The patient is usually most comfortable in a sitting position. Drug treatment is as follows:

1. EPINEPHRINE—.3–.5 cc of 1:1000 solution SQ–may repeat every 20 minutes × 2 for a total of 3 doses. Use with caution if the patient is older than 40. In younger individuals, the risk of cardiac dysrhythmias, even if this drug is combined with aminophylline, is low [*Ann Emerg Med,* June 1986, Vol. 15, pp. 699–702]. If the

attack is "broken" and the patient discharged from the Emergency Department, a SQ injection of a long-acting suspension of epinephrine (SusPhrine .1–.3 cc SQ) may prevent recurrence. SusPhrine has a duration of action around 6–8 hours (as compared to epinephrine's 1–2 hours) and is recommended in patients < 40 years old.

2. Inhaled beta-stimulatory bronchodilators. ISOETHARINE (Bronkosol) may be used as an alternative first therapy or as THE first-line drug if the patient is older than 40. Use 1/2 cc mixed in 2.5 cc of NaCl every 2–4 hr via a hand-held nebulizer. Most feel there is currently no role for IPPB (intermittent positive pressure breathing) machines in the acute treatment of uncomplicated asthma. Some literature has described that the presence of sulfur dioxide (in minute concentrations), as well as sodium metabisulfate in isoethrane solutions, may actually aggravate symptoms in sensitive individuals [*JAMA,* June 8, 1984, p. 2982]. Thus, if the patient appears to paradoxically worsen, change to another bronchodilator. Metaproterenol (Alupent) and isoproterenol (Isuprel) solutions designed to be mixed for nebulization may contain the same compound.

    Some experts feel that inhaled beta-aerosols should be the first drug of choice in any asthma attack. Isoetharine has a rapid onset of action and is short-lived in the body. Thus, if side effects occur, they rapidly dissipate. It may be repeated every two hours if necessary as well. For this reason, it has been the agent of choice for many years. Recently, metaproterenol and albuterol have emerged as popular agents. Liquid albuterol for nebulization is now available [*Ped Emerg Care,* 1986, Vol. 2, p. 250]. Though popular in children, isoproterenol is generally avoided in adults due to potential side effects.

3. AMINOPHYLLINE—If the patient has not previously been on the drug, the loading and maintenance doses stated earlier apply. If they have been taking the medi-

cation AND blood levels are readily available, use the same maintenance dose as stated earlier. Calculate the loading dose by the following formula:

$$\text{LOADING DOSE (mg)} =$$
$$\text{Wt (Kg)} \times .7$$
$$[\text{Desired level} - \text{Measured Level}]$$

Studies have shown that it is nearly impossible to predict one's aminophylline level on clinical grounds. Thus, it is optimal to obtain a level on all patients. If no blood levels are available, give one-half the calculated loading dose (3 mg/kg).

Aminophylline can cause serious toxicity if the dose is not properly adjusted. Interestingly, there are significant differences between acute toxicity (such as in a suicide attempt or massive IV overloading) and chronic toxicity. Acute overdose is accompanied by hypotension, hypokalemia, and low serum bicarbonate. Seizures and cardiac arrhythmias are unlikely unless the serum level exceeds 100 mg/L. Patients with chronic toxicity, on the other hand, are more likely to have seizures and serious arrhythmias with lower serum levels (28–70 mg/L) [*Am J Emerg Med*, 1985, Vol. 3, pp. 386–394].

Caffeine, which is chemically similar to aminophylline, has also been reported to have bronchodilatory properties. It, of course, is not indicated as primary therapy in an asthmatic patient [*Chest*, 1986, Vol. 89, p. 335].

4. STEROIDS are optional for mild attacks. Several studies have suggested fewer recurrences with oral methylprenisolone (Medrol) or prednisone given for one week after the acute event, even in a mild attack, though. For the more severe conditions, give Solu-Medrol 125 mg IV followed by decreasing daily doses of oral Prednisone: 60, 50, 40, 30, 20, 10, and 5 mg per day then stop. The regimen of an intravenous bolus, followed by decreasing daily doses of steroid seems to maximize both Emergency Department response as well as to decrease the frequency of recurrent attacks [*N Engl J Med*, 1986, Vol. 314, pp. 150–152]. Inpatients should be kept on IV Solu-Medrol for 24 hours and then weaned to oral steroids.

5. ANTIBIOTICS—Use if purulent sputum, fever, or pulmonary infiltrate are present. The choice depends upon the patient's allergies but is usually one of the following: erythromycin, tetracycline, doxycycline, ampicillin, amoxicillin, or cefalexin.

Evidence has shown that arterial desaturation occurs following inhalation of beta-sympathometic agents in the treatment of asthma. This is due to the fact that these agents increase cardiac output before they have a significant bronchodilatory effect. Thus, pulmonary shunting results. It is likely that similar desaturation occurs following other agents as well. The effect is transient, lasting less than 30 minutes. Nonetheless, with obvious precautions taken for CO_2-retainers, oxygen therapy is initially warranted for all acute asthmatic attacks for this reason [*Chest*, 1984, Vol. 86, pp. 868–869].

By definition, **status asthmaticus** is severe asthma that does not respond to three injections of epinephrine. Patients not responsive to initial inhalations of isoethrane and aminophylline infusion may fall in the same category. These individuals are ALWAYS admitted, given IV fluids, aminophylline, steroids, antibiotics, and inhaled bronchodilators. Blood gases are carefully followed and intubation with mechanical ventilation considered.

If these fail, inhaled ATROPINE may work. The dose is .025 mg/kg in .9% NaCl via nebulizer. This has an anticholinergic effect that leads to bronchodilation via different mechanisms than the previously suggested agents. The easiest way to prepare this is to dissolve a 0.3 mg atropine tablet in 2.5 cc NaCl. A hand-held nebulizer is then used. The dose may be repeated if necessary in 10–15 minutes.

An aerosolized anticholinergic agent used widely in Europe, ipratropium bromide, has just been released in this country, but is not indicated for an acute asthma attack. Generally, 40 to 80 µg of ipratropium is equivalent to 2 mg of inhaled atropine, but neither is as effective a bronchodilator as the newer beta-adrenergic agents [*West J Med*, 1986, Vol. 3, pp. 341–342]. It may be of particular benefit in psychogenic asthma [*Am J Med*, (suppl 5A), 1986, p. 55]. Intravenous salbutamol [albuterol] (available in the United States only in inhaled form as either Ventolin or Proventil) is reported to work well in treating status asthmaticus in children.

Several case reports have demonstrated the efficacy of an intravenous infusion of the general anesthetic ketamine (1.0 to 2.5 mg/kg/h) in reversing status asthmaticus that is refractory to conventional modes of therapy [*Crit Care Med*, 1986, Vol. 14, pp. 514–516]. Isoflurane anesthesia has also been used with success [*Crit Care Med*, 1986, Vol. 14, p. 832]. Table 3-5 summarizes the drug treatment of asthma.

The treatment of an acute attack during pregnancy does not differ radically from conventional therapy. Generally, subcutaneous epinephrine is favored. Data are not available on metaproterenol and albuterol. Ephedrine is also felt to be safe. For status epilepticus, standard regimens including theophylline, aminophylline, epinephrine, and most steroids are considered safe. No data exists for isoethrane [*NEJM*, 1985, Vol. 312, pp. 897–902]. There is one case report of subcutaneously administered terbutaline causing severe hypotension in a pregnant asthmatic [*Am J Emerg Med*, 1986, Vol. 4, pp. 218–221]. It is possible that the beta-1 stimulation caused by this agent could lead to vasodilation and lowering of what is already a normal to low systemic vascular resistance.

Contraindicated treatments

A few contraindicated treatments should also be mentioned. IPPB increases the risk of pneumothorax and pneumonmediastinum and should NOT be used. N-acetyl cysteine (Mucomyst) can actually aggravate bronchospasm. Water is a much better hydrating and mucolytic agent (loosens up secretions). Beta-blockers such as propranolol have effects opposite to most standard asthma therapies and are, thus, relatively contraindicated.

Table 3-5. Drug Therapy of Acute Asthma

Epinephrine
.3–.5 cc (1:1000) SQ—MR every 20 min × 2
(Total: 3 doses)

Susphrine
.1–.3 cc SQ if attack broken and patient sent home

Isoetharine
1/2 cc in 2.5 cc NaCl via nebulizer
(Note: Start here if patient is over 40 years of age.)

Aminophylline
No previous therapy
- .6 mg/kg IV over 20–30 minutes loading dose
- .5–1 mg/kg/hr maintenance infusion
Previous therapy
- Level unavailable—3 mg/kg loading dose and same maintenance
- Level available—same maintenance; loading dose = WT (kg) × .7 (desired level − measured level)

Antibiotics
If purulent sputum

Note: If the above fail consider:
- Atropine (inhaled)
- Intravenous salbutamol (not available in United States)

Pearls to Remember

When treating the asthmatic patient, remember:

1. A quiet chest in an acute asthmatic is a bad sign (too "tight" to wheeze).

2. "Normal" ABGs in a patient with acute asthma are a sign of CO_2 retention and impending respiratory failure.

3. All that wheezes is not asthma—wheezing in older people is frequently due to pulmonary edema NOT asthma. Treat with aminophylline, not epinephrine, if in doubt.

4. Upper airway obstruction (i.e., tumor, foreign body) causes selective inspiratory wheezing.

5. Patients with asthma have an 8–20% chance of experiencing an attack following ingestion of aspirin or nonsteroidal anti-inflammatory agents. If a patient has nasal polyps, the prevalence increases to 30–40% [*Allergy Clin Imuno*, 1984, Vol. 74, p. 617].

6. Asthma attacks can be fatal. Several reasons are possible, including hypoxia, increased myocardial work, arrhythmias, and medication toxicity [*N Engl J Med*, 1986, Vol. 314, pp. 423–429]. Spontaneous pneumothorax can also occur in the face of an acute asthma attack. If this occurs, tension pneumothorax, with attendant cardiorespiratory embarrassment, may be present and require immediate diagnosis and treatment.

CHRONIC OBSTRUCTIVE PULMONARY DISEASE (COPD) EXACERBATION

An exacerbation of COPD may be defined as an acute worsening of a chronic condition characterized by either limitation of airflow secondary to airway disease (chronic bronchitis) or destruction of pulmonary parenchyma (emphysema). Most patients have a combination of both.

The **pathophysiology** of chronic bronchitis involves mucous gland hypertrophy with subsequent mucus plugging and obliteration of airways. This limits airflow markedly and often results in chronic sputum production. In emphysema, there is enlargement of the air passages distal to the terminal bronchioles with destruction of alveolar walls. This leads to loss of elastic recoil in the lung and a marked decrease in expiratory airflow.

Regardless of the underlying pathology, all patients with COPD have the following:

1. Increased airway resistance, with a resultant increase in the work of breathing.

2. Inefficiency of inspiratory muscles due to chronic thoracic hyperinflation.

3. Ventilation-perfusion mismatching leading to impaired gas exchange.

When COPD patients go into respiratory failure, they tend to breathe in a rapid, shallow fashion. Their respiratory drive tends to be increased, rather than decreased. This has been shown to be the case irrespective of whether or not the patient's baseline state is one of CO_2 retention. Thus, great respiratory effort is expended in acute respiratory failure by the patient.

The major **cause** of COPD is cigarette smoking. A significant majority (> 90%) of heavy smokers suffer chronic respiratory symptoms and are at a markedly increased risk for the development of both chronic bronchitis and emphysema [*Am Rev Respir Dis*, 1981, Vol. 123, p. 372]. Air pollution and industrial inhalants (silicone, asbestos) may play a minor role. Widespread tuberculosis can damage enough lung tissue to result in COPD.

Diagnosis

History

The patient may give a history of emphysema or bronchitis. Usually, they complain of severe dyspnea which has been increasing over a number of days. Patients are often still cigarette smokers and may have stopped their medications because they "felt good." A history of cough with sputum production, especially a *change*, should be sought. It is also helpful to know if the patient has been on home oxygen and how much.

Physical examination

On physical exam, the patient will often be sitting and obviously tachypneic. Intercostal and/or supreclavicular retractions may be present. There may be cyanosis of the lips (common) and fingertips. Many patients have a barrel-shaped chest. Quiet breath sounds are the rule in COPD and not as worrisome as in acute asthma. Wheezes and rales may also be present. An extremely quiet chest, though, should be cause for concern.

Laboratory tests

Lab work obtained should include ABGs, CBC, and blood cultures if there is any evidence of pneumonia. The blood gases will usually show mild to severe hypoxia. CO_2 retention may or may not be present. It is always helpful to know the patient's baseline ABGs if available. If they are not, one can usually determine the acuity of a pCO_2 elevation by the pH. If the pH is relatively normal or alkalotic in the face of a markedly elevated pCO_2 (i.e., > 55), there is at least some element of chronic CO_2 retention. Impending respiratory failure is usually suggested if the pH is less than 7.20, the pCO_2 greater than 50 mm Hg, and the pO_2 less than 50 mm Hg.

Chest X-ray will usually show only flattened diaphragms and increased anterior-posterior diameter. Evidence of pneumonia may also be present. This examination may be of particular benefit in obtunded patients or those with organic brain syndromes. Up to 75.8% of these individuals presenting with acute respiratory complaints have concomitant pneumonia [*Arch Intern Med*, 1986, Vol. 146, p. 1321].

An EKG should also be obtained, as both right and left ventricular function can be altered in acute hypoxemic respiratory failure [*Crit Care Med*, 1986, Vol. 14, p. 852]. Table 3-6 summarizes the diagnostic approach to a COPD exacerbation.

Treatment

Treatment involves placing the patient in a sitting position. Low-flow oxygen at 1–3 LPM NP is administered. If the patient becomes more lethargic or combative with oxygen, they may be starting to retain CO_2, and the flow should be decreased. An IV of D_5W at a TKO rate is warranted. The rate and perhaps choice of fluid may need to be changed depending on the patient's state of hydration. Drug treatment is as follows:

1. ISOETHRANE—1/2 cc in 2.5 cc NaCl via hand-held nebulizer; repeat every 2–4 hours. IPPB is contraindicated for reasons previously stated. There is some evidence that inhalation of beta-agonists may improve the clearance of mucus from the airways via the cilia. Some may prefer other inhaled bronchodilators (see page 27 on Asthma).

2. AMINOPHYLLINE—Use the loading dose described for asthma. The maintenance dose is often modified in these patients because they are usually older and sicker than the "pure" asthmatic. Patients > 50 years old, or those with cardiac and/or liver disease, should have the maintenance infusion run at .2–.3 mg/kg/hr. Serum levels should be obtained to ideally manage an IV aminophylline drip. In these patients, aminophylline may improve diaphragmatic efficiency.

3. METHYLPREDNISOLONE (Solu-Medrol): 125 mg IV every 8 hours—This is the IV steroid of choice as it has less fluid retention properties than hydrocortisone (Solu-Cortef).

4. ANTIBIOTICS—Ampicillin (500 mg po every 6 hours) or tetracycline (same dose) should always be given in an acute COPD exacerbation, even if infection is not obvious. It is the MOST common precipitating factor. If there is purulent sputum or an infiltrate on chest X-ray, get a sputum specimen for gram stain and culture. While awaiting results, give cephalothin (Keflin) 1 gm IV every 6 hours—this is the best drug choice because of its anti-*Staph* coverage. Antibiotics are then modified pending the culture results. Table 3-7 summarizes the drug treatment of a COPD exacerbation.

Table 3-6. Diagnostic Approach to COPD

History
> Emphysema or chronic bronchitis
> Severe dyspnea, increasing over past few days
> Cigarette smoker
> Stopped medications—''Cause I felt good''
> Cough, sputum production—especially a change
> Home oxygen

Physical
> Sitting, tachypneic
> Intercostal/supraclavicular retractions
> Cyanosis—lips, fingertips
> Barrel-shaped chest
> Quiet breath sounds—to be expected
> Wheezes, rales

Lab
> ABG—Hypoxia, may show CO_2 retention
> Chest X-ray—flat diaphragms, increased anterior-posterior diameter

Table 3-7. Drug Treatment of a COPD Exacerbation

Isoetharine
> 1/2 cc in 2.5 cc NaCl via nebulizer—repeat every 2-4 hours around the clock (may substitute another inhaled beta-sympathomimetic agent)

Aminophylline
> IV loading dose of 6 mg/kg
> Maintenance infusion = .2-1 mg/kg/hr IV

Methylprednisolone
> 125 mg IV every 8 hours

Antibiotics
> No purulent sputum or infiltrate
> • Ampicillin 500 mg PO Q 6 hr
> • Tetracycline 500 mg PO Q 6 hr
> Purulent sputum and/or infiltrate
> (After sputum gram stain, culture; blood cultures)
> Cephalothin (Keflin) 1 gm IV q 6 hr
> (Modify according to bacteriology studies)

NEAR-DROWNING

Drowning is defined as death due to asphyxiation during an immersion episode. It may occur with or without inhalation of the surrounding fluid medium. Near-drowning occurs when the process of drowning is interrupted or reversed.

Causes of near-drowning are usually swimmer exhaustion, lack of skill, and panic. An acute medical incident during swimming (myocardial infarction, seizure, trauma) can result in acute incapacitation, leading to drowning. Hyperventilation in preparation for a long underwater swim can suppress the respiratory drive sufficiently to result in anoxia while submerged. Suicide attempts are a final way that near-drowning occurs. Often this is in association with jumping from a bridge or ledge and multiple serious traumatic injuries are also present. Despite this, the *single most important factor* in adult drownings is the use of alcohol and mind-altering drugs. Studies have shown that anywhere from 35–75% of drowning victims have elevated blood alcohol levels.

The **epidemiology** of near-drowning is also very interesting. Affected individuals are often the very young and the aged. Males have a 5–8 times greater incidence than females. Similarly, blacks have a 3–5 times greater frequency than do whites. The majority of drownings and near-drownings DO NOT occur in the ocean but rather in lakes, rivers, ponds, and backyard pools. This is thought to be the case due to better surveillance and rescue techniques utilized by ocean lifeguards. Residential pools are a significant cause, especially in children, as are bathtubs. Spas and "hot tubs" are becoming increasingly more involved in drownings. This is likely due to the effects of alcohol usage associated with bathing in them. Interestingly, many victims are competent swimmers—greater than 90% of incidents occur within 10 yards of shore, often in shallow water.

There are three causes of drowning. **"Dry" drowning** encompasses 10–20% of victims. Here, asphyxiation is caused by anoxia as a result of laryngeal spasm which prevents the entrance of water as well as air into the lungs. This leads to cerebral anoxia, edema, and unconsciousness. These victims have the best chance of survival.

"Wet" drowning involves 80–90% of cases. In this type of drowning, the victim makes a violent respiratory effort and fluid fills his lungs. **Secondary drowning** is defined as the recurrence of respiratory distress (usually in the form of pulmonary edema or aspiration pneumonia) after successful recovery from the initial incident. It can occur from a few minutes up to four days later.

Special Considerations for Care

One needs to think about several factors when taking care of near-drowning victims. Many immersion victims are hypothermic. Possible effects of low water temperatures include death secondary to exposure. Cold stimulation of the vagus nerve may lead to decreased heart rate and unconsciousness. This can lead to drowning and is potentiated by the presence of alcohol in the blood. On the positive side, cold may decrease cerebral metabolism and prolong survival.

The mammalian diving reflex may be potentiated by cold water. This reflex occurs when the human face is submerged in water. Respiration is inhibited (possibly secondary to glottic spasm) and profound bradycardia occurs (due to vagal stimulation). The cardiac output is shunted to the heart and brain with severe peripheral vasoconstriction and cyanosis occurring. Because of the diving reflex, a patient may be resuscitated even after prolonged

submersion if ventilation and circulation are maintained immediately upon removal from the water or even before. Table 3-8 summarizes the mammalian diving reflex.

Table 3-8. The Mammalian Diving Reflex

The Reflex
- Occurs with human facial submersion in water
- Potentiated by cold water

Causes
- Inhibition of respiration (? glottic spasm)
- Profound bradycardia (vagal stimulation)
- Shunting of cardiac output to heart/brain
- Severe peripheral vasoconstriction, cyanosis

Seawater vs. freshwater drownings

Differences between seawater and freshwater drownings have been grossly overemphasized in the past and are based upon much animal work. Previously reported massive electrolyte shifts do NOT occur in near-drownings and, in most cases, normal values are present. Transient fluid shifts can occur but are self-correcting in most cases. Lab studies suggest that 22 ml of water per kilogram needs to be aspirated before notable electrolyte changes will occur. It is highly unlikely that any human will aspirate this quantity of water. The only time significant electrolyte changes have been documented in man is near-drowning involving the extremely salty Dead Sea [*JAMA*, 1985, Vol. 253, p. 557].

Though the endpoints are the same, the mechanisms of lung damage from seawater and freshwater near-drowning are very different. Seawater is hypertonic to blood (3–4 times as concentrated in electrolytes and other osmotically active particles). Its presence in the lung causes the influx of hypotonic serum. This fills the alveoli (air sacs in the lung) and leads to a large shunt with profound hypoxemia (i.e., blood cannot exchange oxygen and carbon dioxide with filled alveoli, and they are bypassed). Pneumatocytes are likely injured as well, but salt water aspiration, per se, has no effect on lung surfactant already present. Some evidence exists in animal models to suggest that the pulmonary vascular endothelium is damaged the greatest early on in near-drowning [*Am J Emerg Med*, 1986, Vol. 4, pp. 4–9].

Freshwater aspiration, on the other hand, leads to a washout of surfactant. This compound is required for the lung tissue to maintain its elasticity. Loss of surfactant results in collapse of alveoli with subsequent hypoxemia. Thus, aspiration of either seawater or freshwater decreases pulmonary compliance and results in pulmonary edema with a concomitant intrapulmonary shunt and hypoxia.

Many of the late onset syndromes seen with near-drowning are likely due to lack of surfactant. The fact that these may be delayed for up to 46 hours in salt water near-drowning victims suggests that pneumatocytes are damaged early, and then later, fail to produce adequate quantities of surfactant, leading to alveolar collapse.

Cerebral hypoxia often precipitates neurogenic pulmonary edema which worsens an already bad situation. Thus, the endpoints in near-drowning, no matter WHAT type of water involved, are metabolic acidosis (which may be quite severe), pulmonary edema, and aspiration injuries (i.e., from chemicals and foreign matter). Table 3-9 summarizes the mechanisms of drowning.

When examining victims of near-drowning, it is important to note that they may initially appear to be normal. Usual **signs and symptoms** of problems include progressive dyspnea, wheezing, rales, and rhonchi. The patient may be tachycardic and cyanotic. The temperature (which MUST be taken rectally at some point in time) may be high or low. This is because of either heat loss secondary to hypothermia or hyperpyrexia (increased temperature) due to hypothalamic injury (the hypothalamus is the portion of the brain that regulates temperature) from hypoxia. Chest pains or mental confusion may be present. Coma, respiratory, or cardiac arrest can occur.

Table 3-9. The Mechanisms of Near-drowning

Seawater
> Hypertonic fluid enters the lungs
> An influx of hypotonic serum occurs
> The alveoli are filled, and hypoxia occurs
> A late decrease in surfactant production may occur due to type II pneumocyte damage

Freshwater
> Surfactant is rapidly washed out
> Alveoli collapse
> Hypoxemia occurs

The aspiration of either, thus, leads to:
> Decreased pulmonary compliance
> Pulmonary edema with shunting and hypoxia
> Neurogenic pulmonary edema
> Aspiration injuries from foreign material (if any)

Treatment

The victim should be removed from the water as soon as possible. CPR should be started if required. A technique for in-water CPR has been described which involves the rescuer supporting the victim horizontally from behind and delivering chest compressions by cross-chest hand positioning [*JAMA*, 1980, Vol. 244, p. 1229]. This technique has not been widely taught and is controversial. Some experts feel that it affords no significant advantage over no CPR and is difficult to perform [*Ann Emerg Med*, 1982, Vol. 11, p. 166]. Though interesting, this method is not recommended as standard therapy in the near-drowning victim.

Mouth-to-mouth respirations may be given in the water after clearing the airway. If there is any suggestion of neck injury (i.e., diving accident), stabilize the neck prior to removal of the patient from the water. Additionally, the following measures should be followed:

1. High-flow oxygen (10–15 LPM, mask) REGARDLESS of condition.

2. Salt-water victims only—positional drainage of lungs (head-dependent position). This recommendation is somewhat controversial and not universally accepted.

3. IV—NS or RL TKO; cardiac monitor.

4. Sodium bicarbonate (1 mEq/kg IV) MAY be indicated if the pH is severely acidotic (i.e., < 7.10). Caution should be exercised as this agent has several potential deleterious effects.

5. Some have recommended the immediate application of a subdiaphragmatic thrust (the ''Heimlich maneuver'') to all near-drowning patients. Though still controversial, the current recommendation of the AHA is that this be used only if mouth-to-mouth rescue breathing fails to successfully resuscitate the victim [*JAMA,* 1986, Vol. 256, p. 75].

In the Emergency Department, draw ABGs (even if the patient is alert and oriented since marked hypoxia may still exist), CBC, electrolytes, blood alcohol level, and toxicology screen. Since near-drowning does not significantly lower the hematocrit, internal hemorrhage should be suspected if this finding is present in the absence of significant hemolysis.

One should treat pulmonary edema if it is present using some form of positive pressure breathing. A **chest X-ray** should be obtained on ALL patients. Remember that it may initially underestimate the degree of injury. An EKG, along with cardiac monitoring, should also be performed.

Positive end expiratory pressure (PEEP) or continuous positive airway pressure (CPAP) may be highly effective because of their effect on intrapulmonary shunting. Many studies suggest early institution of PEEP may reverse the acute process in the lungs. If aspiration of particulate matter is suspected, the patient may need bronchoscopy via the ET tube. Prophylactic steroids and antibiotics are NOT indicated. Along the same lines, there is no demonstrated effect of hypothermia or barbiturate therapy (''H.Y.P.E.R.'' therapy) on morbidity and mortality after near-drowning [*Crit Care Med,* 1986, Vol. 13, p. 529].

Comatose victims of cold freshwater submersion should receive vigorous cerebral resuscitation including the use of intracranial pressure monitoring, if available. The use of barbiturates in coma is still considered highly experimental and is not to be recommended at this time outside of a research protocol.

Complications

Several complications can occur following near-drowning. Persistent hypoxemia is common and usually multifactorial in etiology. Infection, especially pneumonia, may occur even several days later. Unusual organisms are to be expected, especially if the victim was swimming in polluted water. Renal failure has been reported but is not overly common.

The most bothersome complication is a persistent neurological deficit. The best predictor of severity is the time to the first spontaneous gasp following removal from the water. The shorter this period, the better the neurological prognosis. Patients taking > 1 hour for this to occur (if it does at all) have a bleak prognosis.

Pearls to Remember

1. Be prepared for vomiting at any time.

2. ALL submersion victims should be transported. Even if the patient initially appears to be fine, they can deteriorate rapidly. Pulmonary edema is especially likely. Late deterioration occurs in about 1 out of 20 near-drowning victims. It usually occurs within 4 hours, but with salt-water immersion, latent periods of up to 46 hours have been reported [*Brit Med J,* 1980, Vol. 281, pp. 1103–1105]. One study has suggested that 4–6 hours may serve as an adequate observation period in that all of their patients who developed respiratory distress did so within that time [*Ann Emerg Med,* September 1986, Vol. 15, p. 1084]. This suggestion is not uniformly accepted.

3. Beware of neck injuries—they often go unrecognized. It is best to treat any unconscious submersion victim with spinal immobilization and proper X-ray evaluation.

4. A hypothermic victim is not dead until they are "warm and dead."

SPONTANEOUS PNEUMOTHORAX

Pneumothorax may be defined as the presence of gas within the pleural space. There are three ways in which this can occur:

1. From the lung via a perforation of the visceral pleura.

2. From outside via a perforation of the chest wall and thus, the parietal pleura.

3. From gas-forming organisms (rare) in the pleural space.

There are several **types** of spontaneous pneumothorax. The most common type, **idiopathic,** will be discussed first followed by a review of the others.

Idiopathic spontaneous pneumothorax is defined as that which occurs without an inciting event. The **etiology** is the rupture of a small, usually clinically undetectable, structurally weak bleb.

The **epidemiology** of idiopathic spontaneous pneumothorax is interesting. The preponderance of affected individuals are males (85%), mostly between the ages of 20 and 40. The most common complication is recurrence, happening in anywhere from 10–60% of patients. There appears to be an increased risk with greater body height. Some authors feel there is a predisposition in men with long, narrow chests. For unknown reasons, most affected persons are cigarette smokers.

Diagnosis

History

The history is usually that of the abrupt onset of unilateral pleuritic chest pain. There may be accompanying shortness of breath and, at times, nonproductive cough. There are many cases of spontaneous pneumothorax reported to occur during exertion but the weight of the evidence does NOT support this as a predictable inciting factor.

Physical examination

The physical examination will reveal the patient to be tachypneic. Decreased breath sounds and hyperresonance may be present over the affected side. In a smaller pneumothorax, these signs are often absent. If a tension pneumothorax is present (i.e., hemodynamic compromise secondarily to respiratory and circulatory embarrassment), the trachea may be deviated AWAY from the affected side, and significant hypotension may be present.

Laboratory tests

Abnormal arterial blood gases, though these are NOT necessary for the diagnosis, may be revealed.

The definitive study is the **chest X-ray.** It is important to remember that small pneumothoraces will NOT show on the standard inspiratory X-ray and that expiratory views may be needed. These should always be obtained in any previously healthy young patient with the sudden onset of chest pain.

The presence of a pneumothorax is verified on X-ray by a distinct separation of the lung edge and the chest wall. This appears as a blackened space that lacks any airway markings whatsoever. The size or "%" of the spontaneous pneumothorax can be determined from the X-ray by measuring this distance (the "interpleural distance") and referring to a standardized nomogram. A rough rule to follow is as follows:

% PNEUMO = INTERPLEURAL DIST (CM) $\times$ 10

Thus, if the distance between chest wall and lung edge is 2.5 cm, the patient has about a 25% pneumothorax. Figure 3.1 illustrates these findings and measurement of the interpleural distance.

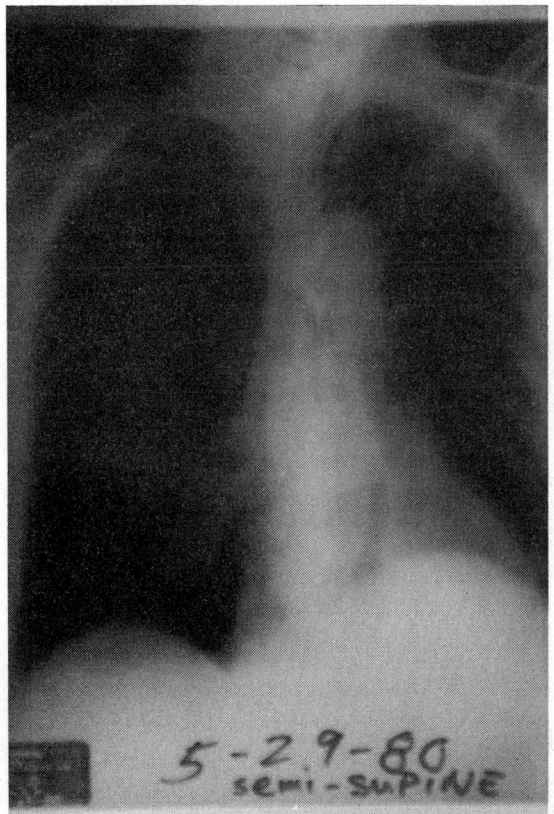

Figure 3.1. The findings and measurements of interpleural distance.

Treatment

Treatment for idiopathic spontaneous pneumothorax consists of the following:

1. Initially treat as any chest pain patient (i.e., oxygen, IV, cardiac monitor, etc.).

2. These patients should be transported and evaluated regardless of age.

3. If the pneumothorax is > 25%, placement of a chest tube for drainage of air is necessary.

4. If the pneumothorax is < 25% and there is no evidence of significant underlying disease, progression, and this is NOT a recurrent spontaneous pneumothorax, the chest tube may not be necessary. Some choose to observe these individuals as outpatients, but the majority should be watched in the hospital for at least 24 hours. The chest X-ray should be repeated in 1–2 days and then at monthly intervals. The rate of reabsorption of air is 1.25% per day. Thus, a 30% pneumothorax would take about 3–4 weeks to completely resolve.

5. Overzealous expansion of a spontaneous pneumothorax greater than three days old can lead to unilateral pulmonary edema on the affected side. Thus, if the decision is made to place a chest tube in this type of a patient, gentle (if any) suction should be employed.

The initial diagnosis and treatment for other types of spontaneous pneumothorax besides the idiopathic variety are similar, though definitive therapy may vary. **Catamenial pneumothorax** is that associated with the menses. It is usually right sided, occurring in women aged 20–30 years old. It is thought secondary to the presence of endometrial implants (intrauterine tissue) in either the lung or pleura that rupture after swelling during the menstrual cycle. Hormonal therapy prevents the recurrence of this problem.

Spontaneous pneumothorax can also be associated with any type of interstitial lung disease. The mechanism in malignant disease is uncertain. Spontaneous pneumothorax is associated primarily with sarcomas that metastasize to the lungs. Certain chemotherapeutic agents (i.e., methotrexate and cyclophosphamide) can also lead to interstitial fibrosis which is associated with spontaneous pneumothorax. Sarcoidosis (an interesting entity that may cause the formation of scar tissue in the lung) and rheumatoid lung disease may also underlie spontaneous pneumothorax by the same route.

Spontaneous pneumothorax associated with COPD is usually secondary to rupture of intact intrapulmonary bullae through intact visceral pleura. These result from the loss of elastic tissue and destruction of parenchyma that result from COPD. Breathlessness and anxiety may be greater than chest pain in these individuals. Often, the degree of shortness of breath is out of proportion to the degree of lung collapse. Thus, it is a good idea to get both inspiratory and expiratory chest films in those with stable COPD who suddenly deteriorate. The treatment is chest-tube drainage. Long periods of this are often required. Table 3-10 summarizes the different types of spontaneous pneumothorax.

Table 3-10. Types of Spontaneous Pneumothorax

Idiopathic
  Occurs without an inciting event
  Usually young, male smoker
  Due to rupture of congenital "bleb"

Catamenial
  Associated with menses
  Young women 20–30 years old
  Due to presence of endometrial
    implants on pleura/lung

Interstitial Lung Disease
  Metastatic sarcoma
  • Methotrexate
  • Cyclophosphamide
  Sarcoidosis
  Rheumatoid lung disease

Chronic Obstructive Lung Disease
  Due to rupture of intraparenchymal
    bullae
  Shortness of breath out of proportion to
    the degree of collapse
  Inspiratory and expiratory films recommended

PULMONARY EMBOLISM

Pulmonary embolism (PE) is defined as the lodging of a blood clot (embolus) in one of the arteries of the pulmonary circulation. This is a common, potentially lethal, and highly underdiagnosed entity. Pulmonary embolism is the third most common cause of death in the United States. There are about 650,000

annually. Of these, 10% die within one hour of the event. Of those surviving, the diagnosis is *missed* in two-thirds with these individuals having a 30% mortality. Ninety-two percent of those who survived > 1 hour in whom the diagnosis was correctly made, lived.

Causes of pulmonary embolism commonly relate to underlying deep venous thrombosis. Small pieces break off and travel, via the vena cava, to the right heart then to the lung. Ninety percent arise from the deep veins of the pelvis and lower extremities. Others originate from infected heart valves (endocarditis), pacemakers, and arteriovenous shunts.

The most common **predisposing factors** in venous thrombosis are venous stasis and hypercoagulability. Stasis is promoted by prolonged immobilization as well as vascular injury. Hypercoagulability is common in many conditions, including: cancer, polycythemia vera, antithrombin III deficiency, pregnancy, use of birth control pills, myocardial infarction, atrial fibrillation, congestive heart failure, obesity, and COPD.

Diagnosis

In terms of **pathophysiology,** several things happen when a blood clot impacts within the pulmonary vasculature. Initially, the platelets break apart, releasing chemical granules ("degranulation"). These "granules" contain such vasoactive substances as histamine, catecholamines, serotonin, and prostaglandins. These lead to constriction of the smooth muscle in both the bronchi and pulmonary arteries. A mismatch of ventilation (due to bronchoconstriction) and perfusion then occurs. If a large main pulmonary artery is blocked (or both of them—"saddle embolus"), a severe strain is put on the right side of the heart. This will often lead to acute right-sided heart failure with circulatory collapse.

History
The patient will usually give a history of chest pain that is often, but not always, pleuritic. There may be dyspnea, apprehension, nonproductive cough, and hemoptysis. In a massive pulmonary embolism, the presenting complaint may be syncope. The patient may relate a story of a long airplane or car ride

or of a previous vascular injury. The presence of a previous pulmonary embolism should be determined, as these patients are at a higher risk of recurrence.

Physical examination

Tachypnea (defined as respiratory rate—16/min) is revealed in 90% of patients. The absence of this sign should strongly reduce the suspicion of pulmonary embolism. Wheezes, rhonchi, and friction rubs are sometimes heard. The patient may have a low-grade temperature (38°C), tachycardia, and an increased pulmonic component of the second heart sound (P2). These three features are present in about 50% of individuals. Less than one-third will have evidence of clinical "phlebitis." Table 3-11 summarizes the clinical features of pulmonary embolism.

Table 3-11. Clinical Features of Pulmonary Embolism

History
    Chest pain—usually pleuritic
    Dyspnea
    Apprehension
    Cough, hemoptysis
    Syncope (massive PE only)

Physical
    Tachypnea (respiratory rate >
       16/min)—90% of patients
    Wheezes, rhonchi, rubs
    Temperature > 38°C ⎱ present in
    Tachycardia > 100 ⎰ 50% of
    Increased P_2 patients
    Clinical phlebitis—< 1/3 of patients

Laboratory tests

Lab studies of most interest are the ABGs. The pO_2 is often decreased BUT 10-15% of patients with proven pulmonary emboli have a pO_2 > 80 mm Hg. More sensitive is a rough estimate of the A-a (alveolar-arterial) gradient. This is a measure of the extraction of oxygen from the air sacs (alveoli) in the lungs versus the percentage of oxygen presented them

from inspired air. Widening of this gradient suggests a problem in oxygenation. This is estimated as follows:

$$\text{A-a gradient} = 140 - [pO_2 + pCO_2]$$

The normal value is between 15, in younger people, and 25, in the elderly. This equation assumes the patient to be on room air.

In the past, the triad of an elevated LDH, SGOT, and bilirubin were thought to be highly suggestive of pulmonary embolism. These are now thought to be of minimal value, and it is NOT recommended that they be obtained for this purpose. The **white blood cell count** averages 11,000 (normal = 5000-10,000) in pulmonary embolism and is, therefore, of no additional value.

The **EKG** is often abnormal but generally nonspecific. Possible changes include:

1. Signs of right heart strain (right bundle branch block, right axis deviation, an "S1, Q2, T3" pattern).

2. Multiple areas suggesting myocardial infarction (this is caused by diffuse myocardial ischemia and right heart strain). Findings mimicking acute anterior myocardial infarction have been described [*West J Med*, 1986, Vol. 145, p. 98].

3. Nonspecific ST and T wave changes are the MOST COMMON findings noted.

The **chest X-ray** is rarely normal with massive emboli but with smaller emboli is much less helpful. Clues such as atelectasis, diaphragmatic elevation (unilateral), pleural effusion (unilateral), and a wedge-shaped infiltrate may be present. Two-dimensional echocardiography may demonstrate a dilated right ventricle, dilatation of the pulmonary artery, and poor intraventricular septal movement [*Am Heart J*, 1986, Vol. 112, p. 1284]. Various tests that confirm the presence of deep venous thrombosis are helpful if positive—Doppler studies, plethysmography, fibrinogen leg scanning, and venography.

A **radionucleotide lung scan** should be obtained early in the patient's management. A normal perfusion scan virtually rules out the diagnosis of pulmonary embolism. A positive scan is less specific. The perfusion scan becomes more accurate when combined with a ventilation scan. Based on published criteria [*Mayo Clinic Proceedings*, 1981, Vol. 56, p. 161], the probability of acute pulmonary embolism can be ranked as low, indeterminate, or high. These criteria utilize findings in both the perfusion and combined perfusion/ventilation lung scans. In most cases, a "high-probability" lung scan is enough evidence to treat the patient. Otherwise, further testing should probably be done.

Pulmonary angiography should be performed in suspected cases of pulmonary embolism with less than a high probability radionucleotide scan or where the patient is at potential high risk for bleeding on anticoagulation therapy (severe hypertension, active GI or genitourinary bleeding, recurrent stroke). This is considered the "gold standard" in the diagnosis of pulmonary embolism. A negative pulmonary angiogram rules out any reasonable chance of significant pulmonary emboli. Some experts would favor impedance plethysmography studies to detect the presence of venous thrombosis before performing an angiogram [*J Am Coll Card*, 1986, Vol. 8, p. 1288]. Table 3-12 summarizes the laboratory and X-ray features of pulmonary embolism.

Treatment

Treatment of the patient with potential pulmonary embolism includes oxygen therapy (2–4 LPM, NP), cardiac monitoring, and pain control. Morphine in doses of 2 mg IV every 5 minutes is helpful in severe chest pain. Dobutamine has been used successfully in shock associated with pulmonary embolism.

Anticoagulant therapy is initiated acutely with HEPARIN. This substance combines with the naturally occurring protein antithrombin III to inhibit certain steps in the blood coagulation system. It has NO effect upon pre-existing thromboses or emboli. The sole purpose is to prevent recurrence.

Heparin may be started if a high index of suspicion is present BEFORE definitive studies are available. Therapy is followed by the partial thromboplastin time (PTT). An initial bolus of 2,000–10,000 units is given IV. This is immediately followed by a continuous intravenous infusion of 1,000 units per hour (mix 20,000 U heparin in 500 cc D_5W—this

---

Table 3-12. Lab and X-Ray Features of Pulmonary Embolism

Arterial Blood Gases
Room air hypoxemia—present in 80–85%
Widened A-a gradient often more helpful

Enzymes (LDH, SGOT, Bilirubin)—Not Helpful

CBC—WBC averages 11,000—Therefore Not Helpful

EKG—Nonspecific But Often Abnormal
Right heart strain
Multiple areas of "infarction"
Nonspecific ST-T changes (most common)

Chest X-Ray—Nonspecific
Atelectasis
Diaphragmatic elevation
Pleural effusion
Wedge-shaped infiltrate

Tests to Rule Out Venous Thrombosis (Helpful If +)
Doppler
Plethysmography
Fibrinogen leg scanning
Venograph

Radionucleotide Venogram
Normal perfusion scan rules out
Rank according to low, indeterminate, or high probability

Pulmonary Angiogram—"Gold Standard"
Indications
Suspected cases with < high probability radionucleotide scan
Patients at high risk for bleeding on anticoagulants
• Severe hypertension
• Active GI/GU bleeding
• Recent CVA

leads to a concentration of 40 U/cc). The PTT is checked 4–6 hours later and the drip adjusted to keep the PTT > 50 and < 80. Heparin should be continued until adequate oral anticoagulation has been achieved. Some groups advocate thrombolytic therapy using streptokinase or urokinase first (see below).

The current thinking is that 7–10 days of heparin therapy is NOT necessary before changing to oral anticoagulants. It may actually be harmful to treat patients longer as the risk of heparin-induced thrombocytopenia (decreased platelets) increases with duration of therapy. Therefore, the current recommendation is to initiate oral anticoagulant therapy (usually Coumadin) within 24 hours of beginning heparin. When adequate oral anticoagulation is achieved as measured by the protime (PT should be 18–25), the heparin should be gradually weaned over several hours. There is much literature which suggests that the *rapid* discontinuation of either heparin OR coumadin can lead to a rebound hypercoagulable state.

Thrombolytic therapy, similar to that described for acute myocardial infarction, has also been used in pulmonary embolism. Both streptokinase (SK) and urokinase (UK) have been used with success. The major indication in pulmonary embolism is hemodynamic instability in the presence of angiographically documented pulmonary embolism. Recommended doses are as follows:

1. SK—250,000 U IV over 20–30 minutes followed by 100,000 to 150,000 U per hour IV × 24 hours; SK should be preceded by hydrocortisone 100 mg IV and then every 12 hours to prevent severe allergic reactions.

2. UK—4,000 U/kg over 20–30 minutes IV followed by 2,000 U/kg/hr IV infusion over 24 hours. One study suggested equal efficacy of a single bolus of UK (15,000 U/kg over 10 minutes directly into the right atrium), followed immediately by systemic heparization [*Circulation,* November 1984, p. 861]. This was a small but interesting study, and this

method cannot be universally recommended at this time.

The thrombin time (TT) is followed by many using this therapy to insure the presence of an adequate thrombolytic state. Others feel this to be unnecessary. The patient should be watched for bleeding problems. It is a good idea to minimize invasive procedures (blood drawing, blood gases, etc.) during the period of thrombolysis.

TOXIC GAS INHALATION

There are three categories of toxic gases—inert/fuel gases, irritant gases, and gases that are systemic toxins.

Inert gases include carbon dioxide (CO_2) and the "fuel gases" (methane, ethane, propane, acetylene). In large enough concentrations, these displace air and oxygen leading to asphyxia. If the inspired air contains < 10% O_2 (remember room air is normally 21% O_2), death may occur with even the slightest exertion.

Irritant gases, in decreasing order of water solubility, include: ammonia, formaldehyde, chloramine, chlorine, nitrogen dioxide (NO_2), and phosgene. The more water-soluble gases dissolve easily in the mucus of the upper airway leading to damage here as well as to the eyes, nose, and mouth. The less water-soluble types travel further into the respiratory tract, leading to pulmonary injury and adult respiratory distress syndrome (ARDS).

Gases that are **systemic toxins** are of two varieties. Carbon monoxide (CO), cyanide (CN), and hydrogen sulfide (H_2S) interfere with the transport and delivery of oxygen for cell energy production. Aromatic and halogenated hydrocarbons (carbon tetrachloride, benzene, toluene vapors) have more direct organ-specific effects. The liver, kidney, brain, and lung are all often involved. These compounds involve the inhalation of vapors rather than gases as we truly think of them. Thus, the aromatic and halogenated hydrocarbons will not be discussed further. Table 3-13 summarizes the categories of toxic gases.

Table 3-13. Categories of Toxic Gases

Inert Gases—Death by Asphyxiation
  Carbon dioxide
  Fuel gases—methane, ethane, propane,
     acetylene

Irritants
  Ammonia   (more H_2O soluble)
  Foramaldehyde
  Chloramine
  Chlorine
  Nitrous dioxide
  Phosgene   (less H_2O soluble)

Systemic Toxins
  Interference with O_2 Transport and
     Delivery
  • Carbon monoxide
  • Cyanide
  • Hydrogen
  Aromatic and halogenated hydrocarbons
  • Carbon tetrachloride
  • Benzene
  • Toluene

Sources of Toxic Gas

Accidental release such as in plant leaks, motor vehicle accidents (involving transporting trucks), and railroad accidents are common sources. Chemical reactions may lead to the release of cyanide and are the commonest source of NO_2 (the oxidation of nitrates in green plants in silos leads to the formation of silo gas).

Fires and the toxic products of incomplete combustion are very common sources of toxic gases. This includes such items as improperly vented gas appliances. Carbon monoxide is released from the burning of any carbon-containing material. Plastics and rayon may release CN and chlorine (Cl_2). The combustion of wool, cotton, and paper can release an extremely irritating substance called acrolein while

nitrogen oxides are common when finished woods, fabrics, and X-ray film burn. Phosgene gas may be produced during a fire involving some plastics and rubber materials. Finally, the combustion of polyurethane products, woods, and silk may lead to the formation of cyanide, ammonia, and formaldehyde gases.

Diagnosis

In discussing the **pathophysiology** of toxic gas inhalation, it is important to examine the factors affecting the type and degree of injury. As mentioned previously, the water solubility of the gas is important. Highly soluble (ammonia, chlorine) gases dissolve in the mucus of the nasopharynx, larynx, and trachea, leading to irritation and large airway injury. Those less-soluble gases (nitrogen dioxide and phosgene) tend to flow deep into lung tissue, resulting in alveolar injury.

The depth and rate of breathing are important as well. A water-soluble irritant tends to be rapidly absorbed during slow, nasal breathing (i.e., there is much time for contact). This same gas may be only 40–50% absorbed with rapid oral breathing. Noxious odors of some gases may serve to warn of problems and avert damage, but several factors must be considered. Many gases are harmful well below their odor threshhold. Others (hydrogen sulfide) produce olfactory fatigue (the rotten-eggs odor seems to fade despite the continued presence of toxic concentrations of gas). Cyanide has a non-noxious odor (sweet, almond-like) as does phosgene (newly mown hay).

The concentration of the gas and the time of exposure are significant. Exposure times less than one minute are unlikely to cause problems. Finally, there may be differences in host susceptibility and smoking habits. Interestingly, cigarette smoking lowers resistance to toxic gases.

The **clinical presentation** differs depending on the type of gas involved. Anoxia-causing gases tend to result in relatively sudden death. Those causing metabolic problems will be discussed on pages 44–47. A few comments are in order currently in reference to irritant gases. Silo gas inhalation (NO_2) will be presented on pages 47–48. Irritant gases may have immediate, delayed, and chronic effects.

Immediate effects occur within 1–2 hours of exposure. They may consist of an irritant reaction, such as that from ammonia, or a bronchospastic response, such as that from sulphur dioxide (SO_2). The irritant reaction is essentially an acute laryngotracheobronchitis. Mucous membranes are red and inflamed. There is eye and nasal irritation with bronchorrhea (copious bronchial secretions), cough, and sore throat. A bronchospastic response consists of dyspnea, chest tightness, and wheezing. Incidentally, carbon monoxide toxicity may precipitate either myocardial infarction or pulmonary embolus (due to hyperviscosity of the blood). Thus, immediate effects noted may be those of these entities.

Delayed effects occur 6–24 hours following exposure. Laryngeal edema with hoarseness, inspiratory stridor, and the complaint of a "lump in the throat" may occur. Soot in the mouth, singed hairs, and stridor are now felt to be rather nonspecific. Flow-volume loops are felt to be much more sensitive indicators of early laryngeal edema. This may worsen 24–48 hours later.

Noncardiogenic pulmonary edema (ARDS) may also occur as a delayed reaction. This results from damage to the alveolar epithelium. The effect is respiratory distress, initially mild with a nonproductive cough and mild chest discomfort. This may or may not progress to full-blown ARDS. If it does, there is a 50% mortality.

Chronic effects are relatively uncommon as complete recovery is the rule from many inhalations if treated properly. Bronchiectasis, damage to the large airways with inadequate clearance of mucus and bacteria leading to copious sputum production and infection, may occur. Recurrent pneumonia is common in this situation. Bronchiolitis obliterans is a result of damage to the respiratory bronchioles with progressive shortness of breath resembling COPD. Steroid administration during the acute phase can markedly decrease the incidence of this complication. Interstitial fibrosis, the formation of fibrous scar tissue in the interstitium between alveoli, is a final potential chronic problem. Table 3-14 summarizes the clinical presentation of irritant gas exposure.

Field evaluation of the toxic gas inhalation patient is as follows:

1. Protect yourself from exposure—use a respirator and appropriate clothing.

2. Remove the victim promptly from the area.

3. O_2—10–15 LPM by mask.

4. IV D_5W TKO; may substitute RL/NS and increase rate if patient is hypotensive (and with medical control approval—too much fluid can precipitate ARDS).

5. Prompt transport.

Table 3-14. Clinical Presentation of Irritant Gas Exposure

Immediate (Within 1–2 Hours)
Irritant reactions—
    laryngotracheobronchitis
- Red, inflamed mucous membranes
- Eye and nasal irritation
- Bronchorrhea, cough
- Sore throat

Bronchospastic reaction—dyspnea, chest tightness, wheezing

Delayed (6–24 Hours)
Laryngeal edema
Hoarseness
Inspiratory stridor
Lump in throat
Noncardiogenic pulmonary edema

Chronic—Complete Recovery Usually the Rule
Late Problems
Bronchiectasis
Bronchiolitis obliterans—prevent with steroids
Interstitial fibrosis

Emergency Department evaluation involves, first, a brief *history*. Is there any eye, nose, or throat irritation? Is there dyspnea, chest tightness, or a history of underlying cardiopulmonary disease.

Physical examination

The physical examination may reveal ocular or facial chemical burns. Stridor may be obvious along with wheezes or rales. Other burns should be looked for (if patient was involved in a fire). Careful attention should be paid to the patient's mental and cardiovascular status.

Laboratory tests

Arterial blood gases (room air if possible), arterial carboxyhemoglobin level, chest X-ray, EKG, and bedside spirometry should be included. Hospital admission is recommended for 24 hours in all inhalation victims, and it is MANDATORY if even a single singed nose hair is noted, if the victims were involved in a closed-space fire, or if soot is found in the pharynx. Arterial carboxyhemoglobin (COHb) levels > 8% in smokers and > 4% in nonsmokers are potentially worrisome.

Treatment

Hospital treatment should be as follows:

1. Frequent vital sign determinations in an ICU.

2. O_2—enough to keep the arterial $pO_2 = 60-70$.

3. Intravenous THEOPHYLLINE and inhaled ISOETHARINE (Bronkosol) are recommended even in the absence of wheezing as they may decrease the incidence of ARDS by decreasing the tendency towards increased capillary permeability. HYDROCORTISONE should be added only if the patient is actively wheezing.

4. Hemodynamic monitoring with a Swan-Ganz catheter is indicated if there is any suggestion of ARDS. The pulmonary artery wedge pressure should be kept at < 12.

5. Prophylactic antibiotics are NOT recommended.

6. Prophylactic STEROIDS are not indicated unless the patient is wheezing OR to prevent bronchiolitis obliterans following NO_2 exposure (silo gas). Gradually decreasing doses of a potent steroid can then be given orally over a six-week period.

Specific Toxins

Carbon monoxide

Carbon monoxide (CO) is a colorless, odorless, tasteless, and nonirritating gas that is a common source of poisoning. The source, incomplete combustion of material containing carbon, is THE major cause of industrial deaths and deaths caused by fire. Domestic sources include indoor barbecues, automobiles, and inadequately ventilated heating systems. Gas furnaces are probably the most common source of nonindustrial CO exposure.

The **pathophysiology** is twofold. Carbon monoxide binds irreversibly with hemoglobin (Hb) leading to the formation of carboxyhemoglobin (COHb). This substance is unable to carry oxygen or CO_2. Thus, the delivery of oxygen to the tissues is severely compromised. The effect is a lower Hb saturation than would be caused solely by hypoxia. Carbon monoxide also directly inhibits the cellular cytochrome (energy transport) system directly. The heart and brain have the highest metabolic rates and are, thus, the most sensitive. Angina, EKG abnormalities, and decreased vision and hearing may occur. Pulmonary edema, disseminated intravascular coagulation (DIC), lactic acidosis, and hypercoagulability are possible.

Symptoms include malaise, weakness, headache, confusion, dizziness, nausea, and shortness of breath. Unconsciousness may occur without premonitory symptoms. Syncope is common with carbon monoxide levels above 24.3% [*J Emerg Med,* 1985, Vol. 3, p. 443]. As mentioned previously, complaints referable to acute MI or pulmonary embolism may be present.

The **physical exam** only rarely reveals the "cherry red" skin and mucous membranes so commonly mentioned. Rales and rhonchi may be present if pulmonary edema is present. Retinal hemorrhages, seizures, and skin lesions (bullae and blisters) may be noted.

Laboratory work obtained should include cardiac enzymes (to rule out subclinical myocardial damage), CBC, and electrolytes. The EKG may show ischemic ST-T changes, infarction, or atrial arrhythmias. A COHb level is a MUST determination, if available. A normal level does NOT exclude the diagnosis, especially if oxygen has been given for a period of time, though. ABGs usually show a normal pO_2 but a marked difference in the measured percentage of saturation and the calculated value. Table 3-15 summarizes the diagnosis of carbon monoxide poisoning.

Table 3-15. Diagnosis of Carbon Monoxide Poisoning

Symptoms
> Malaise, weakness, headache
> Confusion, dizziness
> Nausea, shortness of breath
> Unconscious—can occur without
>   premonitory symptoms
> Symptoms of myocardial infarction,
>   pulmonary embolism

Physical
> Cherry red skin, mucous
>   membrane—rare
> Rales, rhonchi (if pulmonary edema
>   present)
> Retinal hemorrhages
> Seizures
> Bullae, blisters

Lab
> EKG—ischemic ST-T changes, infarction, atrial arrhythmias
> COHb level—normal does not exclude diagnosis!
> ABG—difference in measured VS calculated % saturation, pO_2 usually normal
> CBC, lytes, cardiac enzymes

When considering **treatment,** it is important to remember that the patient's course may fluctuate. The half-life of COHb at room air is 5–6 hours. With 100% O_2, it decreases to 45–90 minutes and even further if hyperbaric O_2 is used (23 minutes). If available, a hyperbaric chamber is, thus, the optimal first choice. Normally, most patients are treated with as high a concentration as possible. If they are awake and alert, endotracheal intubation just to achieve 100% FIO_2 is unnecessary. Hypothermia is *contraindicated* as it shifts the oxygen-hemoglobin dissociation curve to the left, further decreasing the availability of oxygen to the tissues. A mass effect of 100% oxygen will eventually displace COHb from the body.

Criteria for admission include the following:

1. COHb levels > 25%; also if > 15% in a patient with cardiovascular disease or > 10% in a pregnant woman.

2. Presence of acute EKG changes.

3. Abnormal neuropsychiatric presentation.

4. Metabolic acidosis (suggesting severe tissue hypoxia).

5. Arterial pO_2 < 60 on room air.

Many feel that hyperbaric oxygen therapy is warranted even in less serious cases. Minor alterations in the level of consciousness upon Emergency Department arrival may be associated with neuropsychiatric sequelae and are felt by some experts to indicate a need for aggressive therapy. Without hyperbaric oxygen many patients have detectable neuropsychiatric deficits. Over 10% are severely disabled. At least two studies suggest benefit [*Ann Emerg Med*, 1985, Vol. 14, p. 1163; *Ann Emerg Med*, 1985, Vol. 14, p. 1168]; unfortunately, no randomized controlled work is available.

Thus, the general consensus is that patients should be referred for hyperbaric oxygen therapy if the carboxyhemoglobin levels are greater than 20%, if they have lost consciousness, or have neurological deficits or cardiac toxicity. More liberal guidelines may be necessary in pregnancy due to the susceptibility of the fetus to carbon monoxide. The effects of hyperbaric oxygen on the fetus are unknown, and each case should be considered individually by a hyperbaric medicine expert [*Am J*

Emerg Med, 1986, Vol. 4, p. 516].

Cyanide

Cyanide (CN) is present either as hydrogen cyanate (HCN), cyanogen (CN_2), or cyanogen chloride (CNCl). The **source** is fires, metallurgy and photo labs, combustion of rubber products, amygdalin (Laetril), and potentially from long-term nitroprusside infusion. It has a sweet, almond-like odor.

In terms of **pathophysiology,** CN inhibits cytochrome oxidase, which is the terminal enzyme in the mitochondrial electron transport chain. At a microscopic level, the chain "moves" electrons from substance to substance, enabling the cell's metabolic processes to utilize oxygen. CN poisoning prevents this, resulting in the complete inability for the cell to utilize oxygen.

With inhalation, such as during prison executions, death is usually instantaneous. Studies have shown that these individuals could not have been saved even if the circumstances were different, and they were promptly transported to a hospital. When CN is absorbed through the skin or orally the onset of **symptoms** is delayed for a few minutes. Things then gradually progress with death occurring in 3–4 hours. Acute headache, vertigo, drowsiness, convulsions, and coma may be noted. The patient may also complain of tongue burning, excessive salivation, and nausea with oral ingestion.

Often, an early excitation phase, resembling anxiety-hyperventilation, occurs first. This progresses rapidly to coma and possibly seizures.

On **physical examination,** the odor of bitter almonds may be noted on the breath. The ability to detect this odor is genetically determined, being absent in about one-half of the population. Altered mental status, tachypnea, and bradycardia may be noted. The patient's blood may appear bright red due to the inability of cells to utilize oxygen. Later on, cyanosis will invariably be present. The blood pressure is initially elevated then decreases as the severity of the intoxication progresses. On fundoscopic examination, the venules and arterioles may appear equally red, indicating inability of the tissues to utilize oxygen.

Laboratory findings may resemble those in carbon monoxide poisoning. ABGs will show a metabolic acidosis and a narrowed A-a gradient due to the inability of the tissues to use 0_2. Arterial and venous oxygen saturations may be very similar—normally they differ anywhere from 20–50%. In addition, there may be a difference of > 5% between the measured and calculated arterial oxygen saturation. A widened anion gap from lactic acidosis is present on the electrolyte screen. Hyperglycemia may also be noted. EKG abnormalities range from simple tachycardia to peaked T-waves and decreased ST-intervals with the T-wave almost "on top of" the QRS complex.

Rapid institution of **treatment** is mandatory. A regional Poison Control Center should be contacted as soon as possible, BUT this should NOT delay treatment of suspected cyanide intoxication. The principle behind treatment of CN poisoning involves administration of nitrite compounds to oxidize hemoglobin, forming methemoglobin ($Hb\text{-}Fe^{3+}$). $Hb\text{-}Fe^{3+}$ binds with the cyanide-cytochrome oxidase complex, displacing the CN. CN is then complexed with methemoglobin, freeing the cytochrome oxidase. Sodium thiosulfate is given and binds with CN-Hb-Fe^{3+} to form thiocynate, which is excreted. Methemoglobin is then metabolized by the red blood cell back to reduced hemoglobin ($Hb\text{-}Fe^{3+}$). Table 3-16 summarizes how the treatment regimen works.

Table 3-16. Treatment of Cyanide Intoxication

- CN + cytochrome oxidase (C-OX)
  → CN-C-DX
- Amyl nitrate + sodium nitrite + $Hb\text{-}Fe^{2+}$ → $Hb\text{-}Fe^{3+}$ (methemoglobin)
- $Hb\text{-}Fe^{3+}$ CN-C-OX → CN-Hb-Fe^{3+} + C-OX (cytochrome oxidase freed)
- CN-Hb-Fe^{3+} + sodium thiosulfate → thiocynate + $Hb\text{-}Fe^{3+}$

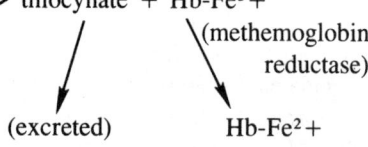

(methemoglobin reductase)

(excreted) $Hb\text{-}Fe^{2+}$

The patient is first placed on 100% oxygen. The easiest way to treat CN poisoning is with the Lilly

Cyanide Poisoning Kit (No. M-76) which is specially prepared for this. Alternatively, the required chemicals may be kept together in the Emergency Department. Amyl nitrite needs to be replaced at least once year each year. The following steps are then performed rapidly:

1. Break the pearls of AMYL NITRITE onto gauze and hold them under the patient's nose or over the ambu-Bag intake valve for 30 seconds to one minute while someone is preparing the sodium nitrite.

2. SODIUM NITRITE, 10 cc of a 3% solution at 2.5–5 cc per minute IV in an adult. Be prepared to treat hypotension (due to vasodilation) at this stage.

3. SODIUM THIOSULFATE, 12.5 gm (50 ml of a 25% solution) IV.

4. Induce emesis in a conscious patient if recommended by the regional Poison Control Center.

Methylene blue should be available (see below) for treatment, but this can also release previously bound cyanide.

Some researchers have suggested the use of hyperbaric oxygen [*Emerg Med,* August 15, 1986, p. 191]. It should be considered if the patient does not seem to be improving after use of the standard antidote kit.

Experimentally, hydroxocobalamin (a form of vitamin B_{12}) has been used, combined with sodium thiosulfate, for cyanide toxicity. It is currently under investigation in this country. Some authorities feel that this may become the drug of choice in acute cyanide intoxication.

Nitrites

Sources of nitrite poisoning include amyl nitrite, butyl nitrite, isobutyl nitrite, and isoamyl nitrite. These compounds are often used as aphrodisiacs, stimulants, and psychedelic agents. Many can be bought either in pharmacies or in so-called "head shops." The various trade names include: Locker Room, Rush, Heart-On, and Joc Aroma Bullet. In large doses, nitroglycerin can also induce methemoglobinemia.

In terms of **pathophysiology,** nitrites may have their effects either when inhaled in excess or ingested. This leads to the formation of methemoglobin (Hb-Fe^{3+}) or oxidized hemoglobin. This molecule is incapable of binding either oxygen or carbon dioxide. Thus, intracellular metabolism is severely hampered due to the lack of oxygen. Certain individuals with hereditarily abnormal hemoglobins may actually oxidize their hemoglobin more readily than others and are thus more sensitive to the effects of nitrites. The other effects of these substances, both "recreational" and potentially toxic, are related to the marked smooth relaxation they can cause.

Symptoms depend on the Hb-Fe^{3+} level and the degree of smooth muscle relaxation. They include dizziness, headache, syncope, lethargy, and stupor. Angina may be precipitated in individuals with coronary artery disease.

On **physical exam,** the ABG will show chocolate-brown discoloration to the blood. The pO_2 is often normal or increased due to the inability to deliver oxygen to the tissues. If available, methemoglobin levels (which will be increased) should be obtained.

Treatment depends upon the severity of the symptoms. If they are mild, oxygen administration and careful observation are warranted. The body's own mechanisms will reverse the problem within 24–72 hours. This is due to the activity of an intrinsic red blood cell enzyme, methemoglobin reductase. The presence of stupor, coma, angina, or a methemoglobin level > 40% indicates significant symptomatology and warrants specific treatment. METHYLENE BLUE, 1–2 mg/kg (as a 1% solution) IV over five minutes should then be administered. If no improvement is noted in one hour, the same dose should be repeated. Larger doses should NOT be used as a paradoxical effect of methylene blue may actually increase the Hb-Fe^{3+} level.

Nitrogen dioxide

Nitrogen dioxide (NO_2) gas can be generated from several **sources.** Industrial exposures have been reported. The more common variety is "silo gas." Here, NO_2 is formed from the oxidation of the nitrates in green plants and fertilizers stored in a silo. Exposure occurs when the individual enters an inadequately ventilated silo.

The **pathophysiology** of NO_2 exposure stems from the fact that this compound is not highly water-soluble. Thus, only slight irritation of the upper respiratory tract occurs during inhalation. It is carried deep into the pulmonary tissues where vapors cause parenchymal lung damage due to the formation of nitric and nitrous acids upon contacting the respiratory epithelium (cell lining). Toxicity is usually triphasic with an initial acute bronchiolitis. A few hours later pulmonary edema may occur. In some, bronchiolitis obliterans and chronic interstitial lung disease may develop several weeks later. Initial exposure to very high concentrations may lead to rapidly fatal bronchiolarspasm, laryngospasm, or simple asphyxiation.

In obtaining the **history,** the greatest danger to the patient to keep in mind is the fact that serious effects are not often felt until several hours following exposure. A typical sequence of events is as follows:

1. Immediately following inhalation: either no reaction or only slight respiratory discomfort, headache, or dizziness. Occasionally, there are nausea and vomiting, but the victim frequently continues his work.

2. Within 5–8 hours after exposure, the worker may notice cyanosis about the lips and ears.

3. Rapidly increasing respiratory difficulty follows with irregular respirations, choking, dizziness, headache, and chest tightness. Occasionally, nausea, vomiting, and palpitations accompany this stage.

4. Late-stage intoxication is characterized by progressive dyspnea and cough.

On **physical exam,** increased respiratory rate, decreased vital capacity and breath sounds, with occasional moist rales and rhonchi, are present. The patient may be hypotensive.

Laboratory studies reveal an increased platelet count (unknown as to why). ABGs show a respiratory alkalosis with hypoxemia.

The **chest X-ray** may or may not show infiltrates typical of adult respiratory distress syndrome or pulmonary edema.

Treatment of nitrogen dioxide inhalation was discussed briefly earlier (page 44). Bronchodilators (theophylline and isoethrane) are used as described previously. If significantly impaired oxygenation is present, mechanical ventilation with positive end expiratory pressure (PEEP) may be helpful. Steroids should definitely be given in an attempt to prevent the development of bronchiolitis obliterans.

Pearls to Remember

When treating any victim of toxic gas inhalation, remember:

1. Don't assume the patient to be all right even if they are currently without symptoms, have normal ABGs, and a normal chest X-ray. Several agents may cause delayed reactions up to 12–24 hours later (i.e., acrolein, acetaldehyde).

2. Don't wait for carboxyhemoglobin levels before giving 100% oxygen for suspected carbon monoxide inhalation. The high concentration of O_2 decreases the half-life of carboxyhemoglobin from six to one and one-half hours.

3. Don't insist on the seriously ill patient breathing room air just to get a "room air" ABG. The A-a gradient can be calculated (requires a different formula than presented earlier, which assumes room air) on any known FIO_2.

Neurological Emergencies

The neurological examination is a key part in any patient assessment. Nontraumatic neurological problems are less common than traumatic considerations, with the possible exception of stroke. Nonetheless, there are a few significant conditions that medical personnel must be familiar with. The approach to the comatose patient will be discussed on page 159 under the "Synthesis" section. The following nontraumatic neurological emergencies will be dealt with in this section:

- Seizures
- Cerebral ischemic syndromes.

SEIZURES

A seizure is defined as a sudden, paroxysmal episode of exaggerated activity or abnormal behavior caused by excessive electrical discharge of cerebral neurons. There are several classifications of seizure disorders. Regardless, the basic mechanism is always the same—rapid and abnormal firing of brain cells. The activity seen in a seizure is directly related to the area of the brain in which the discharge occurs.

Focal seizures are those produced from isolated foci in the cerebral cortex. This discharge may result in several phenomena:

1. Generalized (grand mal) seizures—focal discharge spreads, eventually involving the entire cortex leading to whole-body involvement. Conversely, though, a generalized seizure DOES NOT absolutely require a primary focus first. All brain cells may discharge simultaneously initially, especially in metabolic events.

2. Focal motor seizure—one side of the body or one limb is involved.

3. Sensory seizure—tingling, numbness, or visual disturbances may occur.

Subcortical seizures are those that do not involve motor activity but do result in a transient change in the level of consciousness (LOC). Speech loss or vague actions may occur. These are more frequent in children and teenagers. They are often referred to as "petit mal" seizures.

Temporal lobe seizures lead to personality alterations, syncope, bizarre behavior, hallucinations, and fear. Often referred to as complex partial seizures, even chest pain mimicking angina has been noted [*Am J Med,* February 1986, Vol. 80, pp. 195–202].

Status epilepticus is the presence of repeated seizures without interruption and is discussed further beginning on pages 52–53. Table 4-1 summarizes the classification of seizure disorders.

In evaluating **causes** of seizures, it is important to remember that these events are only a symptom of an abnormality. Seizures may be caused by factors both inside and outside of the central nervous system (CNS). Non-CNS originating seizures can be classified as follows:

1. Metabolic—electrolyte, hypoglycemia, toxemia.

2. Drug or alcohol withdrawal/overdose.

3. Organ related—renal/liver failure, cardiovascular, heart block, hypertension.

Seizures of CNS origin may be caused by or related to the following factors:

1. Infection—meningitis, subdural empyema, brain abscess, encephalitis.

2. Febrile convulsion (children).

3. Epilepsy—defined as a state of recurrent idiopathic seizures.

4. Trauma.

5. Stroke.

6. Tumor—either primary or metastatic.

Table 4-1. Classification of Seizure Disorders

Focal Seizures
From isolated focci in cerebral cortex
- Generalized
- Focal motor
- Sensory

Subcortical Seizures
Transient change in level of consciousness—petit mal

Temporal Lobe Seizures
Behavioral manifestations

Status Epilepticus
Repeated seizures without interruption

Large studies of seizure patients presenting to urban Emergency Departments have suggested, in terms of frequency, the following causes of seizures:

- Anticonvulsant noncompliance—59%
- Unknown—8%
- Alcohol withdrawal—8%
- Breakthrough—5% (i.e., current medications not working)
- Febrile—4%
- Hypoglycemia—less than 1%
- Other (including new onset seizures of unknown etiology)—12%.

Diagnosis

History

In making the diagnosis of a seizure, it is very important to remember that loss of consciousness is NOT an essential feature.

Important features to look for in the history may be easily remembered by the mnemonic "FACTS":

1. **F—Focus:**
   In what part of the body did the seizure begin? In what sequence and to what parts did it spread?

2. **A—Activity—Was there:**
   Twitching? Jerking? Tonic posturing? Tonic-clonic movements? Lapse of attention? Repetitive movements or speech? Thrashing or flailing? Changes in activity when being watched?

3. **C—Color**
   Cyanotic? How long?

4. **T—Time:** When did the seizure start? Duration?

5. **S—Secondary facts:**
   - What was patient doing immediately before the seizure?
   - Was there an aura?
   - Incontinence of urine or stool?
   - Did patient bite his mouth or tongue?
   - Did patient hit head or fall?
   - Seizure history? Medications? Personal physician?
   - Fever?
   - Postictal state? Duration?

Physical examination

During the physical examination of an individual who may have had a seizure, one first ascertains if a postictal state exists. If so, the patient will be unable to give much information. Clothing is checked for loss of urine or feces and the mouth is examined for tongue-biting. The spinal column is examined for tenderness, and a neurological examination is done.

Laboratory tests

Laboratory studies should include ABGs, CBC, electrolytes, glucose, BUN/creatinine, urinalysis, toxicology screen, and anticonvulsant blood levels (if the patient has been on medication). Drug levels should be obtained before giving additional phenytoin, if possible, as up to 12% of patients may have therapeutic levels, despite recurring seizures [*Ann Emerg Med,* January 1986, Vol. 15, pp. 33-39].

Virtually all patients who have had a generalized seizure will exhibit a metabolic acidosis for up to one hour postictally. This is due to the release of lactic acid during massive muscular contractions. A STAT blood sugar should be obtained, especially in status epilepticus. Serum calcium levels should also be expeditiously ordered.

Despite these "standard" recommendations, a large university hospital Emergency Department study revealed that only 2.4% of all seizures were due to derangements in serum chemistries, including hypoglycemia. These commonly occurred in alcoholics and were rare in nonalcoholics unless they had preexisting renal failure or diabetes [*Ann Emerg Med,* May 1985, Vol. 14, pp. 416-420].

X-ray films of the skull are rarely helpful unless there is a history of trauma. Occasionally, shift of a calcified pineal gland is present and helpful. (The pineal gland is a mid-skull structure on X-ray and is calcified in about 60% of normal adults. If there is increased intracranial pressure due to some type of mass effect, it may be shifted from the midline.) Seizures immediately following head trauma are actually fairly unusual. They occur secondary to the effects of impact and have no effect on long-term prognosis. CT scans and EEGs may or may not be necessary, depending upon the situation.

Assessment Guidelines

In considering the seizure patient, it is helpful to first review some assessment guidelines. Keeping these in mind while treating the patient will prevent overlooking eminently treatable causes of seizures. The mnemonic is "AEIOU-TIPS":

1. **A—A**lcoholism—withdrawal seizures are quite common; many alcoholics on anti-seizure medications forget to take them, especially during drinking bouts.
2. **E—E**pilepsy, **E**lectrolytes—90% of all grand mal seizures are due to idiopathic epilepsy; decreased serum concentrations of sodium or calcium can lead to seizures.
3. **I—I**nsulin—decreased blood sugar can cause seizures.
4. **O—O**verdose—sudden stoppage of barbiturates can lead to seizures.
5. **U—U**nderdose—a common cause for a seizure is patients who fail to take their anti-seizure medications.
6. **T—T**rauma, **T**umor—old head trauma may lead to a chronic seizure disorder; tumor may also cause seizures. There is 20% chance of a tumor being present when a seizure presents for the first time in a patient over 21 years old.
7. **I—I**nfection—meningitis or brain abscess may lead to seizures. Up to 43% of seizure patients have an elevated temperature for 48 hours afterwards with less than 10% having evidence of infection [*Arch Int Med,* 1987, Vol. 147, pp. 1153-1155].
8. **P—P**sychiatric—pseudoseizures ("fake seizures") do occur—the essential thing about a grand mal seizure is the unconscious state; if the patient is taking purposeful swings at you, it is NOT a grand mal seizure!

   Pseudoseizures are suggested when the event occurs indoors, often in front of witnesses, many times per day, and if the patient attempts to hide the eyes or keep the eyelids closed. The patient may respond to ammonia salts and exhibit suggestibility. NONE of these features are commonly present with true seizures [*Emergency Medicine,* July 1985, p. 41].

9. S—Stroke—strokes can lead to seizures; also, a transient hemiparesis may appear following a seizure—Todd's paralysis.

Table 4-2 summarizes the treatable causes of seizure disorders.

Table 4-2. Treatable Causes of Seizures

A—Alcoholism
E—Epilepsy, electrolytes
I—Insulin
O—Overdose
U—Underdose
T—Trauma, tumor
I—Infection
P—Psychiatric
S—Stroke

Treatment

The treatment for a self-limited seizure is straightforward. As a general rule, the less you do, the better:

1. Assure airway patency—a nasopharyngeal airway is preferable. NEVER force anything between the teeth.

2. Oxygen, 4–6 LPM via NP.

3. Suction PRN.

4. DO NOT RESTRAIN the patient unless it is absolutely necessary to prevent injury. Instead, move hazardous materials out of the patient's way.

5. Provide reassurance as the patient "wakes up."

6. If the patient "clears" completely, is taking his medications, has his own physician, and is experiencing his usual frequency of seizures, transport/admission may be unnecessary—refer to local protocol.

Status epilepticus can be a life-threatening emergency. Permanent brain damage can occur after only 60 minutes of uncontrolled seizure activity. The principles listed above also apply here. Additionally, EKG monitoring should be instituted, as cardiac arrhythmias are a common cause of death. Centrally mediated pulmonary edema has also been noted in several cases of death occurring in otherwise healthy epileptic patients [*Ann Neur,* May 1981, Vol. 9, pp. 458–464].

After blood is drawn for STAT glucose, an IV of D_5W at a TKO rate should be initiated. If a history is unobtainable, or the blood glucose is not readily available, one ampule of D_{50} should be given IV. If this fails to stop the seizures, **drug therapy** should be instituted as follows:

1. DIAZEPAM (Valium)—2 mg/min IV until seizures stop or a total dose of 20 mg has been given.

2. PHENYTOIN (Dilantin)—start at the same time as diazepam. Give 18 mg/kg using 500 mg phenytoin in 50 cc normal saline. This should be run at a rate between 20–40 mg/min using a constant infusion pump. Ongoing blood pressure and EKG monitoring are required. If there is a decrease in the blood pressure or increase in the PR-interval (so that the total interval is > .2 msec), stop the infusion. Be wary if the patient is already on medication, as mentioned earlier. This method has been shown to be a rapid and safe means to rapidly load a patient intravenously with phenytoin [*Ann Emerg Med,* November 1984, p. 1027]. Intraosseous administration of phenytoin has been reported to be successful in children, though no adult studies exist [*Am J Emerg Med,* 1986, Vol. 4, p. 523]. **If seizure is still present:**

3. PHENOBARBITAL—100 mg/min IV until seizures stop or to a total dose of 20 mg/kg. If this stops the seizure, the patient usually needs endotracheal intubation to control their airway and secretions. **If seizure is still present:**

4. General anesthetic with HALOTHANE and neuromuscular junction blockade. **If an anesthesiologist is not immediately available:**

5. PARALDEHYDE—5 cc (4% solution) in 500 cc D_5W IV, titrated to control seizures **or**

6. LIDOCAINE—50–100 mg IV push—if this works, run a 4:1 drip at 1–2 mg/min. This may be especially good in uremic seizures.

7. If paraldehyde or lidocaine hasn't stopped the seizure within 20 minutes from the start of the infusion, **general anesthesia is mandatory!**

8. Rectally administered VALPROIC ACID has worked as a last-resort drug in children with refractory status epilepticus. No adult studies are available at this time [*J Peds*, 1986, Vol. 106, p. 323]. A retention enema was prepared by diluting the commercially available syrup with tap water in a 1:1 ratio. A loading dose of 20 mg/kg is used followed by a maintenance dose of 10–15 mg/kg three times per day.

9. Animal research has demonstrated that the calcium channel blocker nimodipine is capable of reversing some types of seizures in rabbits. There is no human data on this interesting finding [*Mayo Clin Proc*, April 1986, Vol. 61, pp. 239–247].

Table 4-3 summarizes the drug treatment of status epilepticus.

Seizures in the pregnant patient are treated similarly to those in the nonpregnant woman. Concomitant fetal monitoring is felt to be helpful, as well as prompt OB-GYN consultation. Some have suggested an IV diazepam drip (50–100 mg in 500 cc D_5W run at 40 cc/hour) if diazepam and phenobarbital fail to control seizures. Their algorithm did not include phenytoin. This is not recognized as standardized therapy at this time though [*NEJM*, 1985, Vol. 312, pp. 559–563].

Table 4-3. Drug Treatment of Status Epilepticus

Diazepam
 2 mg/min until seizures stop or total dose = 20 mg

Phenytoin
 18 mg/kg IV infusion (20–40 mg/min)

 If seizures still persist:

Phenobarbital
 100 mg/kg IV until seizures stop or total dose = 20 mg/kg

 If seizures still persist:

General Anesthetic
 Halothane/neuromuscular blockade

 If no anesthetist immediately available:

Paraldehyde
 5 cc (4%) solution/500 cc D_5W IV drip—titrate

 or

Lidocaine
 50–100 mg bolus followed by 4:1 drip

 If seizures still persist:

General Anesthesia Mandatory

Pearls to Remember

Seizures are frightening, both for the patient and medical personnel alike. It is important to remember that most seizures are self-limiting. Some other "PEARLS" are as follows:

1. Trauma to the tongue is unlikely to cause serious problems. Trauma to the teeth *may*. Attempts to force an airway into the patient's mouth can completely obstruct the airway.

2. Seizures in patients greater than 50 years old are frequently caused by arrhythmias.

3. Don't forget to check for a pulse—seizure activity may be the first sign of cerebral hypoxia from cardiac arrest.

CEREBRAL ISCHEMIC SYNDROMES

Cerebral ischemic syndromes result from the disruption of the cerebral circulation with a subsequent loss of neurological function. Basically, all result in a relatively abrupt focal cerebral deficit. Of these, 95% are vascular in origin. Nonvascular causes include seizures, tumors, demyelination syndromes, and psychogenic causes. They may be classified as either occlusive or hemorrhagic.

Occlusive syndromes comprise roughly 85% of the vascular causes for cerebral ischemic syndromes and include the following:

1. *Transient ischemic attack* (TIA)—a transient neurological deficit of vascular origin that usually resolves within 24 hours; one-third of these patients will have stroke, 20% within the first month after the onset of their first TIA. Some use the term "RIND" (reversible ischemic neurological defect) for a similar problem lasting up to 72 hours.

2. *Stroke in evolution*—the progression of a neurological deficit over 24–72 hours with at least some residual.

3. *Completed stroke*—a stable neurological deficit for greater than 24–72 hours.

The classification of **hemorrhagic syndromes** (15% of acute ischemic syndromes) is as follows:

1. *Intracerebral hemorrhage*—bleeding within the brain itself, usually from small penetrating vessels of the brain that have been damaged by hypertension.

2. *Subarachnoid hemorrhage*—bleeding into the subarachnoid space, usually from the rupture of a saccular aneurysm (defect in the arterial wall) or a vascular malformation (arterio-venous malformation).

3. *Subdural/epidural hemorrhage*—bleeding below the dura or in the space between the bony calvarium and the dural sac.

Table 4-4 summarizes the classification of cerebral ischemic syndromes.

Table 4-4. Classification of Cerebral Ischemic Syndromes

Occlusive
  Transient ischemic attack
  Stroke in evolution
  Completed stroke

Hemorrhagic
  Intracerebral hemorrhage
  Subarachnoid hemorrhage

The **causes of occlusive problems** are either thrombosis (due to artherosclerosis or hypertension) or emboli from the heart (due to atrial fibrillation, mural thrombus), or carotid artery. Approximately one-third of these events are due to emboli. Large and fatal cerebral infarctions occur more often with embolization, especially in association with atrial fibrillation. From 50–70% of these patients can be expected to die or suffer severe disability [*J Intensive Care Med,* 1986, Vol. 1, p. 184]. The sick sinus syndrome, with intermittent episodes of bradydysrhythmias, has been noted in patients with embolic events and may be related [*Stroke,* 1986, Vol. 17, p. 192].

Tumor fragments may embolize in patients having recent pneumonectomy for lung cancer, leading to major cerebral infarction [*Stroke,* 1986, Vol. 17, p. 555]. Painless dissection of the aorta may rarely present with acute neurologic deficits, such as hemiparesis and weakness. Chest radiograph reveals characteristic widening of the mediastinum [*Stroke,* 1986, Vol. 17, p. 644].

Hemorrhagic stroke is caused by hypertension, aneurysm rupture, or vascular malformation in subarachnoid hemorrhage. Vascular malformation is associated with polycystic kidneys and coarctation of the aorta. Ruptured intracranial aneurysms have also been reported to result in subdural hemorrhage [*Ann Emerg Med,* August 1986, Vol. 15, p. 944].

Trauma, of course, may also lead to any type of cerebral hemorrhage. Interestingly, 20% of post-traumatic intracerebral hematomas appear immediately (0–3 hours) following the event. The remainder are delayed, with up to 46% initially presenting later than 24 hours [*J Trauma,* 1986, Vol. 26, p. 787]. This is important in that many potentially operable intraparenchymal clots develop after initial CT scanning has been performed.

Oral anticoagulants may lead to intracranial hemorrhage. Coumadin is associated with bleeding complications in approximately 7–8% of patients, of which only a small fraction are intracerebral [*Arch Intern Med,* 1974, Vol. 133, p. 386]. If the patient is greater than 70 years, the presence of hypertension, and preceding cerebral infarction, may be important risk factors. Excessive prolongation of the prothrombin time is commonly present when anti-coagulated patients present with intracerebral hemorrhage. Interestingly, it has been noted that head trauma does not generally appear to play a role in intracerebral hemorrhage in anticoagulated patients. In one series, only 16% of the patients had a preceding history of trauma which was considered mild in nature and not associated with unconsciousness [*Neurology,* 1985, Vol. 35, p. 943].

The ingestion of amphetamines, as well as other illicit "speed" preparations, may lead to intracranial hemorrhage. Over-the-counter preparations (i.e., phenylpropanolamine) have been well documented as an additional cause [*Current Concepts of Cerebrovascular Disease—Stroke,* July–August 1985, p. 19]. It seems that both transient elevations of blood pressure as well as the development of an actual vasculitis of intracerebral vessels may be responsible [*Stroke,* 1986, Vol. 17, p. 590]. The vasculitis may respond to steroids. Cocaine ingestion has been associated with numerous acute cardiovascular complications, including cerebral infarction and hemorrhage.

Transient ischemic attacks have been reported to occur in relatively young patients who are exposed to high altitudes (i.e., mountain climbing) without other predisposing factors [*Crit Care Med,* 1986, Vol. 14, pp. 517–518]. The "classic" risk factors, such as hypertension, carotid stenosis, and cardiac disease, are less likely to be found in younger individuals as well [*Stroke,* 1986, Vol. 17, p. 662].

Alcohol may double or triple the risk of hemorrhagic stroke, depending on how heavy a drinker the individual is. Moderate and heavy drinkers have a 3–4 times increased risk of subarachnoid hemorrhage as compared with nondrinkers [*JAMA,* 1986, Vol. 255, pp. 2311–2314]. Part of the problem in alcohol-associated stroke may be the fact that ethanol provides a large source of free radicals that may perpetuate damage in ischemic brain tissue [*Crit Care Med,* 1986, Vol. 14, p. 841].

Cigarette smoking has been established as a risk factor for the development of subarachnoid hemorrhage [*Stroke,* 1986, Vol. 17, p. 831]. In patients who also had concomitant hypertension, the risk for this event was increased 15-fold as compared to those without either problem. Stopping smoking has been shown to significantly reduce the risk of either thromboembolic or hemorrhagic stroke [*N Engl J Med,* 1986, Vol. 315, p. 717].

A "warning leak" commonly occurs with subarachnoid hemorrhage. Headache (85%), nausea (44%), vomiting (34%), loss of consciousness (34%), and neck stiffness (14%) are reported. An unusually severe headache is most commonly seen. Thus, this complaint must be paid careful attention, especially in a patient without prior history of severe headaches [*Am Heart J,* 1985, Vol. 14, pp. 68–74].

Table 4-5 summarizes the causes of cerebral ischemic syndromes.

Diagnosis

History
The history depends upon the type of event and its location. Occlusive events are generally characterized by the gradual or rapid onset of dizziness, confusion, loss of balance, hemiplegia (paralysis of one side of the body), sensory loss, and, at times, visual

loss in one eye (amaurosis fugax). The presence of amaurosis fugax is associated with a carotid lesion on the same side in 79% of cases. Of these, approximately 22% will be hemodynamically significant [*Stroke*, 1986, Vol. 17, p. 393].

The "classic" thrombotic stroke occurs at night (60% of patients); the patient awakens with a neurological deficit which has progressed over the preceding minutes to hours. Severe headache is usually not present. Its presence should suggest intracranial hemorrhage as a more likely possibility. Embolic stroke, on the other hand, is more likely to occur while the patient is awake and active. The sudden onset of a neurological deficit occurs and may be associated with a headache, seizure, or a brief period of unconsciousness. Twelve percent of patients suffering an embolic stroke will have a seizure at the onset. Up to 30% may have a transient loss of consciousness at the time of the stroke [*Emerg Med Services*, March/April 1985, Vol. 13, pp. 41–47].

Intracranial bleeding usually presents with the abrupt onset (often during activity) of progressive neurological deficit, decreased responsiveness, and headache. Headache is especially prominent with subarachnoid hemorrhage and may be very severe. It is usually described by patients as the "most severe headache in my life." Nuchal rigidity (neck stiffness) and seizures may or may not be present.

Table 4-5. Causes of Cerebral Ischemic Syndromes

Occlusive
> Thrombosis—atherosclerosis, hypertension
> Embolic
> - Heart—atrial fibrillation, mural thrombus
> - Carotid artery

Hemorrhagic
> Hypertension (intracerebral bleeds)
> Aneurysm, vascular malformation (subarachnoid hemorrhage)

Physical examination

Any or all of the following may show on exam:

- Neurological deficit
- Increased blood pressure
- Nuchal rigidity
- Altered level of consciousness. Pupils may be pinpoint but still reactive to light, suggesting pontine hemorrhage. In subarachnoid hemorrhage, fundal bleeding may be noted on ophthalmoscopy. The carotid arteries should be auscultated for bruits though their presence is not, ipso facto, definitive evidence in favor of an embolic etiology for the event.

Laboratory tests

Laboratory tests should be limited. Blood sugar should be determined rapidly in any patient with an acute neurological deficit. Hypoglycemia can result in reversible neurological deficits which may mimic stroke. Additionally, patients suffering *hyperglycemia* in association with stroke have been noted to have more severe cerebral edema and a worse clinical outcome [*Stroke*, 1986, Vol. 17, p. 865]. Other blood tests that may be helpful acutely include electrolytes and a complete blood count (CBC).

In terms of other evaluative testing, **CT scan** is the procedure of choice, if available, but may miss smaller bleeds. CT scans will be abnormal 90% of the time if performed within five days of a subarachnoid hemorrhage. The percentage of positive scans decreases with longer delays following the acute event. Thus, the preferred time is within the first 24 hours. Acute CT scanning is also helpful in that it may reveal acute hydrocephalus, tumor, or hematoma. If thick blood clots are noted on the initial scan, it is highly likely that the patient will develop severe vasospasm later in their course [*Ann Emerg Med*, March 1986, Vol. 15, pp. 274–279].

Many recommend obtaining a CT scan in a transient ischemic attack, because a small percentage of these may be associated with chronic subdural hematoma or tumors. Possible pathophysiological mechanisms include local ischemia or focal epileptic discharges; the mass effect could cause cortical depression by mechanical stimulation. Regional cerebral edema could cause vascular displacement and ischemia or small, repeated hemorrhages could lead to transient neurologic deficits. CT is recommended for differentiation [*J Trauma*, 1985, Vol. 25, pp. 1113–1114].

If one strongly suspects a subarachnoid hemorrhage and the CT scan is negative, **lumbar puncture** should be done to look for bleeding. Before performing this procedure, one MUST make sure that no signs of increased intracranial pressure are present on funduscopic examination. Additionally, the patient should be conscious and neurologically intact. Otherwise, the spinal tap is dangerous as increased intracranial pressure may be present even *without* the "classic" signs (i.e., papilledema, decreased venous pulsations, hemorrhage). The collection of sequential tubes is necessary to differentiate true intracranial bleeding from a traumatic tap.

Nuclear magnetic resonance imaging (NMR) may delineate cerebral infarction earlier than CT scanning. Lesions in the posterior fossa of the skull are particularly well differentiated. Arteriovenous malformations may be seen, but there is no demonstrated superiority of NMR over CT scanning at this time. Subdural hemorrhage is also well visualized with nuclear magnetic resonance imaging, but there appear to be no advantages over CT scanning in evaluating intracerebral hemorrhage, hemorrhagic infarction, and subarachnoid hemorrhage. For these, CT appears to be more accurate at present [*Stroke*, March–April 1986, pp. 328–331].

Angiography is only performed after obtaining appropriate neurological neurosurgical consultation. It is not without risks and should only be used acutely when the results will directly influence patient management. Transient arterial oxygen desaturation has been reported during radiographic contrast medium administration, perhaps due to bronchoconstriction. The underlying mechanism is poorly understood [*Arch Intern Med*, 1986, Vol. 146, p. 1094].

EKG findings in subarachnoid hemorrhage may mimic those of myocardial infarction. ST-segment elevation in the anterior leads suggesting acute anterior-lateral MI can occur [*Heart & Lung*, July 1984, p. 451]. More commonly, deep and symmetric T-wave inversions in the "V" leads are noted. These are felt to be due to the massive release of

catecholamines and, possibly, coronary artery spasm. Careful monitoring is warranted as significant dysrhythmias are common [*Stroke*, 1987, Vol. 18, pp. 558-564]. The presence of atrial fibrillation should be sought specifically.

It may be advantageous to carefully monitor cardiac function in the face of an acute stroke. Studies have shown that patients with a history of angina tend to respond to acute stroke by lowering their cardiac ejection fraction. Those without concomitant coronary artery disease, on the other hand, have an elevated value during the first two weeks following the event. Patients who die within two weeks after the acute stroke have a significantly lower ejection fraction as well [*Stroke*, 1986, Vol. 17, p. 613].

Echocardiography may be helpful in detecting an intracardiac source for an embolus. The lower limit size for detectability is 2–3 mm. Unfortunately, in patients with atrial fibrillation, the apparent absence of a left atrial thrombus is not reliable enough to exclude this possibility. Contrast two-dimensional echocardiography may be helpful in demonstrating the presence of clinically silent atrial septal defects which may be associated with cerebral embolization in young adults [*Ann Int Med*, 1986, Vol. 105, p. 695]. Table 4-6 summarizes the clinical presentation and evaluation of cerebral ischemic syndromes.

Treatment

Treatment of cerebral ischemic syndromes includes maintaining the airway and positioning the patient to prevent aspiration. Oxygen at 3–4 LPM via nasal prongs is administered. An IV of NS at a TKO rate is begun—plain D_5W should be avoided because it may increase intracranial pressure. Possible medications are:

1. ANTICOAGULANTS (heparin and Coumadin)—many use these for TIA and a stroke-in-evolution; the role of these agents in completed stroke is controversial. Consult with a neurologist first. There is a growing trend in favor of ANTIPLATELET drugs in transient ischemic attacks instead of full-dose anticoagulation (with either heparin or Coumadin) [*Arch Int Med*, 1986, Vol. 146, p. 471]. Recent literature has suggested a 43%

rate of transformation from non-hemorrhagic to hemorrhagic stroke in patients who have suffered large thrombotic OR embolic strokes. Thus, anticoagulant administration should be avoided in the first week following ANY type of large stroke, especially if the patient is hypertensive, as the risk of hemorrhagic transformation (and subsequent worsening of the patient's condition) is highest at this time. Many experts, though, feel that in an embolic stroke, if the CT scan at 24 hours demonstrates nonhemorrhagic infarction and neither a massive infarct or acute hypertension are present, it is safe to immediately anticoagulate using intravenous heparin.

Low-dose heparin (5,000 units subcutaneously every 12 hours) to prevent pulmonary embolism in stroke patients appears to be safe [*Stroke,* March–April 1986, Vol. 17, pp. 179–184].

The risk of major bleeding associated with oral anticoagulation in stroke patients ranges from 2% to 22% per year (2–9% fatality rate). Major bleeding episodes are often intracranial. Cost-risk benefit analysis suggests that in order for such treatment to be beneficial, a greater than 50% reduction in the stroke rate per year must be seen. This has not been proven to occur. Thus, many experts feel that the present evidence does NOT support the use of anticoagulant therapy in minor stroke [*Stroke,* 1986, Vol. 17, p. 111].

Many experts feel, though, that patients with chronic atrial fibrillation should be on oral anticoagulation in hopes of preventing major cerebral (or other systemic) embolism. A significant effect seems to occur irrespective of the underlying etiology of the dysrhythmia. Thus, the presence or absence of mitral valve disease made no difference in anticoagulant efficacy for stroke prevention. Similar findings have also been noted regardless of whether atrial fibrillation was chronic or paroxysmal [*Am Heart J,* 1986, Vol. 122, p. 1039; *Stroke,* 1986, Vol. 17, p. 622].

A few investigators have looked at the administration of the thrombolytic agents via angiographic catheters in acute stroke. At this time, the technique is still considered highly experimental, though potentially promising [*Stroke,* 1986, Vol. 17, p. 595].

Table 4-6. Clinical Presentation and Evaluation

History
Occlusive events—gradual or rapid onset of:
- Dizziness, confusion
- Loss of balance, hemiplegia
- Sensory loss, unilateral visual loss

Hemorrhagic events—abrupt onset of:
- Neurological deficit
- Decreased responsiveness
- Headache—very severe

Physical
Neurological deficit
Increased blood pressure (with hemorrhage)
Nuchal rigidity
Altered level of consciousness
Pinpoint pupils (pontine bleed)
Fundal bleeding (subarachnoid hemorrhage)

Laboratory
CT scan—the first procedure of choice, if available
Lumbar puncture—blood in cerebrospinal fluid
EKG—may mimic MI in subarachnoid hemorrhage
Angiogram—at discretion of neurosurgeon

---

2. STEROIDS—dexamethasone 10 mg IV, then 4 mg IV every 6 hours, for intracranial hemorrhage.

3. LAXATIVES, STOOL SOFTENERS—to prevent straining at stool.

4. TREATMENT OF HYPERTENSION—use caution in occlusive stroke—acutely lowering elevated BP too rapidly may lead to further neurological deficits. This is due to the failure of cerebral autoregulation and great spontaneous fluctuation in the blood pressure following an ischemic event [*Arch Intern Med,* 1986, Vol. 146, pp. 66–68]. There is no evidence that hypertension has a deleterious effect on the outcome of ischemic stroke during the acute phase. Current data suggests that there is a spontaneous blood pressure decline following an acute stroke over a four-day period [*Stroke,* 1986, Vol. 17, p. 861]. This must be taken into account when considering any form of antihypertensive therapy.

Thus, the current recommendation for **nonhemorrhagic stroke** is to avoid antihypertensive medication unless:

a. There is end-organ damage (heart or kidney) *OR*

b. The diastolic blood pressure rises to greater than 130 mm Hg *OR*

c. Hypertensive encephalopathy is present.

In a **hemorrhagic stroke,** most experts prefer reduction of the systolic blood pressure to levels below 160 mm Hg.

5. ANTI-FIBRINOLYTIC THERAPY (Amicar) or ANTI-SPASM AGENTS (calcium blockers) should be used only in consultation with a neurosurgeon. Most neurosurgeons no longer use Amicar, favoring instead early surgery. Amicar has been noted to increase the frequency of vasospasm (producing hydrocephalus) and systemic and venous thrombophlebitis. Thus, antifibrinolytic therapy is used only in a patient who has had a severe subarachnoid hemorrhage and is essentially in a vegetative state.

The peak incidence for cerebral vasospasm is 5–8 days following acute subarachnoid hemorrhage. It occurs in 40–60% of patients and is the most frequent cause of death or serious residual neurological deficit. Calcium blockers should be considered experimental for this indication. One study suggested that methylprednisolone substantially reduced vasospasm, but further data are necessary before this can be widely recommended [*Emergency Medicine,* November 30, 1985, p. 61].

The current therapy of vasospasm includes enhancing the cardiac output, inducing arterial hypertension, and expanding the intravascular volume in hopes of increasing cerebral perfusion. These techniques can only be used, though, once the aneurysm which led to the hemorrhage has been surgically clipped.

6. MANNITOL—a potent diuretic. Should be used only with the recommendation of the consulting neurosurgeon. Some authors have noted acute oliguric renal failure (which spontaneously reversed) in patients given mannitol [*Archives of Internal Medicine,* November 1984, p. 2214].

7. NALOXONE—this drug has been used experimentally with reportedly beneficial results in animal studies. One human study has suggested possible efficacy, urging further therapeutic trials [*Stroke,* 1986, Vol. 17, p. 404]. Large doses were used (10 mg per square meter per minute). The postulated mechanism of action is via alteration of transmembrane calcium flux in the brain. There may also be an effect in terms of preventing free-radical induced damage. At this time, though, this form of treatment cannot be recommended due to inadequate supporting evidence.

8. A couple of newer monitoring devices deserve brief mention. A quantitative measure of cerebral function is obtained by either evoked potential monitoring or compressed spectral array EEG monitoring. These techniques involve electrical

monitoring of raw EEG and other data that provides information relative to cerebral blood flow that many feel is much better than current means [*J Intensive Care Med,* 1986, Vol. 1, p. 179]. These may become the "electrocardiograms of future neurological intensive care." A transcranial Doppler ultrasound device, which allows noninvasive bedside assessment of blood flow direction and velocity, has also been described.

Pearls to Remember

Strokes are common. They can be especially devastating in a young person. Consider the following:

1. Suspect intracranial hemorrhage in cases of persistently increased blood pressure, especially if the patient is unconscious.

2. Syncope, lightheadedness, and vertigo, especially when they appear alone, are not usually indicative of transient ischemic attacks. These symptoms, rather, should suggest disorders of the labyrinthine system (inner ear) or cardiovascular system (orthostatic hypotension or cardiac dysrhythmias).

3. In subarachnoid hemorrhage from rupture of intracranial aneurysms, bleeding amounts to only 5–10 ml—the maximum loss is usually no greater than 25 to 30 ml. This is because rapid rises in intracranial pressure tamponades the bleeding site, a clot forms, and bleeding stops. Acute expansion of the aneurysm occurs in 80% of the patients and often an accompanying small sentinel bleed or leak about 14 days before the rupture. This usually causes a headache, which lasts 6–8 hours, that the patient will describe as the worst he has ever experienced. The greater the amount of bleeding, the higher the risk of subsequent spasm. Thus, early surgery is indicated, not only to "clip" the aneurysm but to irrigate the subarachnoid space and remove blood in the hopes that this will prevent spasm.

4. One-third of patients with subarachnoid hemorrhage die immediately. One-third either die in the hospital or are left disabled, and one-third are functional survivors. Left untreated, 50% of patients with a ruptured aneurysm will rebleed within six months with a 3% chance of rebleeding each year thereafter. Thus, surgical therapy should be undertaken if at all possible.

5. Excluding the occurrence of delayed hemorrhage or cerebral vasospasm, the primary determinant of prognosis in any cerebral ischemic syndrome is the level of consciousness on admission [*Stroke,* 1986, Vol. 17, p. 294].

6. Deterioration in a formerly stable stroke patient may be due to the development of a seizure state known as periodic lateralized epileptiform discharges. The patient may or may not have focal seizures, following which their level of consciousness is depressed and the neurological deficit worse. Evaluation, using laboratory and CT testing, is usually normal. The diagnosis is made by electroencephalogram, which shows a characteristic pattern [*J Intensive Care Med,* 1986, Vol. 1, p. 184].

7. Transient ischemic attacks may be mimicked by migraine-like phenomena. Headaches may accompany neurological deficit in only 40% of cases. Symptoms suggestive of "migraine accompaniments" instead of TIA include:
   - The presence of a visual aura
   - A "march" of symptoms, with serial progression from one to another
   - Headache occurring with a spell (hemorrhage must also be ruled out, of course)
   - A relatively benign course [*Stroke,* 1986, Vol. 17, p. 1033].

Poisoning and Substance Abuse

Though not intended to serve as a substitute to the many superb toxicology texts, this section will review the basic principles of poisoning and substance abuse treatment. Additionally, a section on snakebites is included at the end.

ACUTE TOXIC DRUG REACTIONS

This section will be approached slightly differently than previous ones. General principles or poisoning and overdose will be discussed followed by some "PEARLS." Several common poisonings and drug reactions will then be presented—acetaminophen, phencyclidine, salicylate overdoses, alcohol withdrawal syndromes, and narcotic withdrawal syndromes. Following this, a summary section, "Toxic Syndromes," will be presented.

General Principles in Poisoning and Overdose

Each year thousands of individuals die from either accidental or deliberate ingestion of poisons. Many of these are preventable. Nearly all ingestions in children less than 10 years old are accidental. Most hospital admissions for poisoning involve adult suicide attempts [Spyker, D. A., Acute Poisoning: General Management. In *Current Emergency Therapy* (3rd ed.). Aspen, 1986].

Forty-four percent of poisonings involve medications, with slightly more being prescription agents.

Following this are cleaning agents (12%), plants (9%), cosmetics (7%), pesticides (6%), turpentine and paints (4%), and petroleum distillates (3%).

The majority (90.6%) of exposures reported to the American Association of Poison Control Systems occur in the home, with a single substance being implicated in 93%. Only 1.3% of this patient group had multiple ingestions. These data may have been somewhat skewed in that suicidal-intent ingestions comprised only 5.1% of this series [*Am J Emerg Med*, 1986, Vol. 4, p. 427].

Proper attention to the A, B, C's are the vanguard of poisoning management:

1. Assess and maintain the airway—intubate if respiratory insufficiency, loss of consciousness, impaired or absent gag reflex exists. If the patient is not intubated, place them on their left side with the head down to prevent aspiration.

2. High-flow oxygen (10–15 LPM via mask).

3. Assess cardiovascular status by vital signs and EKG—hypotension in overdose is usually responsive to volume expansion. Therefore, start an IV of NS or RL TKO and increase as necessary (MAST pants may also be considered).

After supportive therapy has begun, it is helpful to try and identify the drug taken. Pills at the scene, and chemical tests on urine, blood, and stomach contents can be helpful. In one study, positive results were obtained in 80% of patients receiving an Emergency Department toxicology screen when an ingestion was suspected. Ethanol was the most common drug found (48%) with an average concentration of 250 mg%. Multiple drug use was documented in 28% of patients. There were *76 cases* of laboratory tests providing additional information on the nature of the intoxication (i.e., two-thirds of the cases) which proved clinically useful [*Am J Emerg Med,* 1985, Vol. 3, pp. 507–511]. Thus, toxicology screening appears to be a reasonable thing to do.

It is very important to **always contact the regional Poison Control Center!** This should be done even if you are *absolutely* certain of the treatment! Standard emergency textbooks and especially remedies printed on containers are usually out-of-date and incorrect. The regional Poison Control Center has monthly updated (Poisindex) information they can give you. Table 5-1 has a list of selected regional Poison Control Centers. The *Physician's Desk Reference* (PDR) also has a current list of centers and their toll-free numbers.

Vital signs

The vital signs may be of aid in diagnosing the type of ingestion. The **blood pressure** tends to be the least helpful because it is subject to many physiological variables and may be stable despite significant poisoning. Some ingestions can, though, lead to hypertension (sympathomimetics, amphetamines, cocaine). The **pulse** tends to be much more valuable. Tachycardia suggests sympathomimetic (cocaine, amphetamine, caffeine) or anticholinergic (atropine, tricyclic antidepressant) ingestion. Bradycardia is compatible with parasympathomimetic (pilocarpine, amanita mushrooms), cholinesterase inhibitor (organophosphate insecticide), beta-blocker, and digitalis intoxication.

The **respiratory rate** may be increased. Usually this goes along with so-called "global excitability" and is not isolated. If an isolated tachypnea is present, especially if the patient has an altered level of consciousness, one should think of salicylate poisoning. Dyspnea and respiratory distress are caused by hydrocarbon and caustic inhalations. Bradypnea and apnea, of course, are most compatible with narcotic or sedative-hypnotic ingestion.

The **temperature** may be elevated with salicy-

late, atropine, or scopalamine ingestion. Toxic psychosis (amphetamine) and delirium tremens are also commonly accompanied by hyperthermia. A lowered body temperature may occur with alcohol, barbiturate, and narcotic ingestion.

Diagnosis

Physical examination

The physical examination will often reveal something suggestive of the etiology of the poisoning problem as well. Obviously, the most important thing to keep in mind when performing the **neurological exam** is to decide if the patient is alert and awake enough to tolerate Ipecac (i.e., to protect his airway). Decreased visual acuity may suggest methanol or atropine poisoning (mydriasis also present). Miosis is, of course, compatible with narcotic, barbiturate, and cholinesterase inhibitor poisoning. Botulism causes paralysis of the extraocular muscles. Phencyclidine (PCP) is the only agent that will lead to both horizontal and vertical nystagmus.

The **cardiovascular exam** may reveal the presence of an arrhythmia if the agent was a tricyclic antidepressant or phenothiazine. The presence of a heart murmur should alert the examiner to the possibility of endocarditis in a drug addict. Rhonchi and wheezing may be caused by numerous agents, usually irritant inhalants, though narcotic, anticholinergic, and cholinesterase inhibitors can lead to pulmonary edema and bronchorrhea.

Other potentially useful findings of the physical exam include liver tenderness (acetaminophen ingestion—takes hours to days for development), decreased bowel sounds (narcotics, anticholinergics), cyanosis (nitrites), flushing (atropine), and needle marks (narcotics). Bullae at pressure points may occur in overdose with barbiturates, opioids, and other sedatives. Table 5.2 summarizes the physical examination in poisoning.

Some experts recommend plain abdominal radiography to determine whether or not ingested tablets are still in the stomach. Depending on the drug taken, up to 64% may not be detectable [*Am J Emerg Med,* 1986, Vol. 4, p. 302]. A guide to the expected radio-opacity of commonly ingested substances is as follows:

Table 5-1. Selected List of Regional Poison Control Centers

State	Telephone Number
Alabama	800-462-0800 (Statewide)
Arizona	602-626-6016 or 800-362-0101 (Statewide)
Arkansas	800-482-8948 (Statewide)
California	916-453-3692 or 800-852-7221 (Northern California)
Colorado	303-629-1123 or 800-332-3073 (Statewide)
Connecticut	203-674-3456
Delaware	302-655-3389
District of Columbia	202-625-3333
Florida	813-251-6995 or 800-282-3171 (Statewide)
Georgia	800-282-5846 (Statewide)
Hawaii	800-362-3585 (Statewide)
Idaho	800-632-8000 (Statewide)
Illinois	217-753-3330 or 800-252-2022 (Statewide)
Indiana	317-630-7351 or 800-382-9097 (Statewide)
Iowa	319-356-2922 or 800-272-6477 (Statewide)
Kansas	800-228-9515 (Statewide)
Kentucky	502-589-8222 or 800-722-5725 (Statewide)
Louisiana	800-535-0525 (Statewide)
Maine	800-442-6305 (Statewide)
Maryland	301-528-7701 or 800-492-2414 (Statewide)
Massachusetts	800-682-9211 (Statewide)
Michigan	313-494-5711 or 800-572-1655 (Statewide)
Minnesota	612-221-2113 or 800-222-1222 (Statewide)
Mississippi	601-354-7660
Missouri	800-392-9111 (Statewide)
Montana	800-525-5042 (Statewide)
Nebraska	402-390-5400 or 800-642-9999 (Statewide) or 800-228-9515 (Surrounding states)
New Hampshire	800-562-8236 (Statewide)
New Jersey	201-926-8005 or 800-962-1253 (Statewide)
New Mexico	505-843-2551 or 800-432-6866 (Statewide)
New York	516-542-2324
North Carolina	800-672-1697 (Statewide)
North Dakota	800-732-2200 (Statewide)
Ohio	800-682-7625 (Statewide)
Oklahoma	800-522-4611 (Statewide)
Oregon	800-452-7165 (Statewide)
Pennsylvania	412-681-6669
Rhode Island	401-277-5906
South Carolina	800-922-1117 (Statewide)
South Dakota	800-228-9515 (Statewide)
Texas	800-392-8548 (Statewide)
Utah	801-581-2151
Vermont	802-658-3456
Virginia	804-924-5543
Washington	800-732-6985 (Statewide)
West Virginia	800-642-3625 (Statewide)
Wisconsin	414-433-8100
Wyoming	800-442-2702 (Statewide)

NOTE: Only numbers for designated state or regional poison control centers are given in this listing. Though this listing was correct at the time of this writing, no responsibility is assumed for the current and/or accuracy of any number in this chart.

Table 5-2. Physical Findings in Poisoning

VITAL SIGNS

Blood Pressure—Least Helpful

Sympathomimetics, amphetamines, cocaine can cause hypertension

Pulse

Tachycardia—sympathomimetics, anticholinergics

Bradycardia—parasympathomimetic, cholinesterase, inhibitor, beta-blocker, digitalis ingestion

Respiratory Rate

Tachypnea—if isolated, salicylate ingestion

Dyspnea—hydrocarbon, caustic inhalation

Bradypnea/apnea—narcotic, sedative-hypnotic

Temperature

Elevated—salicylate, atropine, scopalamine

Decreased—alcohol, barbiturates, narcotics

PHYSICAL EXAMINATION

Neurologic Exam

Is patient alert/awake enough for ipecac?

Decreased visual acuity—atropine, methanol

Miosis—narcotics, barbiturates, cholinesterase inhibitors

Extraocular muscle paralysis—botulism

Cardiorespiratory Exam

Arrhythmia—tricyclics, phenothiazines

Heart murmurs—endocarditis in a drug addict

Rhonchi/wheezing—narcotics, anticholinergics, cholinesterase inhibitors can cause bronchorrhea and pulmonary edema

Other Significant Findings

Liver tenderness—acetaminophen

Decreased bowel sounds—narcotics, anticholinergics

Cyanosis—nitrites

Flushing—atropine

Needle marks—narcotics

Bullae at pressure points—barbiturates, narcotics

1. *Highly radiopaque*—chloral hydrate, ferrous sulfate, haloperidol, spironolactone, vitamins.

2. *Moderately radiopaque*—allopurinol, antacids, albuterol, amitriptyline, amoxicillin, aspirin, desipramine, ethchlorvynol, fluphenazine, lithium, pentazocine, procainamide amitriptyline, and thioridazine.

3. *Not or minimally radiopaque*—acetaminophen, amphetamine, ampicillin, chlorpromazine, diazepam, digoxin, diphenhydramine, diphenoxylate/atropine, doxepin, hydromorphone, lorazepam, loxapine, oxycodone/acetaminophen, phenytoin, and theophylline.

It should be noted that not all preparations of each mentioned drug have been studied in detail and the above are only rough guidelines. If tablets or fragments are seen on an abdominal X-ray, the findings are helpful. Of course, a negative film does not necessarily exclude a significant ingestion. A positive film is helpful in estimating the amount of drug taken and the efficacy of gastric emptying by lavage or emesis.

Generally, any adult patient who presents with a depressed level of consciousness should have the following done:

1. Dextrostix or Chemstrip-BG of fingerstick blood.

2. If blood sugar < 60 or if you are unable to determine the blood sugar, give 1 ampule D_{50} IV. Thiamine 100 mg IV should precede the administration of glucose. If there is no response, give:

3. NALOXONE (Narcan)—.8 mg IV (2 cc—2 amps). Observe for increased respirations or responsiveness. Titrate every 3–5 minutes to maximum dose of 4 mg according to *respiratory status*. If you completely awaken the patient, there is a good chance they will refuse help or transport. When the naloxone wears off, the narcotic effect may persist, leading to recurrent coma. Larger doses may be necessary in certain cases, such as

proproxyphene (Darvon) ingestion. Naloxone is also available in 2 and 10 mg ampules and may be given by intralingual injection or via an endotracheal tube.

Naloxone has been given in healthy volunteers via continuous intravenous infusion. Adequate blood levels appear to be maintained with administration rates equal to two-thirds of the bolus dose which resulted in reversal each hour [*Ann Emerg Med*, May 1986, Vol. 15, pp. 566–570].

The standard approach to any poisoning is to promote gastric emptying, decrease absorption of the poison, and induce catharsis. Termination of exposure to environmental substances is also vital. If approved by the Poison Control Center, and if the patient is awake *with a gag reflex:*

1. IPECAC—30 cc + 16 oz water— may repeat in 20 minutes if not successful in inducing emesis. Larger amounts of fluid should NOT be given. These do not appear to enhance vomiting and may actually promote gastric emptying and further absorption of the poison.

2. ACTIVATED CHARCOAL—50–100 gm—orally or via NG tube. Delete if an oral antidote is to be given.

3. MAGNESIUM CITRATE—150–300 cc orally (acts as a cathartic). If a combination of activated charcoal and sorbitol (Actidose—see page 66) has been used, magnesium citrate is not necessary. Though uncommon, cathartic-induced magnesium toxicity with acute neuromuscular deterioration and respiratory depression requiring dialysis has been reported [*Ann Emerg Med*, 1986, Vol. 15, p. 1214].

Recent evidence has suggested that emetic response to ipecac is not affected by early (10 minutes) administration of charcoal [*Ann Int Med*, February 1987, Vol. 16, pp. 164-166].

If the patient has a depressed level of consciousness, *and* it is recommended by the Poison Control Center:

1. Intubate the trachea.
2. Gastric lavage with a large bore (36F) Ewald tube. Use isotonic saline with 300 cc per instillation. Continue until the return is clear. Follow the lavage with charcoal and a cathartic (or sorbitol-charcoal).

There is some work suggesting that acutely poisoned patients may be managed successfully without gastric emptying. The clinical outcome of patients who were awake and alert on presentation to the Emergency Department did not appear to be altered by ipecac administration. Gastric lavage in obtunded patients led to a better outcome only if begun within one hour of the ingestion [*Ann Emerg Med*, June 1985, Vol. 14, pp. 562–567].

Many experts feel that activated charcoal by itself is the most effective agent in terms of clearing a poisonous substance from the body. There is a "super-activated" form that is four to five times as absorbent as the standard agent. Absorption of many poisons is inhibited to a significant degree [*Ann Emerg Med*, November 1986, Vol. 15, p. 1301]. Multiple doses of activated charcoal may actually increase the clearance of certain substances (salicylates, digoxin, phenobarbital, theophylline, carbamazepine) from the body as well.

Though not uniformly accepted at this time, the reader should be aware that several groups are not using gastric emptying (ipecac or lavage). Instead, they are relying on the repeated administration of activated (or super-activated) charcoal, with apparent good results [*Arch Int Med*, 1986, Vol. 146, pp. 969–973]. On balance, the majority of current work suggests that gastric lavage is more efficacious than is ipecac-induced emesis in cleaning the stomach. The question of whether or not either is actually necessary is unanswered at this time [*J Emerg Med*, 1985, Vol. 3, pp. 133–136; *Ann Emerg Med*, June 1986, Vol. 15, pp. 692–698; *Am J Emerg Med*, 1986, Vol. 4, pp. 205–209], though it appears that activated charcoal administration may become the primary gastrointestinal decontamination procedure after acute poisoning [*Ann Emerg Med*, August 1987, Vol. 16, pp. 838–841; *Am J Em Med*, 1987, Vol. 5, pp. 305–310].

A reasonable compromise, in light of currently

available information, is to use one or more large oral doses of a high-surface-area activated charcoal (50–100 gm) and a cathartic (instead of ipecac or lavage) in most poisoned patients (if the poison is adsorbed by charcoal). A gastric emptying procedure "should be considered in patients ingesting massive quantities of poison and presenting within the first hour after ingestion if spontaneous emesis has not occurred," as well as if the poison is not absorbed by activated charcoal [*Arch Intern Med,* 1986, Vol. 146, p. 1381].

It is always difficult to "interest" the patient in activated charcoal. A preparation is now available in which the charcoal is premixed in a sorbitol solution (Actidose, 50 gm activated charcoal in 240 ml 70% sorbitol, Paddock Laboratories, Inc., Minneapolis, MN). This actually serves a twofold purpose—the solution is sweet (and actually rather palatable). Additionally, sorbitol is a large carbohydrate molecule which is not absorbed in the GI tract. This leads to significant osmotic diarrhea. Thus, is is not usually necessary to give another cathartic (such as magnesium citrate) as well.

If an additional cathartic is to be given, though, the "saline cathartics" ($MgSO_4$, Sodium Sulfate, Mg citrate) are preferred because they do not interfere with the adsorptive activity of charcoal. Also, if these are aspirated, there is no risk of developing a lipoid pneumonia as there might be if mineral oil were used.

Activated charcoal alone produces a GI transit time of 23.5 hours. Sorbitol is the most rapidly acting cathartic: Mg citrate— 4.2 hours; $MgSO_4$—9.3 hours; sorbitol—0.9 hours. It is also the most predictable with an average total action time of one hour. Mg citrate is the most palatable (lemon-flavored).

Sorbitol can lead to severe abdominal cramps before catharsis. Patients and their families need to be advised of this. In the elderly (as well as in young children), there is also a potential for fluid/electrolyte depletion when massive diarrhea is induced by sorbitol [*Ann Emerg Med,* December 1985, Vol. 14, pp. 1152–1155].

Pearls to Remember

1. Product labels with "antidotes" and "home antidote" packages or kits are dangerous. **Do not use these.** Follow the directions of your regional Poison Control Center. Studies have proven that a regional Poison Control Center official is the ONLY reliable source of up-to-date information!

2. The history in ingestions is always poor and usually unreliable.

3. *Assume* multiple drug ingestions, especially in suicide attempts. This *includes* ingestions with alcohol—people often mix pills with alcohol. Toxicology screening may be helpful.

4. DO NOT induce vomiting in patients without a gag reflex, who have a decreased level of consciousness or who are actively seizing. Also omit if ingestion was of a strong acid/base or hydrocarbons (i.e., gasoline), unless approved by the Poison Control Center.

5. Some compounds are not absorbed by charcoal. These include elemental metals (iron, lithium, boron), some pesticides (malathion, DDT), and cyanide [*Arch Intern Med,* January 1985, Vol. 145, pp. 43–44].

6. A waxing and waning level of consciousness should be a clue to either glutethimide intoxication or a naloxone effect that is wearing off.

7. Active removal is indicated for certain poisonings in which there is a high probability of tissue damage. These include: ethylene glycol, methyl alcohol, theophylline, and salicylates (in appropriate toxic levels).

ACETAMINOPHEN OVERDOSE

Acetaminophen is found in over 20 varieties of over-the-counter analgesics and antipyretics. It is also present in many prescription-only remedies. A partial list of these many products includes: Tylenol, Datril, Anacin-3, Bayer Nonaspirin, BromoSeltzer, Darvocet-N, Excedrin, Liquiprim, Novahistine, NeoSynephrine Compound, Nyquil, Parafon Forte, Romilar, Sinutab, Tempra, Vanquish, Wygesic, and Super Anahist.

As few as 20 tablets of acetaminophen can produce fatal liver damage (> 10 grams in adults). Peak plasma levels are generally reached within one hour of ingestion. Alcohol seems to potentiate acetaminophen toxicity—lower doses of acetaminophen are required to cause comparable problems during periods of heavy drinking than in "dry periods" or nondrinkers [*Ann Int Med,* 1986, Vol. 104, pp. 399–404]. The onset of toxicity is slower (16–18 hrs) if Darvocet-N (propoxyphene HCL + acetaminophen) is ingested.

Signs and symptoms of a toxic ingestion vary according to the amount taken and the time interval:

1. *Early (12–24 hours)*—anorexia, nausea, vomiting, pallor, sweating.

2. *Intermediate (1–3 days)*—milder early-phase symptoms, right upper quadrant abdominal pain (liver tenderness), decreased urine output.

3. *Late (3–5 days)*—liver failure, death.

Diagnosis

The diagnosis of potentially lethal ingestion is made in consultation with a regional Poison Control Center. The Rocky Mountain Poison Control Center in Denver specializes in this area and maintains a toll-free line specifically for acetaminophen overdoses (1-800-525-6115).

Serum acetaminophen levels are drawn at least four hours after the ingestion. This level correlates well with toxicity. If the exact number of pills taken is known (difficult information to obtain accurately!), there exists a nomogram to predict toxicity. Under some cases, a serum level may not be necessary. Either way, consultation with a Poison Control Center is mandatory.

Treatment

To be effective, treatment must start within 10–16 hours following the ingestion. It is given as follows:

1. ACETYLCYSTEINE (Mucomyst)—140 mg/kg orally followed by 70 mg/kg every 4 hours for a total of 17 doses.

2. If the plasma level is within the toxic range, the full number of doses is given; if not, antidote therapy is stopped.

3. Standard therapy (i.e., Ipecac) may be used but many feel that activated charcoal should be omitted, as it would absorb the Mucomyst. This is considered controversial at this point. Definitive studies are not as of yet available [*Ann Emerg Med,* June 1985, Vol. 14, p. 568].

PHENCYCLIDINE (PCP) INTOXICATION

Phencyclidine, or PCP, is one of the most common dangerous street drugs available today. It goes by various "street" names including angel dust, PCP, peace pill, supergrass, and TAC. Originally, it was used as a veterinary anesthetic until taken off the market because it was deemed too dangerous.

Signs and Symptoms

The signs and symptoms of PCP ingestion are dose related:

1. *General (seen at any dose)*—vomiting, hyperreflexia, tachycardia, tachypnea, hypertension, nystagmus, hypersalivation.

2. *Low dose (from smoking or "snorting" the drug)*—blank stare, may/may not speak; quiet or restless; poor orientation, euphoric or fearful; regressive, self-

destructive or homicidal behavior. This may last *six to eight hours.*

3. *Moderate and high dose (ingestion)*—stupor/coma, tachycardia, HBP, myoclonus, hypertonicity; hyperpyrexia, convulsions, and bronchorrhea.

4. *Massive overdose*—hypotension, apnea, areflexia, and status epilepticus with rhabdomyolysis (destruction of muscle tissue); secondary renal failure often follows (myoglobin is released from damaged muscle tissue during rhabdomyolysis, which is very toxic to the kidneys).

Treatment

First, assess the airway and treat any obvious problems appropriately. All treatment, if possible, should take place in a quiet nonthreatening environment. The number of caretakers should be limited. Bright lights should be avoided, and tactile stimulation minimized. "Talking down" the patient, as is commonly done in LSD intoxication, is *not indicated* in PCP poisoning. The regional Poison Control Center should be contacted. **Drug treatment** may be helpful:

1. DIAZEPAM (Valium)—5–10 mg IM or IV to manage seizures or agitation. An alternative is HALOPERIDOL (Haldol)—2.5–5 mg IM. *Avoid* phenothiazines (Thorazine), as they can potentiate the effects of PCP.

2. If the patient is awake, use ASCORBIC ACID (vitamin C) to acidify the urine. Give this for one week. PCP is a weak base and, therefore, ionized. It will be "trapped" in acidic urine. Emesis and lavage are NOT recommended!

If the patient is comatose, the following regimen should be used [*JACEP*, February 1979, Vol. 8 (2), p. 68]:

1. Intubate the trachea.

2. Gastric lavage, activated charcoal, and cathartic via NG tube.

3. FUROSEMIDE, 40 mg IV every 4–6 hours.

4. Ascorbic acid, .5–1.5 gm IV every 4–6 hours.

5. PROPRANOLOL (Inderal) may be used to counteract severe adrenergic effects, and NITROPRUSSIDE (Nipride) may be used to treat severe hypertension.

SALICYLATE OVERDOSE/POISONING

Most salicylate ingestion involves aspirin but methyl salicylate (oil of wintergreen) can provoke a crisis—any ingestion of this latter substance is dangerous! One teaspoon of oil of wintergreen contains five grams of salicylate. This is the equivalent of 22 adult strength aspirin tablets. If aspirin only is taken, the ingested dose is calculated as follows:

$$\text{DOSE IN MG/KG} = \frac{[\text{\# TABLETS INGESTED}] \times \text{MG ASA PER TABLET}}{\text{PATIENT WEIGHT (IN KG)}}$$

In a single ingestion, if the calculated ingestion is less than 150 mg/kg and there exists no concurrent febrile illness, dehydration, or renal disease (which could further toxicity even at lower doses), probably no further treatment is needed. **Verify with the Poison Control Center.**

Treatment is indicated if the ingestion is greater than 400 mg/kg or if any of these **signs and symptoms** of salicylate intoxication appear: unexplained hyperpnea, especially if accompanied by vomiting, tinnitus, fever, confusion, lethargy, seizures, and coma.

Salicylates initially cause respiratory stimulation, leading to a respiratory alkalosis. As time progresses, they cause a metabolic acidosis with an elevated anion gap. These items should be sought on arterial blood gases and electrolyte determinations.

Treatment

Treatment consists of the following measures (again, verify with the Poison Control Center first):

1. Induce emesis, charcoal administration, catharsis.

2. Correct systemic acidosis if present with IV NaHCO$_3$. The dose can be estimated by the following formula:

   mEq NEEDED = [25 − CALCULATED HCO$_3$] × (.5 × WT IN KG)

   One-half this amount should be given initially and the rest according to blood gases.

3. Forced alkaline diuresis—NaHCO$_3$—DO NOT USE acetazolamide (Diamox) as this alkalizes the urine but leads to systemic *acidosis!* Add 2 amps NaHCO$_3$ to one liter NS and give IV at 150–500 cc/hour. Give furosemide as necessary to maintain urine output at 3–6 ml/kg/hr. Urinary pH should be maintained at 7.5–9.0.

Dialysis or hemoperfusion is indicated in the following circumstances:

1. Coma, respiratory, or cardiovascular insufficiency.

2. Severe, unresponsive acidosis.

3. Plasma salicylate level greater than 100 mg/dl at 6 hours.

4. Renal failure.

5. Inability to induce an alkaline diuresis.

NARCOTIC WITHDRAWAL SYNDROMES

The signs of narcotic withdrawal are those of sympathetic nervous system overactivity. **Signs and symptoms** have been graded according to severity:

1. *Grade 1*—lacrimation, rhinorrhea, diaphoresis, yawning, restlessness, insomnia.

2. *Grade 2*—mydriasis, piloerection, muscular fasciculations, myalgias, arthralgias, abdominal pain.

3. *Grade 3*—tachycardia, hypertension, tachypnea, fever, anorexia, nausea, extreme restlessness.

4. *Grade 4*—diarrhea, emesis, dehydration, hyperglycemia, hypotension, "fetal posturing."

The syndrome ordinarily starts at the time when the next dose of narcotic would be due. This averages four to six hours following the last ingestion. Symptoms peak at 36–72 hours and are usually over within seven to ten days. Methadone withdrawal leads to a more prolonged course, starting at 36–72 hours, peaking in six days, and lasting up to two weeks.

Laboratory findings are generally unremarkable, though the white blood cell count is often elevated as is the 17-ketosteroid level (both are likely elevated due to stress).

Treatment

Keep in mind that though uncomfortable, narcotic withdrawal is RARELY dangerous to the patient. Alternatives include the following:

1. METHADONE—Though used in outpatient treatment programs, this is NOT an alternative for the emergency treatment of narcotic withdrawal.

2. PROMAZINE (Sparine)—This phenothiazine is helpful and can be given either orally or as an injection. The dose is 25 mg every 30 minutes as necessary to a maximum dose of 125 mg. This agent seems to have less euphoric side effects than some of the other phenothiazine drugs.

3. CLONIDINE—has a central effect that is

highly effective when given orally. It may be necessary to control nausea and vomiting initially with an injectable phenothiazine, though. The recommended dose is .2 mg initially, then .2 mg every four to six hours for seven days. The patient should then be weaned off the drug over three days, as rebound hypertensive crisis can occur if this is not done.

Before concluding this section, it is worth briefly mentioning some common "street" treatments for narcotic withdrawal (referred to as "cold turkey"). An ice bag placed on the "patient's" groin is the most common. The exact purpose of this is not well elucidated in the scientific literature. Administration of milk, at times intravenously, is another popular folk remedy. This is also highly dangerous as pulmonary fat emboli may result.

ALCOHOL WITHDRAWAL SYNDROMES

Alcohol is probably the most commonly abused drug in this country. The prevalence of alcoholism in both the general hospital and Emergency Department patient population averages 20%, irrespective of the class setting of the institution [*Am J Psychiatr*, 1968, Vol. 125, p. 681]. There are several well-defined syndromes of withdrawal toxicity that can occur in addition to the well-known problems associated with acute intoxication. The *classification* of these syndromes is as follows:

1. *The "shakes"*—occurs within 24 hours of cessation of drinking. The patient appears shaky, tremulous; a mild sleep disturbance is present accompanied by blood pressure elevation and conjunctival injection.

2. *Withdrawal seizures*—occur 24–48 hours following the last ingestion; they are usually grand mal in nature. The EEG following the event is normal. One-third of the patients with withdrawal seizures will progress to full-blown delirium tremens (DTs). These seizures DO NOT need treatment unless they are ongoing. *But* the first seizure, even if suspected to be due to alcohol withdrawal, in any patient should receive a full workup! **Remember to rule out head trauma and meningitis.**

3. *Delirium tremens (DTs)*—occur 72 hours or later after the last ingestion. Consist of delirium, hallucination, and signs of automatic nervous system hyperactivity (fever—very common, tachycardia, diaphoresis, tremor, and hyperexcitability). There is a 15% *mortality* associated with this entity.

Table 5-3 summarizes the alcohol withdrawal syndromes.

Table 5-3. Summary of the Alcohol Withdrawal Syndromes

The "Shakes"
Onset within 24 hours of cessation
Shaky, tremulous
Mild sleep disturbance
Hypertension
Conjunctival injection

Withdrawal Seizures
Occurs 24–48 hours after cessation
Grand mal with normal EEG afterwards
⅓ of these patients will → DTs
Full workup first time around
No treatment unless ongoing
Rule out head trauma!

Delirium Tremens (DTs)
Occur > = 72 hours after cessation
Delirium, hallucinations
Signs of autonomic nervous system hyperactivity:
• Fever—common
• Tachycardia
• Diaphoresis
• Tremor
• Hyperexcitability
15% mortality!

Treatment

The treatment of mild withdrawal symptoms consists of oral CHLORDIAZEPOXIDE (Librium), 25 mg four times per day. This may be increased as needed. Multivitamins and thiamine are also given. The treatment of withdrawal seizures is as covered previously under "Seizures." The full-blown syndrome of DTs is a life-threatening emergency and must be rapidly dealt with as follows:

1. *Well-lit room.*

2. *Restrain prn*—heavy leather restraints usually are necessary.

3. *Lab*—electrolytes, calcium/phosphorous, CBC, blood sugar.

4. *IV fluid replacement*—depends on electrolyte measurements.

5. *Look for alternative sources of fever* (especially pneumonia).

6. *Drugs*—DIAZEPAM (Valium)—5 mg IV every five minutes until sedation is achieved; after 6 doses (and no resultant sedation), then increase the dose to 10 mg. Repeat every hour to maintain the patient in a slightly drowsy state. *Large* initial doses are often required. After 24–48 hours, decrease the dose by 25% each day (since the metabolites of diazepam persist for 24–36 hours). This regimen has been well documented to be safe. Over 1,000 mg have been given acutely IV to patients in DTs without any adverse problems. In fact, one report described a 34-year-old male who required 2,640 mg of IV valium over 56 hours to sedate him. No significant side effects were noted [*Crit Care Med*, 1985, Vol. 13, p. 246].

Some workers have given atenolol (Tenormin) 50 mg daily to patients in the DTs, in addition to the above therapies. There appears to be a reduction in the length of hospital stay, as well as more rapid normalization of the patient's vital signs. This is still to be considered experimental [*NEJM*, 1985, Vol. 313, pp. 905–909].

Cloridine [*Arch Int Med*, 1987, Vol. 147, pp. 1223–1226] and intravenous phenobarbital have been reported to work well in alcohol withdrawal. Early studies suggest that both IV phenobarbital [*Ann Emerg Med*, August 1987, Vol. 16, pp. 847-850] and oral chlordiazepoxide may prevent alcohol withdrawal [*West Jrnl Med*, seizures June 1987, Vol. 146, pp. 695-696].

In evaluating the mental status of any intoxicated patient, it is helpful to estimate, based on their blood alcohol level, when they should be "baseline." Nonalcoholics metabolize ethanol at a rate of 10–20 mg/dl/hr while chronic abusers metabolize it at 30–50 mg/dl/hr. Thus, one can roughly calculate when the patient's mental status should no longer be altered by alcohol.

Mention should be made of disulfiram (Antabuse) reactions. This substance is commonly prescribed as an adjunct to alcohol treatment. Ingestion of alcohol within seven days of taking this substance leads to nausea, vomiting, palpitations, and anxiety. It can also lead to very severe problems such as arterial hypotension, flushing, and cardiovascular collapse. Refractory shock, only responsive to norepinephrine (Levophed) infusion has been reported [*Am J Emerg Med*, 1986, Vol. 4, p. 323].

TOXIC SYNDROMES

There are several constellations of findings common to certain poisonings. These are grouped into six common "toxic syndromes":

- Narcotic-opiate
- Sedative-hypnotic
- Cholinergic
- Anticholinergic
- Sympathomimetic
- Methemoglobinemia.

Again, please remember that maintenance of Airway, Breathing, and Circulation are still your first priority. The Poison Control Center should **always** be contacted before beginning any therapy other than maintenance of A, B, C's (with very few exceptions—such as cyanide poisoning).

The **narcotic-opiate syndrome** is due to ingestion (orally or intravenously) of morphine, demerol, heroin, propoxyphene, or similar agents. There is respiratory depression, miosis, and often coma. Neurogenic pulmonary edema may also occur. The treatment is naloxone. It is now well recognized that at least three opiate receptors exist in the central nervous system. Naloxone antagonizes primarily "mu"-receptor sites (the classic morphine receptor) in the brain.

The **sedative-hypnotic syndrome** is caused by barbiturates, benzodiazepines (Valium, Ativan, etc.), chloral hydrates, methaqualones (Quaaludes), and phenothiazines (antipsychotic drugs). Symptoms begin with mental confusion progressing to coma with respiratory and/or cardiovascular depression. Pulmonary edema has also been reported. Quaaludes may produce tonic-clonic spasms, myoclonus, and seizures. Treatment consists of supportive care.

The **cholinergic syndrome** is secondary to exposure to organophosphate or carbamate insecticides, physostigmine, or nerve gas. Pathophysiologically, acetylcholinesterase is inactivated leading to unopposed parasympathetic stimulation. The mnemonic use for this syndrome is SLUDGE:

S—Salivation
L—Lacrimination
U—Urination
D—Defecation
G—GI cramping
E—Emesis.

The patient may also have sweating, bradycardia, miosis, bronchorrhea, and seizures. Atropine is the standard treatment and should be given in a dose of 2 mg initially in adults. The initial dose for children is .05 mg/kg. A specific antidote, pralidoxime chloride is indicated for muscular weakness and/or muscular fasciculations. The dose is 1 gram for adults IV.

The **anticholinergic syndrome** is caused by scopolamine, atropine, belladonna, jimsonweed, Lomotil, and tricyclic antidepressants. Sufficient quantities of anticholinergics are in some over-the-counter cold remedies as to precipitate significant toxicity. As you'd suspect, the symptoms are opposite those of the cholinergic syndrome, and the mnemonic is "ANTI-SLUDGE":

Anti/S—dry mouth and mucous membranes
Anti/L—lack of tears
Anti/U—urinary retention
Anti/D—constipation
Anti/G—constipation
Anti/E—(not present).

Additionally, tachycardia, hypertension, hyperthermia, psychosis, and hallucinations may be present. Patients with atropinism have been described as being "red, hot, hyper, and mad!" Usually, supportive care is sufficient, though physostigmine treatment may be warranted, especially in the face of life-threatening problems with tricyclic antidepressant overdoses. Alkalinization with bicarbonate is usually tried first, though. Many consider this to be the mainstay of tricyclic antidepressant overdose therapy.

The mechanism by which bicarbonate works in tricyclic overdose is uncertain. It is felt that the change in pH may lead to increased protein binding, with a reduction in the amount of "free" drug in the blood. Some animal studies suggest that it is actually the sodium moiety, rather than the bicarbonate anion, that slows the rate of rise of the phase 0 action potential.

Phenytoin is the recommended antiarrhythmic (following bicarbonate therapy) in tricyclic antidepressant overdose. Its electrophysiological actions are opposite to those of tricyclics. Any patient with signs of toxicity should receive 15 mg/kg of this agent (not to exceed 1 gram). Of course, procainamide and quinidine are contraindicated, as they have similar effects to tricyclics on the cardiac conduction system. Atropine is contraindicated in bradydysrhythmias because of its own anticholinergic effects.

Norepinephrine is the vasopressor of choice, as tricyclic antidepressant overdose causes hypotension via total body depletion of this substance. This occurs due to drug inhibition of norepinephrine uptake and its subsequent degradation by various enzyme systems. Ipecac administration is, of course, *contraindicated* due to the potential for both rapid absorption of ingested tricyclics as well as ongoing enterohepatic circulation. It is highly possible that the conscious patient could be comatose by the time ipecac-induced emesis occurs [*Ped Emerg Care,* 1986, Vol. 2, pp. 28–35]. Late deaths (up to 24 hours postingestion) have been reported, despite apparently normal early recovery in tricyclic poisoning. This may be due to myocardial cell binding of the drug [*Ann Emerg Med,* 1986, Vol. 15, p. 1349].

Some of the newer tricyclic-like agents differ pharmacologically from the "classic" types. Thus, significant differences (and similarities) in toxicity may occur. Salient differences for the most commonly used agents are as follows [*Ann Emerg Med,* 1986, Vol. 15, p. 1039]:

1. AMOXAPINE (Ascendin)—lack of cardiovascular toxicity but a higher incidence of seizures, acute renal failure, and mortality.

2. MAPROTILINE (Ludiomil)—basically the same as the older tricyclic drugs (i.e., CNS and cardiotoxicity).

3. TRAZODONE (Desyrel)—very little anticholinergic effects. Generally very safe as compared to the other agents.

The **sympathomimetic syndrome** can be caused by a variety of agents, including amphetamines, thyroid, and caffeine. Symptoms consist of hypertension, tachycardia, and agitation. Superficially, this syndrome is similar to anticholinergic poisoning *except* that sympathomimetic overdose also causes nausea, vomiting, abdominal pain, and moist skin and mucous membranes. Beta-blockers may be used in treatment.

The **methemoglobinemia syndrome** was briefly discussed in Chapter 3 on Respiratory Emergencies. Causes are numerous and include nitrates/nitrites (food preservatives, recreational drugs, nitroglycerin), local anesthetics, sulfa drugs, some dyes, photochemicals, and antifungal drugs. Cyanosis refractory to oxygen therapy occurs due to the conversion of ferrous iron (Fe^{++}) to the ferric state (Fe^{+++}, methemoglobin). Blood levels > 10% are symptomatic. A quick laboratory test is to compare a drop of the patient's blood next to a known normal sample on a piece of filter paper. If significant levels of methemoglobin are present, the patient's blood appears a chocolate-brown color. Treatment is with high-flow oxygen and methylene blue [*JEMS,* August 1983, pp. 60–61].

SNAKEBITE

There are over 7,000 venomous snakebites annually in the United States. The majority of these are rattlesnakes. Though the toxicity of snakebites is not solely neurological, this entity is discussed here because of its relationship to the "poisoning" section. The severity varies widely from puncture wounds to death. Despite a large number of species of snakes in the United States, only two families are of great concern—coral snakes (Elapids) and vipers.

Coral snakes are found in the more Southern states from Arizona to Florida. They are brightly colored with alternating black, white (or yellow), and red bands that encircle the entire body. Their nasal area is totally black. These features distinguish them from several nonpoisonous snakes with similar markings. The old adage may be helpful: "Red on yellow will kill a fellow; red on black, venom lack." They may be up to three feet in length.

Vipers include the cottonmouth, copperhead, massasuaga, pigmy rattlesnake, and the "true" rattlesnakes. Most are widely distributed across the United States with the cottonmouth limited to the southeastern states and Texas. These reptiles characteristically have a triangular head, vertically slit pupils, heavy bodies, and movable folding upper fangs. The famed rattle is lacking on copperheads and cottonmouths. The skins of these animals may be very attractive. In fact, 30–40% of rattlesnake bite victims each year are engaged in collecting or marketing the snakes when they are bitten. Though uncommon, there are reported cases of persons being "bitten" by removed snake heads that have been preserved for several weeks [*Ann Emerg Med,* 1986, Vol. 15, p. 955].

Snake venoms have several physiological properties—neurotoxicity (paresthesias, paralysis, neuromuscular transmission disturbances), hemotoxicity (coagulant, anticoagulant, hemolytic, platelet problems), and cardiotoxicity (decreased cardiac output and blood pressure). Additionally, enzymes in the venom lead to tissue destruction. Most venoms are a complex mixture of proteins with mixed effects.

Diagnosis: Coral Snakebite

Fang marks from the coral snake may be difficult to locate, and, initially, there may be no pain around the wound. The venom is primarily neurotoxic. Though rarely fatal, the following may be observed:

1. Euphoria, drowsiness, nausea, vomiting.

2. Increased salivation—mostly from a decreased ability to swallow.

3. Paresthesias, headache.

4. Ptosis (droopy eyelid), blurred vision.

5. Shortness of breath, abnormal reflexes.

6. Generalized paralysis.

No laboratory work is necessary.

Treatment: Coral Snakebite

In terms of treatment, incision, suction, and ice are ill-advised. Unless the animal is known to be a Sonoran coral snake for which no antivenin exists, early administration of antivenin is recommended. It should be repeated later if symptoms of envenomation actually occur. This should all be done in consultation with the regional Poison Control Center!

Diagnosis: Pit Viper Bites

Clinically diagnosing these bites is somewhat easier because there will almost always be a visible puncture wound, often oozing blood. Despite this, 20% of patients with a true fang mark will show no evidence of envenomation. This may relate to the size of the snake or the interval between bites—if the snake

has just struck, the "poison sacs" may have not adequately "recharged" for a bite to envenomate.

Signs and symptoms of envenomation may be any or all of the following:

1. Rapidly occurring pain and numbness locally in the vicinity of the bite—if a limb, this may travel proximally.

2. Early edema traveling up the extremity. Despite what is often massive swelling, arterial compromise is rare. The amount of fluid that pours into the tissues with this edema may account for some of the hypotension a patient may have.

3. Local ecchymoses initially, which then spreads and leads to a bluish hue around the bite area.

4. Local blebs filled with hemorrhagic transudate.

5. Signs of lymphangitis/lymphadenitis—red streaking up and down the extremity, swollen/tender lymph nodes.

6. Paresthesias, muscle fasciculations, generalized weakness.

7. Unresponsive hypotension, petechiae, conjunctival hemorrhage and bleeding—this constellation of findings suggests a widespread coagulopathy.

Laboratory work obtained should include a CBC, PT, PTT, fibrinogen level, platelet count (decreased in 42% of patients), urinalysis, and electrolytes. The hemoglobin is decreased in 37% of patients with glycosuria (sugar in the urine) and proteinuria (protein in the urine) being present in 20% and 16% of the victims, respectively. An abnormal EKG (nonspecific findings) is present in 26%.

The **severity of envenomation** is a continuum. Anywhere between 10–25% of patients bitten are NOT envenomated. The severity is classified as follows:

1. *Minimal*—local manifestations, no systemic signs, no laboratory abnormalities.

2. *Moderate*—manifestations beyond the im-

mediate bite area, significant systemic signs/symptoms, decreased fibrinogen and platelets, signs of hemoconcentration (elevated hematocrit and sodium levels).

3. *Severe*—manifestations throughout the entire extremity or body part, serious systemic signs and symptoms (such as hypotension), marked and widespread laboratory abnormalities.

Treatment: Pit Viper Bites

The general treatment of viper bites is as follows:

1. Basic life support as needed.

2. Oxygen, 10 LPM by mask.

3. IV NS—titrate as per blood pressure.

4. If there is evidence of envenomation AND the person is seen within 10 minutes of the bite AND transportation time is greater than 1 hour to an Emergency Department or clinic:
   - Apply a constricting band 5–10 cm proximal to the bite. This is designed to occlude lymphatic flow only, NOT arterial or venous flow. The band should admit two fingers.
   - Make small, shallow (no longer than 5 mm or deeper than 4 mm) parallel incisions through the fang marks.
   - Apply suction—use your mouth only if you do not have any open sores within!

5. Immobilize the affected part at heart level.

6. Give the patient a tetanus shot.

7. Provide local wound care as you would any other ''dirty'' wound.

Antivenin treatment of viper bites has its greatest effect if given within four hours. It should be reserved for life-threatening envenomations as the risk of serious sensitivity reactions, including anaphylaxis to the horse serum used, is high. This is NOT recommended for field use. Consultation should be obtained through the regional Poison Control Center before antivenin is used. The protocol is as follows:

1. Skin test the patient for sensitivity to horse serum—inject .1 ml of a 1:10 dilution intradermally. A (+) reaction is redness at the site within 10–15 minutes. If the patient is (+), do not proceed without talking to the Poison Control Center. If negative at 20 minutes, proceed but remember that life-threatening anaphylaxis can still occur with a negative test.

2. The dose of antivenin is calculated based on the severity of the envenomation as discussed earlier:
   - *Mild*—1–5 vials
   - *Moderate*—6–12 vials
   - *Severe*—15–30 vials.

3. Antivenin (Crotalidae) polyvalent is first diluted—each vial in 50 cc NaCl and given via continuous infusion. Antivenin should be administered slowly at first. Occasionally, the BP may drop transiently for no apparent reason early on—in this case, wait a few minutes and try again (as long as there are no other signs of anaphylaxis). Attempt to give the total dose within the first four to six hours of treatment.

4. Monitor therapy by symptoms, laboratory tests, and the circumference of the extremity (if involved) just proximal to the bite and a point 10–20 cm above. These parameters should be recorded every 15 minutes during antivenin administration and then every four hours thereafter.

5. Antivenin for exotic species may be obtained through the Oklahoma City Zoo (24 hour number: 405-271-5454).

Pearls to Remember

When dealing with poisonous snake bites, keep in mind the following:

1. Do not chill or apply ice to the wound—severe tissue damage can occur.

2. Do not apply a tourniquet—if others before you have applied one (prior to your arrival), place a less constricting band more proximal and with an IV in place, slowly remove the original tourniquet.

3. Do not use steroids except in a severe hypersensitivity reaction.

4. Never inject antivenin into a finger or toe directly.

5. Heparin is not recommended for coagulopathies.

6. Do not consider fasciotomy unless objective evidence of a true compartment syndrome exists.

7. If the patient is pregnant and has a hypersensitivity reaction to the antivenin, consider using ephedrine 20–50 mg IV push instead of epinephrine. Epinephrine may further decrease the blood flow to the uterus and compromise the fetus [*Southern Medical Journal*, 1985, Vol. 77, p. 402].

8. Preliminary studies have suggested that local electric shock therapy may markedly decrease limb edema and pain, in some cases eliminating the need for antivenin therapy [*Outdoor Life*, June 1987, pp. 55–58, 110–112]

Endocrine and Metabolic Emergencies

Emergencies involving the endocrine and metabolic functions of the body can be devastating and, some, rapidly fatal. In this section, we will learn about:

- Hypoglycemia
- Diabetic ketoacidosis
- Hyperosmolar hyperglycemic nonketotic coma
- Addisonian crisis.

HYPOGLYCEMIA

Hypoglycemia may be defined as a state of decreased blood glucose that may result in a decreased level of consciousness. Prolonged hypoglycemia may lead to neurological dysfunction and death. It appears that severe hypoglycemia causes the production of an endogenous neurotoxin which is released by the brain into tissue and cerebrospinal fluid. This interrupts interneuronal connections leading to hyperexcitation of cells and subsequent rupture. It is felt that this mechanism may explain the tendency toward seizure activity seen clinically [*Stroke*, 1986, Vol. 17, p. 699].

Hypoglycemia can be classified as reactive or fasting.

Reactive hypoglycemia is a decreased blood sugar level which results in symptoms within five hours of food ingestion. There has been a recent "craze" in the lay press concerning hypoglycemia. Unfor-

tunately, this also appears to be a catchall diagnosis used by many physicians for "spells" of unknown etiology. This *incorrect* usage of the diagnosis stems from the transitional low blood glucose state which is commonly found on a five-hour glucose tolerance test (GTT). Up to 50% of the individuals taking a GTT will have blood sugar levels of less than 50 mg% but *without symptoms;* this DOES NOT diagnose true reactive hypoglycemia. The diagnosis is only made when the patient exhibits Whipple's triad—symptoms, plasma glucose values in the hypoglycemic range, and amelioration of the symptoms by restoring plasma glucose to normal levels with the ingestion of food. A low blood glucose MUST be at the time of the patient's symptoms.

A few individuals have true reactive hypoglycemia. The measured blood sugar levels on a five-hour glucose tolerance test may be used to classify patients as follows:

1. *Prediabetes*—The blood sugar (BS) is abnormally elevated in the first two hours of post-glucose ingestion. It is then low at the 3–5 hour marks, which *may* predict the development of overt diabetes in some individuals.

2. *Alimentary hypoglycemia*—There is a rapid rise in the blood sugar followed by hypoglycemia 90–180 minutes later. This is most common in patients who have had gastric surgery, but others may show this same pattern. Intravenous glucose tolerance is normal in these individuals.

3. *Functional*—There is a normal early rise in the blood sugar level but hypoglycemia occurs 2–4 hours after the oral glucose load. In truly functional hypoglycemia, symptoms accompany this low blood sugar. Additionally, if special blood tests are done to indicate the presence of stress-related hormones (i.e., cortisol, epinephrine) in the blood, these are present and elevated at the time of symptoms. Symptoms are relieved by the administration of glucose. Some patients exhibit this pattern with an oral glucose load but not with a test meal; recent literature has questioned totally the existence of true functional hypoglycemia.

Figure 6.1 shows some typical curves from five-hour glucose tolerance tests in various conditions.

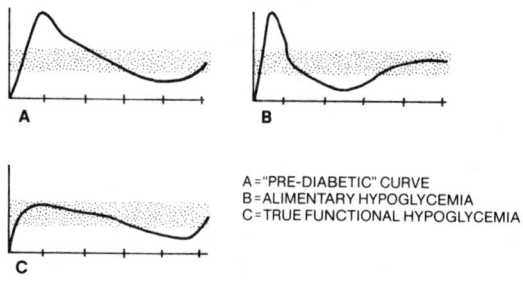

A = "PRE-DIABETIC" CURVE
B = ALIMENTARY HYPOGLYCEMIA
C = TRUE FUNCTIONAL HYPOGLYCEMIA

(HASH MARKS REFER TO 1, 2, 3, 4, AND 5 HOURS)

Figure 6.1. Typical five-hour glucose tolerance test curves.

Fasting hypoglycemia may be defined as a low blood sugar state after the patient passes from the fed to the fasted state. **Causes** of fasting hypoglycemia are as follows:

1. *Drugs*—alcohol, salicylates, insulin, oral diabetes medicines. Hypoglycemia, with an accompanying anion-gap acidosis, has been reported in acetaminophen toxicity (see page 82 on Diabetic Ketoacidosis) [*Ann Emerg Med*, October 1984, Vol. 13, pp. 956–959]. Pentamidine treatment of *Pneumocystis carinii* pneumonia in the acquired immunodeficiency syndrome has been associated with severe hypoglycemia

at times [*Clin Pharmacol Ther*, 1986, Vol. 39, p. 271].

2. *Hormone deficits*—steroids, growth hormone, thyroid hormone.

3. *Extensive liver damage*—the liver is then unable to mobilize glucose reserves or create new ones.

4. *Severe exercise.*

5. *Tumors* that produce insulin or an insulin-like substance.

In the hospitalized patient, up to 45% of hypoglycemic episodes occur in diabetic patients, usually due to administered insulin. Many of these patients have chronic renal insufficiency, with or without concomitant diabetes. The mortality of hospitalized patients who suffer hypoglycemic attacks is high (27%) and likely related to the severity of the underlying illness. It is important to note that iatrogenic insulin overdose is a significant cause of hypoglycemia in this patient population. Thus, blood sugars should be watched carefully, even in persons on previously well-established outpatient insulin regimens [*N Engl J Med*, 1986, Vol. 315, p. 1245].

A rare cause of fasting hypoglycemia in diabetics is the occurrence of spontaneous pituitary infarction. It is recognized by the sudden appearance of a severe headache, which is usually retro-orbital, and frequent episodes of hypoglycemia [*J Intensive Care Med*, 1986, Vol. 1, p. 336].

Diagnosis

History

In making the diagnosis of hypoglycemia, there may be a history of anxiety, hunger, weakness, or shakiness. The onset may be sudden or gradual. It is important to note when the patient last ate. If the patient is on insulin or an oral diabetic medicine, the type, dose, and when it was last taken should be noted. A history of diabetes and the presence of a Medi-Alert tag should be searched for.

Physical examination

The physical examination reveals symptoms

primarily due to the outpouring of adrenalin by the body. Some patients *may not* exhibit these classic symptoms and may only show a decreased level of consciousness. Subtle impairment of mentation and behavioral changes may be present, including slurred speech and combativeness. The patient is often, though not always, diaphoretic and tachycardic. Tremor and hypothermia may be present. Seizures can occur, but true grand mal seizures are rare in adults. Gastric aspiration with the adult respiratory distress syndrome has been reported in suicide attempts using an insulin overdose [*Medicine,* 1985, Vol. 64, pp. 323–332].

Focal neurological deficits may be present, especially in the elderly or alcoholic patients. These defects may include decerebrate posturing, anisocoria (unequal pupils), and abnormal plantar reflexes. Interestingly, they often reverse within a couple minutes of IV glucose administration. Many feel that this supports the notion that these deficits are actually seizure phenomena, which reverse with treatment of hypoglycemia, rather than fixed neuronal damage that should take much longer to return to normal [*Am J Med,* June 1985, p. 1036].

Laboratory tests

Laboratory testing will reveal a fingerstick blood sugar that is usually less than 40 mg%. Impairment of cerebral function has been demonstrated at blood sugar levels of 55 mg/dl [*J Inten Care Med,* May–June, 1986, Vol. 1, p. 149]. It is possible, though, for a patient whose blood sugar was previously very high (> 300 mg%) to exhibit hypoglycemic symptoms with a rapid decrease of the blood sugar to the normal range. Therefore, this must be suspected even if the measured blood sugar is "normal." Table 6-1 summarizes the clinical features of hypoglycemia.

Treatment

Treating the patient with suspected hypoglycemia involves first of all, the A, B, C,'s. A fingerstick blood sugar should be rapidly obtained using either Dextrostix or Chemstrip-BG strips. An IV of D_5W at a TKO rate is begun. Drug treatment is as follows:

1. THIAMINE—100 mg IV should precede the administration of glucose to prevent the development of Wernicke's encephalopathy.

2. DEXTROSE 50%—50 cc orally if patient is awake and able to protect airway, otherwise give IV. The IV administration of a 50 cc bolus of D_{50} leads to an average rise in the blood sugar of 166 mg/dl, though the range is wide. Levels cannot reliably be predicted after an IV glucose bolus [*Am J Emerg Med,* 1986, Vol. 4, p. 504].

3. GLUCAGON— 1 mg IM if unable to start an IV. This will lead to a rapid rise in the glucose via stimulation of the compound cyclic AMP.

4. IV GLUCOSE INFUSION—for severe reactions, the patient should be given at least 375 mg/kg/hr of glucose IV. (The percentage of a solution indicates the grams/100 cc. Thus, a 5% sugar solution (D_5W) contains 5 grams/100 cc or 50 grams dextrose per liter. The amount of sugar required can, therefore, be easily calculated.) The blood sugar should be watched carefully. It has been shown that the absorption and action of insulin is erratic, especially in suicide attempts using massive doses in nondiabetics. Thus, hypoglycemia may persist for hours to days longer than expected [*Ann Emerg Med,* July 1984, p. 505]. Oral glucose is NOT effective under these circumstances.

Pearls to Remember

Hypoglycemia can be a serious condition. It should be suspected in all instances of coma and irrational behavior. Remember:

1. A patient may be disoriented and demanding insulin. DO NOT give this in the field under any circumstances! Give only in a hospital setting and then *only* after checking the blood sugar.

2. Hypoglycemia can present as seizures

(rare), coma, behavior problems, intoxication, confusion, or a stroke-like picture with focal deficits (particularly in the elderly).

3. Elderly patients or those who have hypoglycemia for a long period of time may be slower to awaken.

4. In a diabetic suffering a severe hypoglycemic reaction, expect their blood sugar to be difficult to control for up to one month following the acute episode. This is due to the release of stress hormones ("counter-regulatory hormones") by the body to combat the lowered blood sugar. Many of these compounds remain in the blood for a long time.

Patients who have undergone recent, intensive insulin therapy, such as with an insulin pump, tend to have a decreased counter-regulatory hormone response to hypoglycemia due to "downgrading" of receptor sites. This may decrease their perception of hypoglycemia and make hypoglycemic episodes particulary risky [*Ann Int Med,* 1985, Vol. 103, pp. 184-190]. In addition, they may be more susceptible to the development of diabetic ketoacidosis (see below).

5. If the diabetic is unconscious, it may be difficult to decide between hypoglycemia and diabetic ketoacidosis. It is always safer to assume that the blood sugar is low. Therefore, sugar should be given to any unconscious or semiconscious diabetic. If the condition turns out to be hypoglycemia, sugar will result in rapid improvement and may be lifesaving. If it is coma, little harm will be done by giving sugar.

6. The signs and symptoms of hypoglycemia are those of an adrenalin outpouring (in most patients); diabetic ketoacidosis signs are those of dehydration.

7. Administration of dextrose in the alcoholic with depleted thiamine stores may precipitate acute encephalopathy (brain syndrome).

Therefore, thiamine is given with dextrose in alcoholics.

Table 6-1. Clinical Features of Hypoglycemia

History
  Anxiety, hunger
  Weakness, shakiness
  Sudden or gradual onset
  History of diabetes
  Patient on insulin

Physical Exam
  Decreased level of consciousness
  Sweating, tachycardia
  Tremor
  Hypothermia
  Seizures, focal neurological deficits

Laboratory
  Fingerstick BS < 40 mg%

DIABETIC KETOACIDOSIS

Diabetic ketoacidosis (DKA) is a metabolic disturbance caused primarily by insulin depletion resulting in hyperglycemia and the production of abnormal ketones and acids in the body. Though studies suggest that anywhere from 60–90% of cases should be preventable, diabetic ketoacidosis continues to occur [*Mayo Clin Proc,* 1986, Vol. 61, p. 820].

The **pathophysiology** of diabetic ketoacidosis involves acute insulin deficiency (relative or absolute). Decreased insulin leads to a decrease in the tissue glucose uptake as well as an increase in liver glucose production. Together, these result in an elevated blood sugar level (hyperglycemia).

The elevated blood sugar concentrates in the kidneys, forcing them to excrete extra water. This is referred to as an osmotic diuresis. Dehydration and depletion of vital electrolytes (sodium and potassium) result. With further decrease in insulin levels, adipose (fatty) tissue is broken down to its component-free fatty acids (FFA) and a compound known as glycerol.

The liver then converts FFAs to ketone bodies in an attempt to "feed tissues" starved by inadequate glucose uptake. The most common ketone bodies are hydroxybutyrate and acetoacetate. These are oxidized in the peripheral tissue to form the acids, lactate and pyruvate. These serve as precursors of glucose as well. Finally, muscle protein is broken down to its component amino acids (for additional cellular nutrients) which further contributes to acidosis. This process is summarized in Table 6-2.

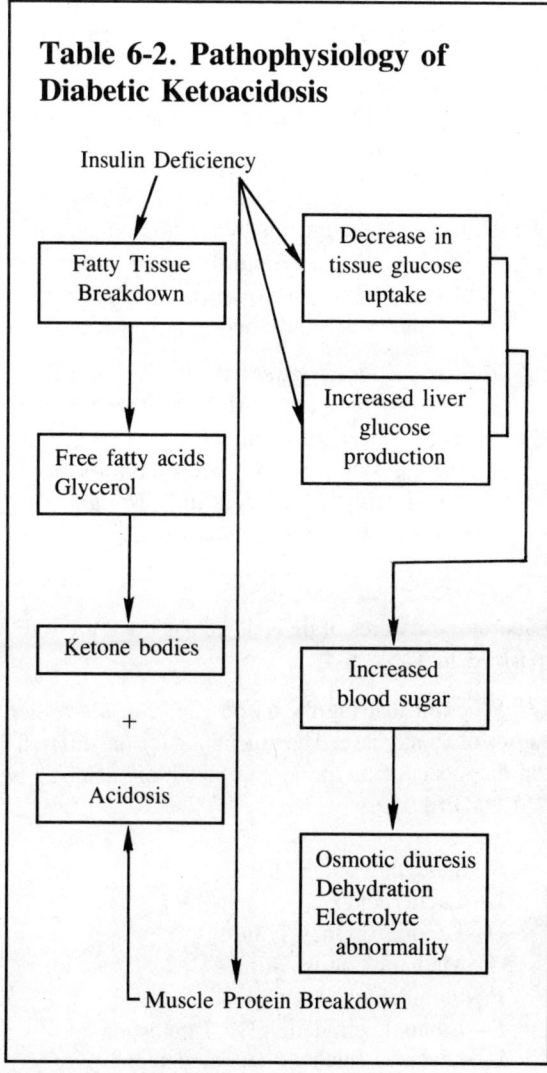

Table 6-2. Pathophysiology of Diabetic Ketoacidosis

Precipitating Factors

In treating the patient with diabetic ketoacidosis, there are several possible precipitating factors that should be ruled out. Infection, most commonly viral gastroenteritis, is the most prevalent. It is important to remember that fever is *uncommon* with infections in diabetic ketoacidosis. An increased white blood cell count (leukocytosis) is common in diabetic ketoacidosis *without* concomitant infection, so the diagnosis is complicated further. Therefore, a high index of suspicion is necessary to identify infection precipitating diabetic ketoacidosis. A left shift (> 10 bands) in the differential count may be helpful in diagnosing infections [*Am J Emerg Med*, 1987, Vol. 5, pp. 1–5]. Omission of insulin, myocardial infarction, pancreatitis, stroke, trauma, and surgery are less common precipitating factors in diabetic ketoacidosis. It is, unfortunately, all too common to see diabetics fail to take the proper amount of insulin during acute periods of nausea and vomiting (or other illness). In reality, they require more insulin, not less, due to the intercurrent illness.

Subclinical brain swelling occurs in most conscious adults who are treated for diabetic ketoacidosis. This has also been demonstrated via CT scan in children as well. Though often a serious problem in children, the significance of cerebral edema in adults is unclear. It is recommended that rapid fluid administration, especially with hypotonic solutions, be avoided when the blood sugar is rapidly falling, thus decreasing the chances of developing clinically evident cerebral edema [*NEJM*, 1985, Vol. 312, pp. 1147–1151].

Diagnosis

History

The history in diabetic ketoacidosis is that of progressive symptomatology over 12–48 hours. This is in sharp contradistinction to hypoglycemia where the onset is relatively sudden. **Symptoms** include polyuria (frequent urination), polydipsia (drinking increased fluids or increased thirst), and occasionally, polyphagia (increased appetite). Progressive weakness, nausea, and vomiting are often seen. Abdominal pain is common. The etiology of this is unknown.

Physical examination

The patient with diabetic ketoacidosis will reveal hyperventilation, often with Kussmaul's respirations—deep, rapid breaths which are nearly always diagnostic of a metabolic acidosis. There is usually evidence of dehydration—dry skin and tongue. The skin is usually warm and flushed. There may be a decreased level of consciousness. A fruity, acetone-like odor is sometimes present on the breath. Table 6-3 summarizes the clinical features of diabetic ketoacidosis.

Table 6-3. Clinical Features of DKA

History
>   Progressive symptoms over 12–48
>   hours
>   Polyuria
>   Polydipsia
>   Polyphagia
>   Weakness
>   Nausea, vomiting
>   Abdominal pain common

Physical
>   Hyperventilation
>   Kussmaul's respirations
>   Evidence of dehydration
>   Warm, flushed skin
>   Acetone-like odor to breath

Laboratory tests

Laboratory findings will reveal increased blood sugar and positive serum ketones (using the Acetest tablet test). Other abnormalities are:

1. *Electrolytes*—Creatinine may be artificially elevated due to increased blood sugar. Potassium (K+) may be high or low. *If* normal or low, WATCH OUT—a serious

K + deficiency exists (see page 83).

2. *Amylase*—Increases in amylase are common, and DO NOT correlate with abdominal pain or pancreatitis. This seems to be a nonspecific reaction to acidemia in general and *not* to either pancreatitis or diabetic ketoacidosis. Hyperamylasemia has been reported in other acidotic conditions as well [*Ann Int Med,* 1986, Vol. 104, p. 362].

3. *Increased anion gap*—This is a measure of extra acids in the blood and is calculated by the following formula:

$$A.G. = [Na + K] - [Cl] + HCO_3]$$

The normal value is 10–18. Any increase suggests the presence of a metabolic acidosis of the so-called "anion-gap" variety (see below).

4. *EKG*—Concomitant hyper- or hypokalemia (high or low potassium), may be reflected. ST-segment depression, prolonged QT intervals, and abnormal T waves.

5. *Arterial blood gases*—Acidosis will be revealed by ABGs. Also pay careful attention to the pO_2 as the adult respiratory distress syndrome has been reported as a complication of DKA [*Cardiovascular Reviews & Reports,* 1986, Vol. 7, p. 801].

Laboratory features of diabetic ketoacidosis are summarized in Table 6-4.

When measuring the anion gap, consider other causes of an increase. The mnemonic for the differential diagnosis of an anion-gap metabolic acidosis is "SLUMPED":

>   **S**—**S**alicylate
>   **L**—**L**actic acidosis
>   **U**—**U**remia (kidney failure)
>   **M**—**M**ethanol intoxication
>   **P**—**P**araldehyde overdose
>   **E**—**E**thanol, ethylene glycol ingestion
>   **D**—**D**iabetes (diabetic ketoacidosis).

Table 6-4. Laboratory Features of DKA

Electrolytes
   Artificial elevation of creatinine
   Potassium—high or low
   Amylase—commonly elevated
   Anion gap elevated

EKG
   May reflect concomitant potassium abnormalities
   ST depression
   Prolonged QT intervals
   Abnormal T waves

Treatment

Diabetic ketoacidosis must be monitored carefully with a flow sheet. It should be noted that several regimens of insulin treatment have been described, including the following continuous infusion method. All are equally effective in decreasing the blood sugar. The following protocol may result in less hypoglycemia and is better tolerated by the patient:

1. Oxygen at 2–6 LPM via NP.

2. IV normal saline at 200 cc/hr (use 1/2 normal saline if Na+ is > 155).

3. IV INSULIN DRIP—Add 5 cc of 25% albumin and 50 U of U100 regular insulin to 500 cc of normal saline. This results in 1 U of insulin per 10 cc of solution.

4. Start the IV drip at .1 U/kg/hr via a constant infusion pump.

5. *After* the infusion has been started, give a loading dose of 10–20 U regular U100 insulin IV push. This may be repeated at double the original dose in 1–2 hours if the blood sugar has not decreased or has increased.

6. *Hourly* blood sugar, potassium, serum ketones, and bicarbonate. Studies suggest that fingerstick blood sugars may be monitored when used in conjunction with a meter to read the strips [*Diab Care,* 1986, Vol. 9, p. 77].

7. When the blood sugar is < 250 mg%, either decrease the infusion rate by 1/2 or greater or change to subcutaneous insulin (regular) hourly.

8. Change to D_5W-containing solutions (i.e., D_2 normal saline, etc.) at a blood sugar = 250 mg%.

Insulin and fluids are the mainstay in the therapy of diabetic ketoacidosis. Close attention, though, should be paid to a few other matters as well:

1. POTASSIUM—With treatment, the serum K+ inevitably falls. If the initial level is normal or high, add 20–40 mEq/L KCL to the IV fluids once urine flow is established; if K+ is < 3.6 mEq/L initially, severe K+ depletion exists. (As acidosis increases, K+ is shifted out of the cells into the serum; with correction of the acidosis, K+ will return to the cells and the serum K+ may drop precipitously.) Add 40 mEq/L, starting with the first bottle of IV fluids in this case.

2. HCO_3 (bicarbonate)—required only if the pH is < 7.10 or if a pH of < 7.20 is associated with hypotension or shock. Give 2 ampules (88 mEq) in 1 liter 1/2 normal saline over one hour IV. Repeat until the pH is > 7.20, and the patient is no longer in shock.

   Despite the long-standing recommendation to use bicarbonate in diabetic ketoacidosis, many experts are now questioning this philosophy. Even in severe DKA, no differences in recovery or outcome were demonstrated despite the administration of bicarb [*Ann Int Med,* 1986, Vol. 105, p. 836]. Potential deleterious side effects include hyperosmolarity, hypernatremia, and metabolic alkalosis. The American Heart Association has markedly curtailed the recommended use of this drug in cardiac arrest. Thus, judicious consideration is warranted before using it.

3. PHOSPHATE—Despite convincing academic arguments as to why phosphate should be given in diabetic ketoacidosis, no evidence exists that routine administration has any significant clinical effect *unless* marked hypophosphatemia (< 1.5) is present. More commonly than not, the serum phosphorous level is elevated due to a similar type of electrolyte shift as affects potassium [*Am J Med*, 1985, Vol. 79, p. 571].

Pearls to Remember

The therapy of diabetic ketoacidosis as described here is, by necessity and experience, very "cookbook." This method works; it works reliably and is easy to follow. In over 200 cases personally treated by this author, I have NEVER seen a serious complication arise from this regimen.

1. Abdominal pain (? etiology) is common in diabetic ketoacidosis. It usually subsides within 6–8 hours following treatment. Suspect a primary intra-abdominal disorder if:
   - The patient is > 40 years old.
   - Acidosis is not severe.
   - Pain persists > 6–8 hours.

2. Acetest tablets (the "nitroprusside reaction") only measure the presence of acetoacetate. Beta-hydroxybutyrate is more commonly present with severe acidosis and NOT measured by this reaction. With correction of the acidosis, a change in the intracellular *redox* potential favors the conversion of beta-hydroxybutyrate to acetoacetate. Therefore, by following serum ketones, one should expect to see a transient increase before improvement due to increased formation of acetoacetate. This is normal and NOT necessarily a sign of worsening. A paper-strip test for

hydroxybutyrate is manufactured, but the product is not as yet commercially available [*Diabetes Care*, September–October 1984, p. 481]. Table 6-5 summarizes the various ketoacid "shifts" in diabetic ketoacidosis.

Table 6-5. Ketoacid Shifts with Treatment of Diabetic Ketoacidosis

There is a reversible reaction as follows:

HYDROXYBUTYRATE $\longleftrightarrow$ ACETOACETATE

1. Hydroxybutyrate is in a higher concentration with acidosis.

2. With correction of acidosis, the reaction equilibrium moves towards the right, leading to an increase in the formation of acetoacetate.

3. The acetest tablet (nitroprusside reaction) tests *only* for acetoacetate. Thus, as acidosis improves and more acetoacetate is formed, it will appear that the measured amount of ketones has increased:

HYDROXYBUTYRATE $\updownarrow$ **ACETOACETATE**	**Acidosis**

$\uparrow$
CORRECTION OF ACIDOSIS
$\downarrow$

ACETOACETATE $\updownarrow$ **HYDROXYBUTYRATE**	**Alkalosis**

4. Thus, until the total ketone concentration decreases, at which time the acetest will reflect it, expect to transiently see an increased concentration of ketones with correction of acidosis.

3. Acute, reversible gastroparesis and gastric dilitation are common in diabetic ketoacidosis. If an altered level of consciousness is present, an NG tube should be inserted; otherwise, a severe aspiration pneumonia may result. Pain from a myocardial infarction may mimic this entity, so it is also important to check an EKG on any patient with diabetic ketoacidosis over age 35. (Remember: Diabetics can have coronary artery disease at very young ages.)

4. Patients who are undergoing intensive insulin therapy, such as with a continuous infusion subcutaneous pump, are at an increased risk for development of both severe hypo- and hyperglycemic reactions. The reason for easier development of diabetic ketoacidosis is that there is a lack of a substantial subcutaneous reservoir of insulin during pump therapy. Any interruption or malfunction of the pump leads to prompt insulin deficiency. Depending on the patient, ketoacidosis may develop rapidly, especially if the malfunction occurs immediately before bedtime [*Mayo Clin Proc,* 1986, Vol. 61, p. 796].

HYPEROSMOLAR HYPERGLYCEMIC NONKETOTIC COMA

Hyperosmolar hyperglycemic nonketotic coma (HHNC) is a syndrome of marked hyperglycemia, dehydration, and coma with a markedly increased serum osmolality (> 350) and minimal, if any, ketosis or acidosis. Though one-sixth as common as diabetic ketoacidosis, HHNC carries with it a 40% mortality! It usually occurs in elderly individuals with mild or previously unknown diabetes mellitus. **Predisposing factors** include: steroid and diuretic therapy, underlying renal disease, pneumonia, and stroke.

Though commonly thought to occur only in elderly patients with severe underlying illness, HHNC has been reported in nondiabetics with burns, heat stroke, acute pancreatitis, infections, surgery, thyrotoxicosis, acromegaly, hemodialysis, and IV hyperalimentation. Phenytoin, propranolol, chlorpromazine, and cimetidine have been associated with the syndrome as well. Though rare, there are case reports of hyperosmolar hyperglycemic nonketotic coma affecting 18-month-old children. [*Am J Med,* 1984, Vol. 77, p. 899].

The **pathophysiology** revolves around depleted insulin reserve. This leads to decreased glucose uptake by the cells as well as an increase in hepatic glucose production (as in diabetic ketoacidosis). An elevated serum blood sugar results. This leads to an osmotic diuresis with concomitant dehydration, severe hypovolemia, hyperviscosity, and possibly thrombosis. Because there exists enough circulating insulin to inhibit the breakdown of fat, no free fatty acids, ketone bodies, or acids are produced. Some muscle tissue may still be broken down, but the released amino acids have little effect on the blood pH. It is perhaps easiest to think of HHNC as a state whereby the liver is "diabetic" and the peripheral tissues "insulinized."

Diagnosis

History

The diagnosis is suggested by the history. Usually the patient is greater than 60 years old. There is often underlying heart, kidney, or infectious disease. The individual may be on either diuretics or steroids and may have a history of Type II non-insulin-requiring diabetes mellitus. Progressively decreasing level of consciousness, at times with seizures, is also reported.

Physical examination

Physical examination reveals a decreased level of consciousness. Seizures, focal or grand mal in nature, may be present. This entity is easily and often confused with stroke. Bizarre behavior may be noted. Dehydration (dry skin and tongue) is present along with shallow respirations without any odor of acetone.

Laboratory tests

Laboratory testing will reveal a markedly elevated blood sugar with negative or only weakly positive serum ketones. The arterial pH is normal. CPK may be markedly elevated, indicating the presence of rhabdomyolysis. The serum osmolality is increased. It can be measured by special equipment or may be estimated by the following formula:

CALCULATED OSM=
2 × [Na] + BUN/2.8 + BS/18

The normal value is 290. In HHNC, the calculated and measured serum osmolalities are usually well over 350.

Lactic acid elevations are common in HHNC and are generally mild. Frank lactic acidosis may be seen, especially if circulatory collapse is present or impending. This is considered an ominous sign [*J Crit Ill,* January 1986, pp. 22–28]. Significant lactic acidosis may be inferred from an increase in the anion gap accompanied by an increase in the *osmolal gap*—the difference between the *measured* serum osmolality and the *calculated* value. Normal ranges are between 0–20 mOsml/L. Obviously, if an institution does not have the facilities to measure actual serum osmolality, the osmolal gap CANNOT be determined.

Other causes of an elevated osmolal gap include: alcohol intoxication, ethylene glycol poisoning, isopropyl alcohol, and methanol intoxication. The osmolal gap rarely exceeds 50. Alcoholic ketoacidosis, unlike alcoholic lactic acidosis, is typically accompanied by low to absent ethanol levels. Isopropanol is metabolized to acetone but not ketoacids. The laboratory findings of an elevated osmolal gap, a normal anion gap, and a positive test for ketones should suggest "rubbing alcohol" intoxication in the appropriate setting [*NEJM,* June 14, 1984, p. 1609]. It should be noted that an osmolal gap in ethanol intoxication can only be reliably determined if the freezing point osmometry method is used. Otherwise volatile alcohols may not be detected [*Arch Intern Med,* 1986, Vol. 146, p. 1843].

BUN and creatinine are usually elevated as well. Often times the BUN is greater than 10× the creatinine, indicating severe dehydration or *prerenal azotemia.*

Treatment

Treating HHNC involves the administration of high-flow O_2 initially. The mean fluid deficit in these patients is 9 liters (versus about 5 L in diabetic ketoacidosis). Therefore, IV fluids must be given as follows:

1. If the patient is hypotensive, use normal saline; if not, use 1/2 normal saline. If you originally start with normal saline, switch to 1/2 normal saline when the shock is reversed. If pulmonary edema develops or increasing hypernatremia occurs, sterile intravenous water can be used safely [*Arch Intern Med,* 1986, Vol. 146, pp. 945–947].

It can be demonstrated that fluid therapy alone can lead to an observed decline in the blood sugar and serum osmolality. This is due to dilution of the extracellular fluid, glucosuria, and what appears to be a change in the rate of glucose metabolism [*Diabetes Care,* 1986, Vol. 9, p. 465].

2. Run fluids at 125 cc/hour.

3. Fluid treatment after hospital arrival should be carefully monitored by a Swan-Ganz catheter or, less ideally, a CVP line.

4. Insulin therapy for HHNC is identical to that for diabetic ketoacidosis. It is important to watch these patients carefully, as they may be extremely sensitive to insulin. Because HHNC represents only a *relative* not an *absolute* insulin deficiency, many patients will require no insulin therapy after resolution of the acute event. Conversely, diabetic ketoacidosis patients almost always will.

5. Potassium reserves are universally depleted in these patients. Replacement should be started at 10–15 mEq/hr with initial therapy. Most of these patients will require a total of 500 mEq of KCL over the first 24–48 hours.

Pearls to Remember

1. Because HHNC commonly presents as a neurological crisis, rapid glucose determination should be an essential part of the evaluation of *all* patients with an acute neurological disorder.

2. A precipitating cause should be sought in

every patient (as with diabetic ketoacidosis). Usually, either an infectious disease (most commonly pneumonia), cardiovascular condition, or metabolic abnormality is found.

ADDISONIAN CRISIS

An Addisonian crisis may be defined as an acute, life-threatening emergency brought about by inadequate production of the hormones cortisol and aldosterone by the adrenal gland during stress. Cortisol and aldosterone are steroids whose function is to help maintain water and salt balance as well as many other vital body functions, especially during stress.

There are several **causes** of Addisonian crisis, though the most common is an acute stress (illness, trauma, myocardial infarction) in a patient with underlying chronic adrenal insufficiency (Addison's disease). An identical state may be induced by stress in a patient who has been on chronic steroid therapy. After about 2–6 weeks, these exogenous drugs suppress the adrenal gland's normal responses. Thus, under conditions of stress, it is unable to respond appropriately. Other causes include acute adrenal gland hemorrhage (often related to anticoagulant medicines), overwhelming meningococcal sepsis (Waterhouse-Friederiksen Syndrome), and failure of the pituitary gland. Patients with hypopituitarism usually have a normal aldosterone response.

The normal adrenal gland secretes 20–30 mg/day of cortisol. This amount can increase 10-fold during stress. Failure of this rise to occur leads to the **pathophysiology** of an Addisonian crisis. There is hypotension due to both decreased vascular tone and perhaps lessened responsiveness to catecholamines (epinephrine and norepinephrine). Aldosterone deficiency leads to decreased renal sodium conservation. The kidneys are unable to clear free water which, combined with decreased Na+ conservation, leads to a low serum sodium concentration. This causes various central nervous system effects including lethargy, coma, and seizures (if low enough). (These will be discussed in Chapter 9.) Lack of mineralocorticoid (aldosterone) effect also leads to hyperkalemia

(increased serum potassium) and a metabolic acidosis. Finally, the absence of the cortisol effect on glucose metabolism may lead to hypoglycemia.

Diagnosis

An Addisonian crisis should be suspected in any patient presenting with hypotension, especially if there is associated nausea, vomiting, and hyperpyrexia (elevated temperature).

History

One should look for a history of primary adrenal insufficiency, hypopituitarism, pituitary/adrenal gland surgery, or exogenous steroid use (drugs such as Prednisone, Cortisone, Decadron, Medrol, or Deltasone). The inhaled steroids (Decadron, beclamethasone) may also lead to dependence.

Symptoms include weakness, apathy, anorexia, weight loss, nausea, vomiting, abdominal pain, and fever.

Physical examination

The patient may be febrile and hypotensive. The presence of hyperpigmentation, especially in the skin folds, should suggest the diagnosis of underlying primary adrenal insufficiency. The examiner should also look for signs of chronic steroid use ("moon facies"—a puffy face that looks somewhat flattened, excess hair growth, Medi-Alert Tag).

Laboratory tests

Laboratory testing will reveal a decreased serum sodium concentration. The potassium may or may not be elevated. If it is, there is often a concomitant metabolic acidosis (non-anion gap type). Hypoglycemia may be present. For some unknown reason, the white blood cell differential count may show a predominance of lymphocytes. The measured serum cortisol level is decreased for the given level of stress. Some authors recommend treating the patient with dexamethasone, which does not affect measured serum cortisol values, and then performing more sophisticated testing. The general consensus at this time is to draw an initial cortisol level before treatment, treat with hydrocortisone (for reasons listed below), and defer formal testing until after the acute event. With current adrenal function tests, it is NOT necessary for the patient to be under a period of high stress for subclinical adrenal gland insufficiency to be detected.

Treatment

Proceed as follows to treat Addisonian crisis:

1. Oxygen 3-6 LPM, NP.

2. IV D_5 normal saline rapidly (at least 250 cc/hour initially)

3. HYDROCORTISONE is the *drug of choice* because it does NOT require conversion in the liver to an active form. It is also the quickest acting. Give 75–100 mg IV every 6 hours.

4. If hydrocortisone alone does not reverse hyperkalemia or hypotension (along with fluids), you should add a mineralocorticoid. Use either DESOXYCOR-

TICOSTERONE ACETATE 5 mg IM two times per day or FLUDROCORTISONE ACETATE (Florinef) .1–.2 mg per day orally.

Pearls to Remember

When dealing with a possible adrenal crisis, keep in mind that:

1. A history of anticoagulant use followed by sudden abdominal pain and collapse suggests an acute adrenal hemorrhage.

2. Both cortisone and prednisone require hepatic conversion to biologically active compounds. This conversion may be impaired in the presence of serious illness. Thus, the drug of choice remains hydrocortisone because it acts the most rapidly and **does not** require hepatic conversion.

Environmental Emergencies

7

This section will deal with emergencies that occur following exposure to heat and cold. The following topics will be discussed:

■ Generalized hypothermia
■ Frostbite
■ Heat-injury syndromes.

GENERALIZED HYPOTHERMIA

Generalized hypothermia is a condition in which the core or internal body temperature is less than 95°F (35°C) due to either decreased production of heat or increased heat loss. There are three primary **causes**—cold water immersion, cold weather exposure, and "urban hypothermia."

Cold water immersion is the principal cause of death following boating accidents. Wet clothing loses 90% of its insulating value (except for wool). Thus, soaked individuals are effectively nude. Cold weather exposure runs a close second in terms of causing problems. Finally, cold stress among the aged, intoxicated, or debilitated can cause fatal hypothermia ("urban hypothermia"). Associated conditions include alcohol, the use of central nervous system (CNS) depressants, infections (i.e., sepsis), endocrine disease (hypoglycemia, hypothyroidism, Addison's disease CNS dysfunction, and burns. Though many are aware of the dangers of hypothermia occurring while skiing and camping, the number of hypothermia victims from these activities is actually very small

as compared to the "urban hypothermia" described previously.

Predisposing factors, then, to hypothermia include any of the following:

1. Any elderly person living alone, especially with chronic disease or who has suffered a stroke.

2. People who are intoxicated with alcohol.

3. Children less than one year old.

4. Victims of submersion injury, especially in cold water.

5. Patients suffering head trauma, especially if the accident occurred outdoors.

6. Any patient with a history of trauma and subsequent blood loss with shock.

7. Getting lost or immobilized in cold weather, especially if the individual is wet.

There are several causes of hypothermia that might not seem immediately obvious. Patients undergoing surgery commonly become hypothermic during the operation. In fact, if they have a normal or elevated temperature, malignant hyperthermia syndrome should be suspected (see page 103). This is due to a combination of a cool operating room and nonwarmed IV fluids. Myocardial infarction may lead to very low cardiac output and hypothermia. This may be reversible with intraaortic balloon pumping.

Finally, sepsis may be associated with hypothermia. Hemodynamic monitoring can be helpful in this circumstance in determining the underlying problem—septic patients tend to have an elevated cardiac index with decreased systemic vascular resistance, whereas hypothermic patients (not from sepsis) tend to have a much higher systemic vascular resistance (SVR) and lower cardiac index [*Ann Int Med,* 1985, Vol. 102, pp. 153–157].

Generalized hypothermia is best described by severity. **Mild hypothermia** (90 °F/32 ° C–95 °F/35 ° C) is reversible if treated. Shivering and vasoconstriction are present. There is a loss of fine manual dexterity (such as that required for fire-starting). The blood pressure, heart rate, and respiratory rates are all increased. The patient may appear oriented with normal posture or may exhibit apathy, poor judgement, memory lapses, and speech difficulty. Lack of coordination may also be present.

Moderate hypothermia (82 °F/27.8 ° C–90 °F/32 ° C) results in the stoppage of shivering (none occurs below 90 °F). Muscular rigidity and stiff distal movements take over. Other **signs and symptoms** are as follows:

1. Progressive decreases in respiratory minute volume (amount of air breathed in a minute), heart rate, and cardiac output.

2. Glassy stare with marked obtundation, progressing to stupor.

3. BP may be undetectable, but the carotid pulse is usually present.

4. Bradycardia, unresponsive to atropine, tachydysrhythmias (especially atrial fibrillation), PVCs and T-wave inversion may occur.

5. Metabolic acidosis is present; blood sugar may be high or low.

Severe hypothermia (less than 82 °F/27.8 ° C) is the most advanced stage. Death usually occurs when the core temperature drops below 78 °F (25.5 ° C). At this stage, deep coma and rigidity are present. The patient appears apneic and pulseless. The pupils are fixed and dilated.

Early EKG changes may include bradycardia with prolongation of the PR, QRS, and QT intervals. Complete heart block is possible at lower tempera-

tures. Atrial fibrillation is extremely common as well. The EKG may show so-called J-wave notching (''Osborne waves'') at the end of the QRS complex as illustrated in Figure 7.1. Originally, the presence of J-waves was thought to portend ventricular fibrillation, but this is no longer felt to be true. The current hypothesis is that they represent late depolarizations or afterpotentials which may predispose to re-entrant rhythms [*Am J Cardio,* March 1985, p. 839]. J-waves appear when the core temperature is below 32° C.

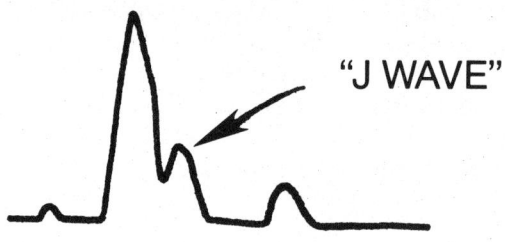

Figure 7.1. ''J waves'' or ''Osborne'' waves of hypothermia.

In severe hypothermia, pulmonary edema with white, frothy sputum can occur. There is a *great* risk of defibrillation-resistant ventricular fibrillation and asystole. **This stage mimics clinical death.** Despite this, with proper therapy, successful resuscitations have occurred. Table 7-1 summarizes the classification of hypothermia by severity.

The **pathophysiology** of hypothermia is interesting. As the body begins to cool, intense peripheral vasoconstriction occurs. The sympathetic nervous system is stimulated with subsequent catecholamine release. Vasoconstriction is most intense in the skin and extremities; blood flow to the fingertips may be reduced by as much as 99%. Shunting of blood from the body surface to the core results in fluid overload in the central vessels, leading to an initial increase in the central blood volume. The kidney senses this, leading to a ''cold diuresis'' with markedly increased urine flow. This ''cold diuresis'' leads, in later stages, to total body hypovolemia and may worsen shock in hypothermia. This is summarized in Figure 7.2.

Table 7-1. Classification of Hypothermia by Severity

Mild Hypothermia (90°F/32°C–95/35)
   Shivering/vasoconstriction present
   Loss of fine manual dexterity
   Increased blood pressure, heart rate,
      respiratory rate
   Apathy or normal mental status

Moderate Hypothermia (82°F/27.8°C–90/32)
   Shivering stops
   Muscular rigidity
   Distal stiff movements
   Decreases in respiratory rate, heart
      rate, and cardiac output
   Glassy stare—obtundation, stupor
   Low or nondetectable blood pressure
   Carotid pulse palpable
   Bradycardia or tachydysrhythmias
   Metabolic acidosis
   BS high or low

Severe Hypothermia (Below 82°F/27.8°C)
   Deep coma, rigidity
   Apnea, pulselessness
   Pupils fixed, dilated
   J-waves on EKG
   Pulmonary edema
   Risk of ventricular fibrillation
   Mimics clinical death!

Cooling — Sympathetic nervous system stimulation
   |
Catecholamine release — Peripheral vasoconstriction
   |
Shunting of blood to the core — Central blood
   volume overload
   |
"Cold diuresis" — Total body hypovolemia:
   possible electrolyte imbalance

Figure 7.2. Pathophysiology of hypothermia.

Increased heat production occurs in the form of shivering. This is the most effective way the body has of producing heat. When the body temperature has decreased to 95°F, the metabolic rate is at its maximum and may be three to six times the basal rate. Shivering stops below 90°F [*JEMS*, November 1985, p. 44].

Diagnosis

Laboratory tests

Laboratory work that should be obtained from any hypothermic patient includes:

1. ABGs—Temperature changes the normal values for pH and pCO_2. Blood samples are often warmed to 37° and the measured results then "temperature-corrected." Some experts feel that so-called "correction nomograms" may be misleading and recommend interpreting the pH and pCO_2 (as determined with the blood warmed to 37°) in a normal fashion. The pO_2 needs to be corrected—the recommended formula: decrease the pO_2 measured at 37° by 7.2% for each degree that the patient's temperature is below 37°.

2. CBC—The hematocrit is usually elevated due to hypovolemia. With very low temperature, the white blood cell count may drop precipitously [*Surgery*, 1965, Vol. 58, p. 607]. Mild hypothermia leads to an increase in the platelet count as well as whole blood viscosity. This may explain noted increases in coronary and cerebral thrombosis in cold weather [*Brit Med J*, 1984, Vol. 289, p. 1405]. Platelet counts tend to drop with decreasing temperature.

3. Blood sugar—often, but not always, elevated.

4. Electrolytes; BUN/creatinine—often increased.

5. Chest X-ray—Rule out aspiration pneumonia.

6. EKG—Multiple arrhythmias may be seen; look for ''J'' waves and signs of muscle tremor. The most frequently observed EKG abnormality is sinus bradycardia. T wave inversion and prolongation of the PR, QRS, and QT intervals can also occur.

Before discussing treatment of generalized hypothermia, it is extremely important to understand the pathophysiology of rewarming. Active external rewarming (hot water immersion, alcohol blankets, etc.) causes peripheral vasodilation which leads to shunting of cooler blood to the core; this may predispose to dysrhythmias. Vasodilation may also contribute to hypotension, causing a shock-like picture (rewarming shock). These phenomena are referred to as ''afterdrop.'' Hypovolemia secondary to cold-induced diuresis may further compound the problem. This method, though, is quick and may be used temporarily especially in the face of severe cardiovascular instability.

Passive external rewarming (covering with a blanket in a warm room) is generally safe for mild cases. It should be noted that body-to-body contact, which is commonly used in the wilderness for rewarming, has been reported to lead to afterdrop phenomena and may be hazardous. Active core rewarming is the most effective (and technically demanding) means.

Treatment

It is *extremely* important to remember to handle these patients with care. **ROUGH HANDLING MAY PRECIPITATE VENTRICULAR FIBRILLATION!** (Handle these patients as you would someone with a known cervical spine fracture.) Do not let the patient exert himself to help you, even if he is able to. This may also precipitate ventricular fibrillation. Initial treatment should consist of the following:

1. CPR as necessary—If the patient is pulseless and apneic, CPR should be performed as usual except that one full minute should be allowed to check for the presence/absence of a carotid pulse.

2. Oxygen—10 LPM via mask—heated if possible. DO NOT give O_2 from a cold bottle. Perform endotracheal intubation if necessary. Even though this maneuver can lead to ventricular fibrillation, it is unlikely if the patient is adequately preoxygenated.

3. Two large bore IVs, NS or RL TKO—Use warm solution only: Delete this step if warm solutions are not available. In an aircraft, electric blankets, heaters, and chemical packs can be used to warm the fluids. Ambulances with inverters will allow the same appliances to be used.

4. Dextrostix/Chemstrip blood—Give one ampule of D_{50} IV if the result is less than 40 mg%.

5. Remove wet clothing and maintain the patient in a warm, draft-free environment.

6. If ETA to the hospital is < one hour, do not attempt rewarming; cover patient with a blanket and transport in a warm ambulance compartment. Wool is a very useful insulating material because of its ability to maintain warmth even when wet.

7. If ETA is > one hour, initiate controlled rewarming during transport as follows. The core temperature should not be elevated greater than 1 °C (2 °F) per hour or ''afterdrop'' may result:

   ■ Use hot packs (not > 110 °F) over carotids, head, lateral thorax, and groin.
   ■ DO NOT attempt to rewarm extremities.
   ■ Administer warm fluids if the patient is conscious. Careful observation to prevent aspiration is necessary. Avoid fluids before and during an aeromedical transport.
   ■ Be aware that hot packs can cause severe thermal injury if allowed inadvertent contact with the skin directly, especially in children.

8. Monitor cardiac rhythm—Attempt defibrillation as appropriate. Some advocate the use of a prophylactic lidocaine bolus and drip.

Active in-hospital rewarming must be monitored by core temperature measurements via a rectal thermoprobe that goes down to 82 °F (27.8 °C). Specific measures that can be undertaken are as follows:

1. Heated, nebulized O_2 either via endotracheal tube or mask.

2. Heated IV fluids (104 °F/40 °C). Fluids in flexible plastic bags may be conveniently heated in a microwave oven (standard 650 watt model). For 1,000 cc bags of NS or RL, 135 seconds at high temperature raises the temperature of a 70 °F bag to 106 °F [*Ann Emerg Med,* May 1984, p. 408]. Glucose-containing solutions should be avoided, as they carmelize at higher temperatures. Two bursts of energy interrupted by shaking and turning the bag for two to three seconds works best. The solution temperature should be measured prior to its infusion into the patient [*Ann Emerg Med,* 1986, Vol. 15, p. 223]. Note that fresh frozen plasma may be thawed similarly (5–30 second exposures) but that packed red blood cells suffer an unacceptably high rate of hemolysis when warmed with a microwave oven [*Ann Emerg Med,* September 1985, Vol. 14, pp. 876–879].

3. Cardiopulmonary bypass—if available, the *method of choice* in patients with cardiovascular collapse (ventricular fibrillation, asystole).

4. Peritoneal lavage—the airway should be secured first, then:
   - Isotonic peritoneal dialysate is heated through a blood warmer at 100 °F.
   - The above solution is exchanged 2 liters at a time every 20–30 minutes.
   - *Goal:* Raise the rectal temperature to 86 °F.
   - The desired effect should be achieved by 6–8 exchanges.

This method appears to be far superior to heated inhalational therapy [*Am J Emerg Med,* May 1984, p. 210]. Some authors have recommended using two trochars (the second for drainage) and running fluid continuously. There are no good human data on this.

Peritoneal lavage is a convenient method to use under most severe situations. It safely raises the core temperature at a rate of up to four degrees per hour.

5. Thoracotomy with mediastinal lavage is rarely used anymore. Mediastinal lavage via a left-sided chest tube was reported to work in dogs. This may be an alternative if peritoneal lavage fails and cardiopulmonary bypass is not immediately available [*Ann Emerg Med,* October 1984, p. 991]. In cases of open abdominal trauma and hypothermia, peritoneal lavage may not be possible. Mediastinal lavage may be helpful under these circumstances [*Am J Emerg Med,* 1985, Vol. 3, pp. 48–54].

6. Intragastric lavage and colonic irrigation with heated solutions (106–110 °F) have been recommended with some, but there is no good animal or human evidence to currently recommend their use.

7. Radio wave hyperthermia treatment, such as that used to provide "deep heat" treatment for cancer, has been used experimentally in dogs for rewarming. No human data exists at this point [*Ann Emerg Med,* January 1987, Vol. 16, p. 50].

When internal rewarming has elevated the core temperature to 86 °F (30 °C), the following measures should be undertaken:

1. A hydraulic hypothermia pad or warm water bath is used to raise the temperature a maximum of 2 °F/1 °C per hour to normal.

2. Keep the limbs insulated or suspended out of the water to achieve a more central warming effect.

3. Brady and atrial dysrhythmias, hypotension, and oliguria may occur during this

stage and usually clear with further increases in temperature.

4. Vasoactive, antiarrhythmic, diuretic, or endocrine drugs should be avoided.

5. A gradual regaining of consciousness and orientation, as the deep body temperature approaches normal, provides the best index to good and effective therapy.

Pearls to Remember

With proper treatment, many victims of hypothermia should recover. Nonetheless, the reported mortality ranges from 20–85%. Mortality is related to the degree and duration of hypotension on admission, associated underlying conditions, and the development of complications. Keep in mind the following:

1. Shivering occurs between 90–98 °F (32–37 °C) but not below.

2. The heart is most likely to fibrillate between 85–88 °F (29–31 °C). It may not convert readily until the patient's temperature is greater than 88 °F (31 °C) and acidosis is corrected, but defibrillation attempts should be made as indicated. No specific recommendation is available at this time because the data are lacking [*JAMA,* 1986, Vol. 255, p. 293].

3. Steroids and prophylactic antibiotics are NOT indicated.

4. Most thermometers do not register below 96 °F (35 °C).

5. Hypothermia may be a sign of hypoglycemia.

6. Avoid stimulating the airway unnecessarily. This may provoke ventricular fibrillation in the hypothermic patient. Other events that may precipitate ventricular fibrillation include: rapid positive pressure ventilation, excess alkalosis, a precordial thump, central line/pacemaker placement, cardiac stimulating medications

(isoproterenol, epinephrine), and physical exertion by the patient. Nonetheless, if adequate preoxygenation is achieved, most authorities feel endotracheal intubation may be safely accomplished if absolutely necessary. The safety of intubation, with adequate preoxygenation, has been established in animal models. The actual risk of precipitating ventricular fibrillation seems greater with the other procedures mentioned above [*Ann Emerg Med,* April 1986, Vol. 15, pp. 412–416].

7. Whenever possible, all treatment of hypothermia should be done in a hospital setting.

8. Do not treat hypothermia-induced hyperglycemia with insulin. These patients tend to be insulin-resistant and may develop serious hypoglycemia during rewarming. Insulin is ineffective at body temperatures less than 86 °F.

9. If proper CPR is used, hypothermia victims can be resuscitated even after 3–4 hours. *A patient is not dead until "warm and dead."*

10. A small minority of investigators are recommending withholding CPR in hypothermia patients who have a rhythm on the monitor *despite* obvious pulselessness and respiratory arrest [*Ann Emerg Med,* 1985, Vol. 14, p. 339]. The general consensus is that this is indeed a rare event and, if noted, essentially a state of electromechanical dissociation exists, and CPR should still be performed as indicated. The chances of precipitating "intractable" ventricular fibrillation in these patients are small [*Ann Emerg Med,* June 1984, Vol. 13, p. 492].

The controversy primarily involves unmonitored, hypothermic patients whose core temperatures are less than 28 °C and who are pulseless and apneic. Some animal evidence suggests that CPR may convert a sinus bradycardia to ventricular fibrillation. There is actually little human data to support this supposition [*Circulation 74* (suppl IV), 1986, IV-29].

Advocates of withholding CPR assume that all unmonitored, severely hypothermic patients who are pulseless and apneic are in sinus bradycardia. They have suggested that it is better to leave them in their "metabolic icebox" than to risk conversion to ventricular fibrillation. If this assumption is wrong, patients in asystole or ventricular fibrillation will not be receiving CPR when they should be.

Of course, those who support performing CPR assume that the patient is in either asystole or ventricular fibrillation. If this assumption is correct, the appropriate therapy has been given. If it is incorrect, there is a small (though undefined) risk of conversion of a nonperfusing bradydysrhythmia to ventricular fibrillation. If this occurred, the fibrillation is being treated appropriately (by CPR). Additionally, the failure to feel a pulse with an electrical complex indicates the presence of electromechanical dissociation, also an indication for CPR.

The current recommendation of the American Heart Association is that these patients receive standard CPR with the exception that up to a minute be used to determine the presence of pulselessness.

11. Cold-induced depression of ciliary activity in the lungs may lead to the accumulation of secretions with the resultant production of frothy sputum and chest congestion. This form of bronchorrhea may be confused with frank pulmonary edema, which can also occur.

12. In elderly victims of hypothermia, there appears to be permanent damage to the hypothalamus, resulting in lower than normal resting body temperatures and a tendency to recurrent hypothermia. Thus, they are at future risk even in the face of only moderately low temperatures [*Int & Crit Care Dig*, 1985, Vol. 4, pp. 12–18].

13. Do not overlook exposure injuries, such as frostbite (see below), though these may initially be less critical than hypothermia.

FROSTBITE

Frostbite is defined as the formation of ice crystals within the tissues. This most commonly occurs in the lower extremities. The **pathophysiology** can be explained in four phases (keep in mind that the worst damage occurs when an area freezes, thaws, then refreezes):

1. *Prefreeze phase*—There is generalized constriction of all blood vessels, followed by selective dilation of veins. Fluid may leak from the walls of vessels during this stage, and capillary walls may fracture leading to the leakage of red blood cells.

2. *Freeze-thaw phase*—Ice crystals begin to form in the extracellular fluid. The intracellular sodium concentration rises markedly as ice is formed, absorbing free water. This, in itself, may cause severe damage. At this stage, though, no actual mechanical damage is done by ice crystals. The formation of ice results in the generation of some heat (due to the exothermic latent heat of crystallization involved) which stabilizes the tissue temperature unless cooling persists.

3. *Vascular stasis phase*—Immediately after thawing, venodilation and arteriolar spasm occur with the resultant flow of slow, viscous cold blood through vessels. Emboli may form, arteriovenous shunting occurs as does tissue hypoxia. In mild cases, the damage may be totally reversible.

4. *Ischemic late phase*—This occurs secondary to vascular occlusion and hypoxia. Nerve damage secondary to ischemic neuritis and ischemic gangrene due to thrombi in blood vessels is prominent.

Symptoms depend upon the stage at which the patient is seen:

1. Initially, there is a painful cold sensation which subsides leading to numbness. The patient may state that the extremity feels ''like a stump.'' This is due to ischemia.

2. Following thawing, there is severe, throbbing pain. This pain may last for several weeks. There may also be tingling and burning, secondary to ischemic neuropathy, which lasts for 3–4 weeks. Post-thawing pain tends to be severe, requiring narcotics for relief.

3. Late symptoms may develop up to four years later. These consist of cold feet, excess sweating, and numbness. They are worse in the winter. Patients who have had one bout of frostbite develop an exaggerated response to cold and are, therefore, more susceptible to another disease again.

Diagnosis

Physical examination
Physical findings, again, depend on the stage at which the patient is seen:

1. The extremity often appears waxy or yellowish-white. It may appear blue-white.

2. It is often hard to the touch, cold, and insensitive to pain.

3. With rewarming, flushing progresses distally down the extremity with either an erythematous appearance or a more worrisome purple/burgundy color.

4. Edema appears within hours of thawing and may persist for days to weeks.

5. Vesicles and bullae may form within hours and last 5–10 days (if they are not ''popped'').

6. A black, hard eschar will form within

9–15 days and an obvious line of demarcation is often present within 22–45 days.

7. Wet, purulent gangrene may set in later.

Table 7-2 is a summary of the physical findings in frostbite.

Table 7-2. Summary of Physical Findings in Frostbite

Appearance of Extremity
Waxy white
Yellow white
Mottled blue-white
Hard, cold, insensitive

Edema
Appears within hours, may last for days to weeks

Vessicles/Bullae
May start within hours, last days

Black Eschar
Appears 9–15 days; demarcates at 22–45 days

Possibility of Wet, Purulent Gangrene

With Rewarming
Flushing progressing distally downward
Erythematous appearance or purple/burgundy color

Treatment

Treat frostbite as follows:

1. Transport without delay. If there is an unavoidable delay, keep the patient warm.

2. Protect the involved site by covering it and handling it gently.

3. DO NOT allow the patient to smoke; this

leads to constriction of blood vessels that will aggravate hypoxemia.

4. Rewarm using the "rapid-thaw" method:
   a. Total immersion of the area in water 37.8–44°C (110°F).
   b. Continually monitor the water.
   c. The process may take anywhere from 30–40 minutes.
   d. Remember, there will often be severe pain upon thawing. Be prepared to use narcotic medicines—intramuscular meperidine (Demerol) works best under these circumstances.
   e. If profound systemic hypothermia coexists, don't thaw a frostbitten extremity until the body's core temperature is normal.
   f. Keep the thawed part clean with meticulous care, which includes sterile linen, caps, gowns, gloves, and masks when changing dressings. Protective isolation may be required in cases with much tissue damage. These injuries are as susceptible to infection as are burns.
5. Unless frostbite is mild, the patient should be admitted and observed for 24–48 hours.

Experimental therapies have been tried to decrease sludging and coagulation. These include dextran, heparin, nonsteroidal anti-inflammatory agents, and arterial vasodilators such as phenoxybenzamine, reserpine, and prazosin. All are without good scientific backing with the possible exception of reserpine. This compound may be helpful especially if slow, instead of fast, rewarming was used which promotes vascular stasis and spasm. In this case, RESERPINE .5 mg is given into the artery supplying the affected extremity (i.e., femoral, radial, brachial) every 2–3 days.

The prognosis in frostbite can be determined by several features. It is a good sign if, immediately after rewarming, the following are present: sensation to pinprick, good color, warm tissues, and large, clear nonhemorrhagic blebs extending to the digit tips. Conversely, a poor prognosis is attended by the presence of small, dark hemorrhagic blebs not extending to the tips of involved digits, the absence of edema, and presence of nonblanching cyanosis.

Pearls to Remember

When dealing with frostbite, keep in mind the following:

1. *Never* rub a frostbitten area.
2. *Never* rub ice or snow on a frostbitten area—severe tissue damage will result.
3. Rewarming is almost always accompanied by *severe* pain, usually requiring narcotics for relief.
4. Patients suffering frostbite are highly susceptible to its recurrence.

HEAT INJURY SYNDROMES

In order to better understand the various heat injury syndromes, it is important to be familiar with the **mechanisms of thermal regulation.** Heat is generated by muscular activity and through metabolic reactions in the body. It is dissipated via four mechanisms:

1. *Radiation*—transmission of heat through space.
2. *Conduction*—transmission of heat from warmer to cooler objects in direct contact.
3. *Convection*—transfer of heat by circulation of heated particles.
4. *Evaporation*—loss of heat at the surface from vaporization of liquid.

In humans, conduction is NOT a major mechanism unless the clothing is removed and the individual placed recumbent upon a cool surface. Convection is also hindered by clothing. At room temperature (68°F), 75% of heat dissipation is via radiation and convection. Evaporation (insensible loss from lungs and skin) accounts for about 25% of heat loss.

As the ambient temperature approaches body temperature, radiation is no longer an effective way to dissipate heat. The body may actually pick up heat via conduction and convection. At high temperatures, evaporation becomes the only effective method of heat dissipation—high humidity seriously impairs heat dissipation since evaporation is much less effective.

Physiological responses to heat occur immediately following exposure. Acclimatization takes about one week. The immediate response to heat is cutaneous vasodilation with shunting of blood from the splanchnic bed and liver to skin. This takes maximum advantage of radiation, conduction, and convection. There is also a marked increase in sweat production—up to 1.5 liters per hour is produced in an unacclimatized person.

Vasodilation leads to a decrease in the peripheral vascular resistance. An increase in heart rate and cardiac output occur as a result of this. These two events are what makes heat injury syndromes so potentially devastating in an elderly population—their cardiovascular system is simply unable to cope with the increased stress.

Acclimatization, as previously mentioned, takes about one week. When accomplished, the individual has a lower pulse, respiratory rate, and temperature with heat exposure. There is an increase in the rate and volume of sweat production with a concomitant increase in plasma volume (6–7%) and a decrease in the sweat concentration of sodium. Thus, they lose less sodium per volume of sweat than the unacclimatized person. These changes are summarized in Table 7-3.

Table 7-3. Changes with Acclimatization

- Decrease in pulse, respirations, and temperature with exposure
- Increase in rate and volume of sweat production
- Increase plasma volume by 6–7%
- Decrease in [Na+] in sweat

These changes can occur with as little as 90 minutes of heat exposure per day. They are maintained for several weeks without re-exposure to heat being necessary. In order to acclimatize properly, an individual's body must be able to successfully adapt and tolerate the above changes. An elderly individual with heart failure would obviously have serious difficulties.

The three heat injury syndromes we will discuss here are heat cramps, heat exhaustion, and heat stroke.

Heat Cramps

Heat cramps are the least common of the heat injury syndromes. They are defined as cramps or pain in the muscles, especially of the abdomen and lower extremities, due to a loss of fluid and salt.

The **cause** is excessive loss of sodium chloride in the sweat. Heat cramps occur usually in the young, unacclimatized individual who engages in exercise or heavy labor in hot climates and sweats profusely. The elderly are *rarely* able to perform the work necessary (even on salt-restricted diets) to achieve a significant salt loss.

The **signs and symptoms** of heat cramps include muscle twitching followed by painful spasms, especially involving the lower extremities and abdomen. Nausea and vomiting may be prominent. Weakness, hypotension, tachycardia, pallor, and/or diaphoresis may be present.

Diagnosis

Laboratory workup will reveal a decreased serum sodium, with absent or low urine sodium, and elevated hematocrit. This indicates hemoconcentration in the face of sodium loss (hyponatremia secondary to loss of sodium and water with relatively more sodium lost).

Treatment

Treatment of severe heat cramps should include O_2 if necessary. The patient should be kept quiet in a cool room. An IV of NS at 125 cc/hr is begun. Massage of the affected muscles may be helpful. In the milder cases, NaCl tablets every 30–60 minutes with water are helpful. In sensitive individuals, these may lead to vomiting. Rest and instruction concerning proper acclimatization are important. Table 7-4 summarizes heat cramps.

Table 7-4. Summary of Heat Cramps

Cause
Excess loss of NaCl in sweat

Signs/Symptoms
Muscle twitching
Painful spasms (especially lower extremities, abdomen)
Nausea, hypotension
Tachycardia, pallor
Diaphoresis

Laboratory
Hyponatremic dehydration

Treatment
Oxygen
IV NS
Massage of affected muscles
NaCl tablets
Instruction in acclimatization

Heat Exhaustion

Heat exhaustion is a more severe result of exposure to heat represented by a more profound fluid and salt loss than occurs in heat cramps.

The **cause** is a profound loss of fluid and electrolytes usually following exertion in a hot, humid environment. There is a high incidence of heat exhaustion in young children, individuals on diuretics, and the debilitated unable to maintain an adequate water intake or having prolonged bouts of diarrhea.

Signs and symptoms of heat exhaustion are: pallor (lack of skin coloration) and profuse sweating. Postural hypotension is often present. Headache with progressive lassitude and thirst are noted. Occasionally, mild temperature elevations (10–103 °F) are present.

Diagnosis

Laboratory workup reveals an increased hematocrit and decreased serum sodium (Na+) value. The urine is concentrated (high specific gravity). Again, this indicates a loss of both Na+ and water, with relatively more salt being lost.

Treatment

Treatment involves rest in a cool environment and IV NaCl. Initially, normal saline, 150 cc/hr, is given. The rate may be increased, depending on the underlying medical condition of the patient. In a young patient (in the Emergency Department), 2–3 liters may be given IV over 2–3 hours. Of course, more caution should be used in the elderly. Table 7-5 summarizes heat exhaustion.

Table 7-5. Summary of Heat Exhaustion

Cause
Profound loss of fluid and electrolytes

Signs/Symptoms
Pallor
Profuse sweating
Postural hypotension
Headaches with lassitude
Marked thirst
Mild temperature elevations
(100–103 °F)

Laboratory
Increased hematocrit
Hyponatremic dehydration

Treatment
Rest in cool environment
IV NaCl

Heat Stroke

Heat stroke is an extreme medical emergency. It is defined as a failure of the body's heat dissipation mechanisms. This leads to an accumulation of body heat and hyperpyrexia (elevated body temperature). A patient suffering heat stroke once is much more likely to suffer from it again since somehow, the body's thermoregulatory mechanisms appear to be permanently damaged.

Causes of heat stroke can be divided into exercise and nonexercise induced. *Nonexercise induced* heat stroke is more likely in certain individuals. Susceptible persons include those with water and salt depletion, cardiovascular disease (diuretic use), diabetes, alcoholism, and children left in a poorly ventilated auto in the hot sun. Patients taking certain medicines are also likely victims: antihistamines, phenothiazines, propranolol, and anticholinergics (common in the elderly for Parkinson's disease). The dehydration associated with some of these conditions is particularly significant since, in and of itself, it can lead to an elevation of the body temperature purportedly due to an increase in the work of the cellular sodium pump which accounts for 20–45% of the basal metabolic rate (BMR) of the body. Hypokalemia, common with diuretic use, decreases muscle blood flow and may decrease sweat gland function [*J Inten Care Med*, 1986, Vol. 1, pp. 5–14].

Thus, the susceptible individual is often afflicted with a condition that impairs their normal regulation of heat. This is not always the case, though, as 25% of individuals using a sauna for 20 minutes have a rectal temperature of greater than 102.2 °F and cases of heat stroke have been reported following hot tub bathing. Accompanying this may be impaired voluntary environmental control—the individual may not perceive a temperature rise and, thus, fail to move to a cooler location or change into lighter clothes. Patients having drug-induced hyperthermia tend to have a poor prognosis [*Crit Care Med*, 1986, Vol. 14, p. 964].

Exercise-induced heat stroke occurs during strenuous exercise in a hot environment in nonacclimatized individuals. For some unknown reason, these persons are simply unable to dissipate heat. Both types are more frequent in humid weather. Table 7-6 summarizes the causes of heat stroke.

In both types of heat stroke, there may be prodromal **signs and symptoms.** These develop over 1–2 days with the nonexertional variety and consist of lethargy, fatigue, weakness, nausea, vomiting, and dizziness. With exertional heat stroke, the prodrome (if it occurs at all) is brief—confused, irrational be-

havior followed by loss of consciousness. Actually, this is unusual—more often the exertional heat stroke victim simply collapses with a sudden loss of consciousness.

Marked temperature elevations are usually noted (> 103 °F)—tissue damage begins at 107 °F. There is obvious impairment of the victim's level of consciousness. Seizures may occur and can be precipitated by therapeutic measures. Anhidrosis (lack of sweating) is usual in nonexertional heat stroke though patients with the exertional variety typically sweat profusely.

Table 7-6. Causes of Heat Stroke

Non-exercise Induced
    Underlying water and salt depletion
    Cardiovascular disease
    Diabetes
    Alcoholism
    Children left in hot, poorly ventilated
      cars
    Medicines:
    • Antihistamines
    • Phenothiazines
    • Propranolol
    • Anticholinergics (Benadryl, Cogentin)

Exercise Induced

Hyperventilation is common. Hypotension is often present. Virtually every organ system is affected:

1. *Skeletal muscle*—Muscle necrosis can occur as a direct result of heat. This is worsened in exertional heat stroke due to the additive effects of lactic acidosis associated with exertion. Rhabdomyolysis may also occur.

2. *Cardiovascular*—The cardiac output is often elevated. This may lead to high output failure. Direct myocardial damage has also been reported, which can lead to

failure. Accompanying dehydration may further decrease the cardiac output.

3. *Central nervous system*—Cell death, cerebral edema, and local hemorrhage have all been reported. These changes result in the nearly universally noted change in level of consciousness. Ataxia may be noted due to the exquisite sensitivity of cerebellar cells to heat. This may persist in survivors as may premature cataract formation due to dehydration.

4. *Kidneys*—Acute renal failure occurs 5% of the time in nonexertional heat stroke and has been reported in up to 35% of exertional heat stroke cases. Dehydration, failure of the cardiovascular system, and rhabdomyolysis may all be contributing factors.

5. *Gastrointestinal system*—Ischemic intestinal ulcerations, which may lead to bleeding, can occur due to heat damage of the mucosa. The liver is *commonly* affected (see below for laboratory changes). Though nausea, vomiting, and massive GI bleeding have been seen in heat stroke, pancreatitis has NOT been reported. The pancreas, in fact, seems to be the *only* organ in the body that is spared. The reasons for this are unknown.

6. *Hematologic system*—The white blood cell count is often elevated due to the release of catecholamines and associated stress. Blood viscosity has been reported to increase, as may the total red blood cell count. The platelet count tends to rise during heat stress. These factors together may account for the increased mortality noted during hot weather from arterial thrombosis [*Am J Med*, 1986, Vol. 81, p. 795]. Anemia and/or bleeding problems may occur (see laboratory section below). Disseminated intravascular coagulation (DIC) is present in most fatal cases.

7. *Endocrine/electrolyte system*—Hypoglycemia may occur in exertional

heat stroke. There appears to be little evidence of adrenal cortical dysfunction in survivors. Numerous electrolyte abnormalities may be noted.

8. *Respiratory system*—The adult respiratory distress system may occur as a result of direct parenchymal damage. Pulmonary hemorrhage with hemoptysis may be present. Estimates of the frequency of pulmonary embolism in heat stroke range from 25–80%. Pulmonary edema (often cardiogenic in nature) may occur.

Diagnosis

Laboratory testing reflects concomitant systemic dysfunction:

1. The BUN/creatinine are elevated, suggesting prerenal azotemia and, at times, acute renal failure.

2. Abnormal liver function tests are noted in 80% of patients. They peak at 24–48 hours and may be abnormal for up to 28 days. The serum total bilirubin is markedly elevated in fatal cases. The height of the peak is of prognostic significance.

3. CPK is almost ALWAYS elevated. Cardiac isoenzymes may be increased, indicating myocardial damage.

4. PT, PTT, and platelet counts are abnormal 50% of the time. Frank disseminated intravascular coagulation (DIC) may occur, as mentioned earlier.

5. Blood gases show a metabolic acidosis (due to lactic acid) and the serum HCO_3 is decreased. The same comments made on page 91 under "Hypothermia" apply here in terms of interpretation of blood gases.

6. The urine has been described as looking like "machine oil" with protein and occasionally casts. The microscopic exam, except for the color, is most often normal

though. Acute renal failure may occur.

7. Hypophosphatemia (decreased serum phosphorus) is common and may lead to respiratory failure.

8. Lumbar puncture (spinal tap) is usually normal, though occasionally there may be slightly elevated protein and glucose concentrations.

9. The EKG may show ST-segment depression, increased QT intervals, and intraventricular conduction defects. These all revert to normal with cooling.

The **prognosis** of heat stroke victims depends on the stability of their cardiovascular system. Reported mortality is 17–70%, depending on the population. Greater than 80% of the deaths occur in patients who are greater than 50 years old. Additionally, mortality seems related to the duration and degree of hyperpyrexia. It markedly increases with core temperatures over 108 °F, age, hyperkalemia, shock, and SGOT > 1,000 in the first 24 hours. Coma of greater than 10 hours' duration is likely to result in a fatal outcome.

Treatment

The keystone to treatment is rapid cooling. The following measures should be expeditiously undertaken:

1. O_2, 2–4 LPM via NP.

2. IV NS at a TKO rate.

3. Cool with wet sheets only if there is good ambient airflow.

4. Valium, 2.5–10 mg IV to control seizures.

5. Cardiac monitor.

In the Emergency Department, using constant rectal temperature monitoring, the patient needs to be cooled rapidly. This is clearly the most important factor. If rapid cooling is not delayed (i.e., the achievement of a temperature of 102 °F or less within

an hour of presentation), mortality is low (15%). Otherwise, mortality may double [*Am J Emerg Med*, 1986, Vol. 4, p. 394]. Several alternative methods are available from which to choose:

1. Cover the patient with crushed ice in a room with a drain in the floor. Remove the patient from the ice (or vice versa) as the body temperature approaches 101 °F.

2. Iced saline gastric lavage is an alternative if the patient is seizing or hemodynamically compromised [*Ann Emerg Med*, May 1984, p. 407]. Studies have shown that lavage reliably decreases the temperature as well.

3. Spraying the patient with tepid water (40 °C) while taking advantage of evaporation through the use of a large ventilation fan may turn out to the most practical means of cooling a heat stroke victim. More data is desirable before widely recommending this technique as current studies are limited to the combination of this method with ice immersion [*Arch Intern Med*, 1986, Vol. 146, pp. 87–90].

4. High-frequency jet ventilation has been shown to result in uniform body cooling when employed in animal models. There is no human data on this method as of this writing. In ventilated patients, this is an interesting potential mode of adjunctive therapy [*Ann Emerg Med*, June 1986, Vol. 15, pp. 680–684].

Several other points need to be kept in mind:

1. CHLORPROMAZINE (Thorazine) 25–50 mg IV may be given, if necessary, to control shivering.

2. Avoid atropine and anticholinergics (Benadryl, Cogentin); aspirin should also be avoided because of its antiplatelet effect. Both aspirin and acetaminophen decrease fever via their influence on the hypothalamus. In heat stroke, this area of the brain is already improperly function-

ing. Thus, these drugs are unlikely to have much of an effect.

3. Steroids and mannitol have no proven benefit.

4. HEPARIN for disseminated intravascular coagulation (DIC) is relatively controversial but preferred by many in this situation.

5. NOREPINEPHRINE (Levophed) should be avoided because it leads to vasoconstriction and may aggravate already-present, heat-induced damage.

6. If muscular rigidity persists despite the above treatment, there is likely an abnormality in the muscular system itself. DANTROLENE SODIUM, which acts directly on the muscular contractile mechanism, should be considered. The dose is 1–2 mg/kg IV repeated at 1–2 minute intervals until symptoms subside or a maximum dose of 10 mg/kg has been given. Though there appears to be a lack of efficacy of this agent in dog studies [*Am J Emerg Med,* 1986, Vol. 4, p. 399], human data is a bit more encouraging. There has been one case report of its success in exertional heat stroke, as well as its established use in malignant hyperthermia [*JAMA,* 1981, Vol. 246, p. 41].

7. As an adjunct, a NITROPRUSSIDE drip containing .5 mg/kg and titrated to have only minimal effect on the blood pressure will increase blood flow to the skin and allow for external cooling.

There are two potentially life-threatening conditions that may be confused with heat stroke: neuroleptic malignant syndrome and malignant hyperthermia. Both are fairly uncommon, but should be recognized as soon as possible when present.

Neuroleptic malignant syndrome is an unpredictable complication of major neuroleptic medications such as haloperidol and the phenothiazines. It may also be seen following acute withdrawal of anti-Parkinsonian drugs (levodopa, carbidopa, and amantidine). It occurs in 0.5% to 1% of patients receiving neuroleptic medications.

Symptoms include stiffness, difficulty articulating and swallowing, fever, and altered level of consciousness. Autonomic dysfunction may be the first indication, including diaphoresis, incontinence, tachycardia, and hypotension. A leukocytosis, markedly elevated CPK, and liver function tests are noted.

Treatment is with bromocriptine or dantrolene. Identification of this disease is essential because there is a 20% mortality if untreated, usually due to respiratory failure, renal failure, arrhythmias, or cardiovascular collapse. Neuroleptic malignant syndrome is felt to be a variant of malignant hyperthermia syndrome.

Malignant hyperthermia syndrome (MHS) is a hypermetabolic state of skeletal muscle that develops due to an idiopathic increase in the muscle sarcoplasmic calcium concentration. MHS is due to an inherited abnormality and occurs usually in response to halothane anesthesia combined with succinylcholine (depolarizing) muscle relaxants. The body temperature may increase 1 °C every five minutes.

Patients develop tachycardia and other dysrhythmias as an early sign. Any unexplained tachycardia during general anesthesia should prompt suspicion of the diagnosis. Since the core temperature is commonly decreased during general anesthesia, a normal or increased temperature is suggestive of the onset of this problem. Limb-muscle rigidity is common but a late sign. Rhabdomyolysis may occur in severe cases as well as metabolic acidosis, hypoxia, hyperkalemia, and disseminated intravascular coagulation. Treatment is with dantrolene IV in the operating room. An oral form, which may be used prophylactically in high-risk patients, is also available [*NEJM,* 1983, Vol. 309, pp. 416–418]. Nitroprusside has been reported to work in refractory cases [*Ann Int Med,* 1986, Vol. 104, pp. 56–67].

Pearls to Remember

Though life-threatening, heat stroke is treatable if recognized and treated properly. Keep in mind:

1. Heat stroke is a medical emergency. Differentiate it from heat cramps or heat

exhaustion. Be aware that heat exhaustion can progress to heat stroke.

2. Wet sheets over a patient without good airflow will tend to *increase* their temperature.

3. Do not let cooling in the field delay transport. Cool the patient if possible while in route.

4. Since signs and symptoms of heat stroke are not always obvious, suspect it in any individual with loss of consciousness under hot conditions.

5. Be sure to rule out other diseases causing severe hyperpyrexia and decreased level of consciousness—meningitis, encephalitis, cerebral malaria (rare!), epilepsy, severe dehydration, and thyroid storm.

6. Especially in the elderly, look for associated disease—pneumonia is very common in this population.

Gastrointestinal Emergencies

8

Though many medical ailments involve the gastrointestinal (GI) tract, only some commonly present as emergencies. Virtually any organ in the vicinity of the abdominal cavity, though, can potentially suffer a crisis resulting in one or both of the emergencies we will discuss in this section:

- Gastrointestinal bleeding
- Acute nontraumatic abdominal pain.

GASTROINTESTINAL BLEEDING

Gastrointestinal bleeding (GIB) is defined as the loss of blood from any portion of the GI tract due to a lesion of the mucosa (lining) itself. Swallowed blood (such as from a nosebleed) may mimic this. For diagnostic and therapeutic purposes, GI bleeding is divided into upper GI (UGI) bleeding (bleeding proximal to the duodenojejunal junction) and lower GI (LGI) bleeding (bleeding located more distally).

Principles of Acute Management

There are several basic principles that must be remembered. One must first determine whether or not an actual GI bleed (GIB) has occurred. If a bleed has occurred, one needs to know if there is current active bleeding. The location, upper gastrointestinal versus lower gastrointestinal, is the next priority. Be-

fore going further, the caretaker must evaluate the medical status of the patient on which the bleed is superimposed and then judge the amount of blood lost and the patient's response. Following this, blood volume replacement and efforts to stop bleeding are initiated. Only then are efforts undertaken to precisely identify the bleeding source. Table 8-1 summarizes this approach to GI bleeding.

Table 8-1. Approach to GI Bleeding

Proceed in this order:
- Has a GI bleed occurred?
- If so, is there currently active bleeding?
- Is the bleeding upper gastrointestinal or lower gastrointestinal?
- Medical status of the patient?
- Amount of blood lost? Patient's response to this loss?
- Blood and volume replacement
- Efforts to stop bleeding
- Efforts to precisely identify the bleeding source

Causes of upper gastrointestinal bleeding

Peptic ulcer disease with bleeding in the duodenum or stomach is quite common. One out of six patients who bleed from a peptic ulcer have had no prior symptoms or history of ulcer disease. **Acute gastritis** results from erosions of the stomach lining, often caused by a recent excessive ingestion of alcohol, salicylates, or exposure to stress (burns, mechanical ventilation—stress ulcers). Nonsteroidal anti-inflammatory agents are also important causes of GI bleeding [*Arch Intern Med*, 1986, Vol. 146, p. 2365].

Esophageal varices are dilations of the veins of the esophagus secondary to increased intraportal pressures. Alcoholic varices are secondary to cirrhosis caused by alcohol ingestion. Patients with alcoholic cirrhosis and varices may bleed from varices (40% of the time) but are as likely to have bleeding from gastritis, gastric ulcer (30%), or duodenal ulcer (20%).

Patients with nonalcoholic cirrhosis and varices are four times as likely to bleed from varices than peptic ulcer. Gastritis in these patients is rare.

Esophagitis is caused by erosion or irritation of the esophagus and may be a source of bleeding. **Paraesophageal hiatal hernia** has been associated with upper GI bleeding, though the more common sliding hiatal hernia has not. A **Mallory-Weiss tear** is diagnosed by the presence of hematemesis following prolonged or forceful vomiting, retching, or hiccups. This is due to a mucosal tear at the gastroesophageal junction. These patients usually stop bleeding spontaneously and seldom rebleed. GI bleeding is *NOT* a prominent symptom in transmural rupture of the esophagus (Boerhaave's syndrome).

Angiodysplasia is the formation of small arteriovenous fistulas which bleed. These are more likely to be found in the lower GI tract (see below) but have been reported as a common cause of upper GI bleeding in patients with chronic renal failure. In fact, angiodysplasia of the stomach or duodenum was the most common source of recurrent upper GI bleeding in patients with chronic renal failure while peptic ulcer disease was the most common rebleeding source in patients without renal failure [*Ann Int Med*, 1985, Vol. 102, pp. 588–592].

Aortoenteric fistula is a fistula from an abdominal aneurysm or prosthetic aortic graft to the intestine. This can result in massive (and often fatal) GI bleeding. A smaller "herald" bleed can occur hours to weeks before the catastrophe. Seventy percent of patients survive six or more hours after this initial hemorrhage. Though upper GI bleeding with hemorrhage into the duodenum is most common, any presentation may occur—hematemesis, melena, or hematochezia. Any patient with an abdominal aortic graft who presents with GI bleeding *must* be assumed to have a fistula until proven otherwise. The consequence of missing this diagnosis is rapid exsanguination. Table 8-2 summarizes the causes of upper GI bleeding.

Table 8-2. Causes of Upper Gastrointestinal Bleeding

- Peptic ulcer disease
- Acute Gastritis
- Esophageal varices—alcoholic, nonalcoholic
- Esophagitis
- Mallory-Weiss tear
- Angiodysplasia
- Aortoenteric fistula

Causes of lower gastrointestinal bleeding

The causes of lower GI bleeding are a bit less extensive but equally as important. **Diverticulosis** is the presence of numerous small outpouchings in the colon called diverticuli. Over 70% of lower GI bleeding is from this source, yet only 3–5% of patients with diverticulosis ever have bleeding from them. Bleeding will continue in 20%, stop and restart in 20% during the same hospitalization, and cease in 60%. A second common cause of lower gastrointestinal bleeding is **angiodysplasia.** These are small arteriovenous malformations, usually in the right colon. These are found in the elderly and are often associated (for an unknown reason) with disease of the aortic valve, especially aortic stenosis.

Blunt abdominal trauma has been reported as a cause of lower GI bleeding. This usually occurs several hours following the event and results from bowel contusion [*Jour of Trauma*, 1984, Vol. 24, p. 1057].

Hemorrhoids, fissures, tumors, and polyps may also serve as sources of lower gastrointestinal bleeding. Massive hemorrhage with these is rare. A final potential source, especially in young women, is **Meckel's diverticulum.** This is the embryonic remnant of the omphalomesenteric duct (which is near the ileum) which persists in a few individuals. It is often lined with ectopic gastric tissue and is susceptible to the same types of bleeding, ulceration, and pain as is the stomach. Meckel's diverticulitis can also mimic appendicitis. Table 8-3 summarizes causes of lower GI bleeding.

Table 8-3. Causes of Lower Gastrointestinal Bleeding

- Diverticulosis
- Angiodysplasia
- Blunt abdominal trauma
- Hemorrhoids
- Fissures
- Tumors
- Polyps
- Meckel's diverticulum

Diagnosis

History

The history can be one of the most helpful features in making a proper diagnosis in GI bleeding. There may have been an ingestion of alcohol, salicylates, or nonsteroidal anti-inflammatory agents. A history of a prosthetic aortic graft should be sought.

Common **symptoms** include hematemesis (vomiting blood), hematochezia (bright red blood in the stool), and melena (tarry, sticky black stools). The patient may have vomited coffee ground-like material (suggestive of digested blood in the stomach). Pain may or may not be prominent. Estimates of the amount of blood lost from reports of stool and vomitus volume are likely to be unreliable. It takes only a drop of blood to turn the entire toilet bowl red.

Background medical problems of possible concern in GI bleeders include coronary artery disease and other cardiovascular disease, especially vascular grafts. Chronic renal disease, cirrhosis, emphysema, and diabetes are also of concern.

Distinction of the *location by history* of bleeding depends on the amount and rapidity of bleeding, the source, and the transit time through the gut. Some guidelines follow:

1. Hematemesis (vomiting of blood)—almost always an upper GI source.

2. Hematochezia (bright red blood in the stool)—may be seen with upper GI bleeding and rapid transit or left colon/sigmoid colon bleeding.

3. Dark red blood—usually bleeding from the ileum to the right colon.

4. Black stool or blood (melena)—suggests at least 100 cc of rapidly lost blood. The source is usually duodenal or jejunal. It must be retained in the gut for eight hours to turn black.

5. Silver stools—caused by biliary obstruction (such as cancer of the ampulla of water) plus GI bleeding.

Physical examination

Physical examination may reveal signs of shock. Orthostatic blood pressure and pulse changes are useful in determining if significant intravascular volume depletion has occurred. Orthostasis usually occurs with a 15–20% loss of circulating volume. Shock is almost invariably present when the patient loses more than 30% of the blood volume.

Significant changes are an increase in the heart rate of 10–20 beats per minute and/or a decrease in the systolic blood pressure greater than 20 mm Hg. Some experts feel that a pulse increase of 30/minute upon standing is the most sensitive and specific test for volume loss of at least one liter [*Am J Emerg Med,* 1986, Vol. 4, pp. 150–162]. If hemodynamic monitoring is available, the first sign of bleeding is an increase in the pulmonary artery pressure [*Surg Gynecol Obstet,* 1977, Vol. 145, p. 685].

Normovolemic children, up to age 12, may show a heart rate increase of up to 30 or 40 beats per minute upon standing. The blood pressure may drop as much as 27 mm Hg. Thus, these parameters are not helpful in patients under 13 years old [*Ped Emerg Care,* 1985, Vol. 1, pp. 123–127]. A recent review of adult data may also suggest possible problems in interpretation of adult values. The following changes occurred when going from lying to standing in normal adult patients [*Heart & Lung,* 1986, Vol. 15, p. 611].

1. Heart rate—increased up to 30 beats/minute.

2. Systolic blood pressure—decreased 0 to 26 mm Hg.

3. Diastolic blood pressure—decreased 10 to 15 mm Hg.

Thus, it appears that orthostatic changes, by themselves, are difficult to interpret. Of course, when combined with an appropriate clinical picture, they mean far more.

The color of the palmar crease, when the fingers are forcibly extended, is a useful bedside measurement for anemia. When the hemoglobin level is below 1/2 normal, the creases do not turn red. The rectal examination will often reveal blood in the stool, either grossly or via special home-testing solutions. The abdominal exam is usually nonspecific though tenderness, decreased bowel sounds, and surgical scars (possibly from graft placement) may be noted.

Laboratory tests

Laboratory work obtained should include: CBC, PT, PTT, platelets, electrolytes, liver functions, and type and crossmatch for blood. Initially, the hematocrit may be normal or elevated. Allow 12–36 hours for changes to occur in acute hemorrhage. An EKG should be done, as acute myocardial infarction is present as a complication in 1–2% of patients with GI bleeding.

An abdominal X-ray is optional at this stage. One should keep in mind, though, that a small proportion of gastric and duodenal ulcers that bleed perforate at the same time. Free air may be noted, best seen on an upright or lateral recumbent view.

Treatment

Initially any patient with GI bleeding, regardless of location, should progress as follows:

1. High-flow O_2—Be aware of continued vomiting, bleeding; in these cases, nasal prongs with lower flows are preferred.

2. Large bore peripheral IV, RL at 150 cc/hour. The patient should have two lines if the blood pressure is < 90 mm Hg. If there is a possibility of endoscopy being performed in the near future, it is best to place IV lines on the patient's right side, as they will need to lie on their left for the procedure.

3. Consider the use of MAST pants. These nicely tamponade bleeding from a ruptured aortic aneurysm.

4. Patients with hematemesis should be transported with the head and trunk elevated to prevent aspiration.

While in the Emergency Department, the patient should have an NG tube placed. If the return is pink or bloody (bright red blood or dark aspirate that is grossly heme-positive) and *not* coffee grounds alone, lavage with iced saline. Bleeding not controlled by 30 minutes of constant lavage should prompt surgical consideration. Of course, if the return is negative or coffee grounds in nature, the tube may be withdrawn.

Tests for occult blood (guiac, "Heme-Occult," etc.) are unreliable and can produce both false-positive as well as false-negative results. Nasal trauma, from passage of the NG tube, commonly contributes to a false-positive test. Urine dipsticks (used to test gastric aspirate for blood) tend to be overly sensitive and are thus not helpful either.

It is important to keep in mind that up to 15% of patients with active upper GI bleeding will have a negative aspirate in the NG tube. Thirty percent with "coffee-ground" returns also had active ongoing bleeding. Thus, the results of NG tube aspiration are not uniformly reliable [*Gastrointest Endosc*, 1981, Vol. 27, p. 73].

Many investigators now feel that tap water is sufficient for lavage in place of normal saline. Whether or not the solution need be iced is still a matter of controversy. Cold causes vasoconstriction which should decrease the rate of bleeding. On the other hand, it also inactivates platelets, which may be detrimental. This issue remains to be proven, one way or the other. The standard method at this time is to use iced solutions. Similar controversy extends to whether tap water or saline should be used. No significant changes in electrolyte concentrations seem to occur with tap water [*Ann Emerg Med,* December 1985, Vol. 14, pp. 1156–1159].

IV vasopressin is the initial therapeutic maneuver for treatment of bleeding esophageal varices. It works by decreasing the portal pressure and is effective in 50–70% of patients. The rebleeding rate, though, may be as high as 42%. One should mix 100 units of vasopressin in 250 cc D$_5$W (.4 U/cc) and run it in as follows:

.3 U/minute × 12 hours *then*
.2 U/minute × 24 hours *then*
.1 U/minute × 24 hours.

Note that this drug causes coronary arterial constriction and should be used with caution in patients with vascular disease. This may be minimized by adding a concomitant nitroglycerin infusion. The nitroglycerin reverses the adverse effects of vasopressin on the heart and systemic circulation. In addition, this agent seems to further decrease portal pressure via a reduction of the portal vascular resistance. Intravenous, sublingual, and transdermal preparations of nitroglycerin have been shown to have similar beneficial effects [*Clinics Crit Care Med,* 1986, Vol. 9, pp. 124-143]. Large studies on combined therapy are currently ongoing.

A new vasopressin analogue, terlipressin, is available experimentally which appears to be more effective without the cardiovascular side effects [*Arch Int Med,* 1985, Vol. 145, pp. 1263–1267]. Some investigators have noted that somatostatin infusion also reduces portal blood flow and may also decrease variceal bleeding. This agent does not seem to have the cardiovascular side effects of vasopressin [*Hepatology,* 1984, Vol. 4, p. 442].

IV vasopressin may successfully stop other types of severe upper GI/lower GI bleeding refractory to available methods—a 20 U infusion over 15 minutes is used. A drip as outlined above may then be used if necessary. Remember, this is only to be used in the case of refractory bleeding in the absence of a trained angiographer who can perform an intra-arterial infusion.

The **Blakemore** (triple-lumen) **tube** is indicated for tamponade of variceal bleeding when vasopressin is contraindicated or unsuccessful. SURGICAL CONSULTATION IS MANDATORY! This tube is illustrated in Figure 8.1.

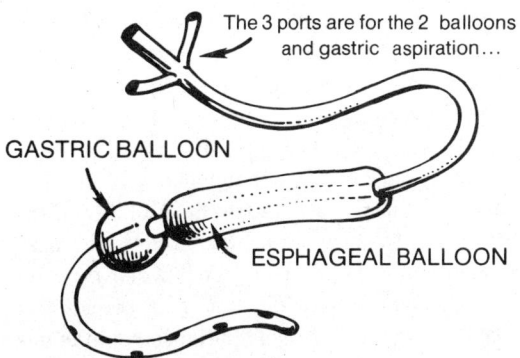

The 3 ports are for the 2 balloons and gastric aspiration...

GASTRIC BALLOON

ESPHAGEAL BALLOON

Figure 8.1. The Blakemore tube for GI bleeding.

Angiography for ongoing bleeding, as well as for diagnostic purposes, is helpful if the bleeding rate is at least 2 ml/minute. If the source is identified, intra-arterial vasopressin or embolization of the artery may be attempted.

CIMETIDINE, 300 mg IV every 6 hours and hourly ANTACIDS are indicated for upper gastrointestinal bleeding. Studies have shown that cimetidine is of no value in stopping acute bleeding, but it may prevent a rebleed. Either antacids or cimetidine (or both) have prophylactic value in prevention of stress ulcers [*Ann Int Med,* 1985, Vol. 103, pp. 173–177]. Some authors have questioned the ability of antacids alone to prevent grossly visible (via endoscope) bleeding [*Crit Care Med,* 1985, Vol. 13, pp. 646–650]. If given rapidly, IV cimetidine may cause hypotension. Thus, it should be infused IV over 20–30 minutes [*Crit Care Med* (abstract), April 1985, p. 314]. Additionally, this drug has been reported as a cause of drug fever [*Arch Intern Med,* 1986, Vol. 146, p. 821].

The data are less clear for the drug ranitidine (Zantac) at this time in GI bleeding. One study showed it to be ineffective unless combined with an anticholinergic agent [*Crit Care Med,* 1985, Vol. 13, No. 13, pp. 651–655]. Other studies suggest that it effectively maintains gastric pH >4 and may be of value in preventing stress ulcer and rebleeding [*Intensivmedizin,* 1984, Vol. 21, p. 15]. Generally, it appears that, depending on the series reviewed, either cimetidine or ranitidine may be effective for both stress ulcer and recurrent GI bleeding. Acutely, neither is particularly helpful. Famotidine is a newly released H_2 blocker that is similar to cimetidine and ranitidine except for markedly increased potency and duration of action. It has not been adequately studied in acute GI bleeding at this time to make recommendations [*Am J Med 81* (Suppl 4B), 1986, p. 49].

The key appears to be maintenance of intragastric pH >4. Antacids seem to do this reliably. If one is to rely on H_2 blockers alone, then frequent intragastric pH monitoring must be done [*Intensive Care Med*, 1985, Vol. 11, p. 295]. It is clear that nasogastric feeding by itself does NOT sufficiently buffer gastric contents to prevent stress ulceration [*Crit Care Med*, 1986, Vol. 14, p. 599].

PROPRANOLOL has been used by some to prevent recurrent hemorrhage from bleeding esophageal varices, but it has not been studied in acute hemorrhage. Theoretically, it should be contraindicated in the actively bleeding because it reduces both the heart rate and cardiac output.

Sclerotherapy (by directly injecting a sclerosing substance into the varices via endoscope) has been used for bleeding esophageal varices. Several studies have suggested that this modality is effective in acute control of bleeding esophageal varices. Survival may be increased, though no definitive advantage of this form of therapy has been established [*West J Med*, October 1986, Vol. 145, p. 481]. The complication rate ranges from 20%. Rarely, life-threatening problems can occur such as esophageal perforation, aspiration pneumonitis, and portal vein thrombosis [*AFP*, 1986, Vol. 34, p. 139].

Many problems are associated with **portocaval shunting** as well, especially if done emergently [*J Inten Care Med*, 1986, Vol. 1, pp. 171–177]. Endoscopic laser treatment has been used for vascular ectasias [*Ann Int Med*, 1986, Vol. 104, pp. 352–354]. Preliminary results with laser coagulation noted a 92% success rate in upper GI bleeding. Mortality was decreased as well. These results are controversial and have not been repeatable [*AFP*, 1986, Vol. 4, p. 139]. There are case reports of patients with postradiation rectal vascular lesions who have had laser therapy with success for rectal bleeding [*Mayo Clin Proc*, 1986, Vol. 61, p. 927].

Transhepatic obliteration of esophageal varices, either percutaneously or via the jugular route, has been described [*N Engl J Med*, 1974, Vol. 291, p. 646]. A catheter is advanced into the involved veins which feed the variceal sites (primarily the left gastric vein) and obliterating substances are injected. This procedure has not been well-studied in the United States, though European studies have reported up to an 80% success rate [*Arch Surg*, 1978, Vol. 113, p. 1331]. Rebleeding, though, is not prevented, due to the development of new collateral vessels or recanalization of previously obliterated vessels. Complications occur in about 20% of patients, including portal vein thrombosis, hemoperitoneum, gallbladder puncture, and fever.

Pearls to Remember

GI bleeding can be a frightening as well as a life-threatening problem. Following the standardized approach shown above will help the health care provided appropriately manage the situation. Some additional helpful "PEARLS" are as follows:

1. Be sure and try to obtain a history of alcohol, aspirin, or nonsteroidal anti-inflammatory drug ingestion; also ask about vascular grafts.

2. About one-third of the people in this country who faint from GI bleeding do so in the bathroom—usually locked in at that. They may not receive attention for some time.

3. The upper GI tract tends to react with irritability and hyperactivity when it fills with blood, so that it quickly empties itself after the bleeding has stopped.

Before moving onto the next section, it is important to review some factors in the **prognosis** of Gi bleeding:

1. The death rate increases 6–25 fold when greater than 10 units of blood are required preoperatively.

2. Recurrent hemorrhage during the same hospitalization is associated with a 4–7 times increased mortality. Except in patients with esophageal varices, nearly all recurrences occur within 48 hours. Rebleeds after five days are extremely un-

usual. Overall, the risk of rebleeding ranges from 6–33%. It differs for each lesion:

Duodenal ulcer	26%
Gastritis	6%
Gastric ulcer	21%
Varices	56%
Mallory-Weiss tear	10%
Esophagitis	10%
Neoplasm	33%

3. A "visible vessel" at endoscopy (i.e., a vessel in an ulcer crater with evidence of recent bleeding) has been shown to correlate with early rebleeding in gastric and duodenal ulcer. This may be an indication for prompt surgery.

4. Mortality in unrecognized or unoperated aortoenteric fistulas is 100%. Bleeding from varices, independent of the therapeutic approach has a mortality approaching 50%.

5. Mallory-Weiss tears have an excellent prognosis with spontaneous cessation of the bleeding in 90% of patients.

6. Blood accumulation within the abdomen is sometimes difficult to estimate. Large amounts are required for a noticeable change in abdominal girth to occur. A rough rule of thumb is that the waist measurement will increase approximately one inch per liter of blood lost into the gut.

7. Alcohol ingestion may lead to vasodilation and bradycardia which might alter the classic picture of hypovolemic shock commonly said to be associated with significant GI bleeding.

ACUTE NONTRAUMATIC ABDOMINAL PAIN

An understanding of the various **types of pain** is key to interpreting the complaint of acute abdominal pain that occurs without prior trauma.

Visceral pain is caused by the sudden stretch or distention of a viscus. It is crampy, gaseous, and usually intermittent. Often, it is referred to the midline of the abdomen. It is diffuse and poorly localized. This type of pain is not well tolerated.

Visceral pain is often accompanied by autonomic symptoms such as diaphoresis, nausea, vomiting, or dysrhythmias. Involuntary contraction of the abdominal musculature may also occur. Most acute intra-abdominal diseases requiring operations are preceded by obstruction (either functional or anatomical). The earliest clinical signs and symptoms will be related to visceral pain. An *example* is the periumbilical crampy pain of early appendicitis.

Somatic pain is caused by stimulation of nerve fibers in the parietal peritoneum by chemical or bacterial inflammation. The patient usually lies quietly with the thighs flexed to relax the peritoneum. Any attempt at palpation is guarded by muscular contractions. This is referred to as involuntary guarding. Reflex cessation of bowel sounds commonly occurs. An *example* of this is the sharply localized right lower quadrant pain of the later phase of appendicitis.

Referred pain is pain from one area that is being sensed in another due to embryological nerve distribution patterns—i.e., the nerves for both areas originated from the same structure in early development. An *example* of this is diaphragmatic irritation being felt in the shoulder. Table 8-4 (page 112) summarizes the three types of abdominal pain.

The **causes** of abdominal pain originating in the *abdomen* are outlined in Table 8-5 (page 113). Causes of abdominal pain originating from extra-abdominal sources are illustrted in Table 8-6 (page 113).

Diagnosis

History
The history is the most important part of the diagnosis in acute abdominal pain. The **onset of pain** is very important. Was it sudden or gradual? Sudden, abrupt pain (when the patient can tell you the precise moment when it started) suggests an acute perforation, strangulation, torsion, or vascular accident. *Examples* include: ruptured ectopic pregnancy, perforated ulcer, mesenteric vascular occlusion, splenic, or renal infarction.

Inflammatory lesions and obstructive phenomena are slower in their development. Examples include: intestinal obstruction, appendicitis, and diverticulitis.

The **severity of the pain at onset** may be helpful. A good general rule is that the most severe entities cause the most intense pain and symptoms. *Examples* include: perforated ulcer and dissecting or ruptured aneurysm. The *exception* to this rule is in conditions where blood loss leads to shock; when this occurs, signs and symptoms of shock overshadow those of the pain.

The **location of pain at onset** as well as **associated symptoms** can be very helpful. Table 8-7 (page 114) lists common entities by the abdominal area they most usually affect.

Changes in the location of pain may be important in the diagnosis. Pain may become localized with abscess formation. On the other hand, perforation of an abscess will lead to generalized pain. Periumbilical pain that moves to the right lower quadrant suggests appendicitis. The sudden cessation of pain may signal perforation. Peritonitis may later develop. This, in fact, is what classically happens in an appendiceal abscess.

There are several characteristic **patterns of referral** of pain:

- *Biliary pain* commonly radiates around the right side to the back and angle of the scapula.
- Pain from the *pancreas* goes straight through to the back in the midline of the lower thoracic area. A posteriorly penetrating duodenal ulcer can present the same way.
- *Blood or pus under the diaphragm* presents as aching pain in the top of the shoulder.
- A *leaking or ruptured aneurysm* will cause pain in the lumbosacral area and occasionally in the upper thighs.
- *Renal colic* pain (kidney stones) will radiate to the groin and external genitalia.
- *Uterine and rectal pain* will often be felt in the lower back. Figure 8.2 (page 114) summarizes some of the commonest types of referred abdominal pain.

Table 8-4. Types of Abdominal Pain

Visceral
Crampy, gaseous, intermittent
Diffuse, poorly localized
Often referred to the midline
Caused by distention of a viscus
Accompanied by autonomic symptoms
Precedes most acute surgical
conditions; Example: Periumbilical
crampy pain of early appendicitis

Somatic
Caused by stimulation of parietal
peritoneum
Patient lies quietly with thighs flexed
Involuntary guarding present
Reflex cessation of bowel sounds;
Example: Well-localized right
lower quadrant pain of the later
phase of appendicitis

Referred
Pain from one area being sensed in
another due to embryological nerve
distribution patterns; Example: The
pain of diaphragmatic irritation
being felt in the shoulder

The presence or absence of **associated symptoms** may be helpful in refining one's diagnosis. When prominent, nausea and vomiting suggest gastroenteritis, gastritis, acute pancreatitis, or obstruction. Pain precedes vomiting in acute appendicitis. Diarrhea is usually present with gastroenteritis.

The failure to pass flatus (gas) suggests obstruction. Chills and fever are compatible with pyelonephritis or generalized bacteremia (of any cause). Other associated events and diagnostic points are as follows:

1. GI distress in others sharing the same meal suggests food poisoning.

2. A recent ingestion of fatty food preceding the pain suggests acute cholecystitis.

3. A history of excess alcohol consumption is compatible with pancreatitis.

Table 8-5. Causes of Abdominal Pain Originating in the Abdomen

Parietal Peritoneal Inflammation
Bacterial contamination—perforated appendix, pelvic inflammatory disease, diverticulitis

Chemical irritation—perforated ulcer, pancreatitis, ruptured ectopic pregnancy

Mechanical Obstruction of Hollow Viscera
Large or small bowel obstruction, including incarcerated hernia

Biliary obstruction (gallstone, tumor)

Urinary tract obstruction (kidney stone)

Vascular Disturbance
Embolism or thrombus

Vascular rupture (aneurysm)

Torsional occlusion (ovary, testicle)

Sickle cell anemia

Abdominal Wall
Trauma or infection of muscles

Distention from visceral surfaces—hepatic or renal capsules

■ Bowel sounds
■ Spasm of abdominal muscles
■ Tenderness
■ Masses
■ Genitorectal
■ Pelvic
■ Special signs
■ Pulmonary and cardiovascular.

Table 8-6. Causes of Abdominal Pain from Extra-abdominal Sources

Other Organ Systems
Thorax—pneumonia, spontaneous pneumothorax, MI

Spine—radiculitis from arthritis, herpes zoster, compression fracture of thoracic or lumbar vertebrae

Metabolic
Exogenous—black widow spider bite, lead poisoning

Endogenous—uremia, DKA, porphyria, allergies (anaphylaxis)

Neurogenic
Organic—tabes dorsalis (late syphilis), herpes zoster, herniated intervertebral disk

Functional

The **age** of the patient is important to consider. Appendicitis usually occurs between ages 5 and 50. Cholecystitis is unusual less than age 20 and colonic obstruction is uncommon in patients less than age 35. One should also try to determine if there was a recent intake of drugs such as steroids, antibiotics, or antacids.

Physical examination

Like the history, the physical examination of a patent with acute abdominal pain needs to be quite detailed. It will be outlined thoroughly, step by step. Note that field evaluation may be limited by the patient's condition. Steps involved in the full abdominal exam are as follows:

■ General appearance

The **general appearance** of the patient is first noted. Vital signs are taken as appropriate. A patient with peritoneal inflammation lies still on the table. A person suffering spasms or colic will usually be writhing in pain. **Bowel sounds** may be difficult to characterize when present, but their absence is very significant and should be noted.

Spasm of the abdominal muscles can be tested by placing the hand gently on the abdomen, depressing it slightly, and gently. The patient is then asked to take in a long breath. During this maneuver, the muscle will be noted to relax if only voluntary spasm (guarding) is present. In true spasm (involuntary guarding), the muscle remains taut. This suggests peritoneal inflammation.

Table 8-7. Diagnosis of Conditions by Location

Left Upper Quadrant

Duodenal ulcer—vomiting, severe pain, shock

Pancreatitis—alcohol, sudden pain, nausea, vomiting

Pyelonephritis—fever

Pneumonia—pleuritic irritation with chest pain on inspiration

Left Lower Quadrant

Ectopic pregnancy—signs of shock

Ovarian cyst—tenderness, rigidity

Kidney stone—severe flank pain, radiation to groin

Pelvic inflammatory disease—fever, nausea, vomiting, vaginal discharge

Diverticulitis—steady pain, diarrhea, rectal bleeding, fever

Right Upper Quadrant

Cholecystitis—pain after food, anorexia, nausea, vomiting, fever

Duodenal ulcer

Pancreatitis

Pneumonia with pleurisy

Pyelonephritis

Right Lower Quadrant

Appendicitis—shifting pain pattern, vomiting, fever, rebound

Diverticulitis (left-sided more common)

Ovarian cyst

Kidney stone

Ectopic pregnancy

Pelvic inflammatory disease

Epigastric

Myocardial infarction

Duodenal ulcer

Gastroenteritis—cramps, vomiting, diarrhea, fever

Periumbilical

Appendicitis, pancreatitis

Abdominal aortic aneurysm—abdominal/back pain, leg weakness, pulsatile abdominal mass, shock

Unlocalized—obstruction, food poisoning, neurological lesion, metabolic problem

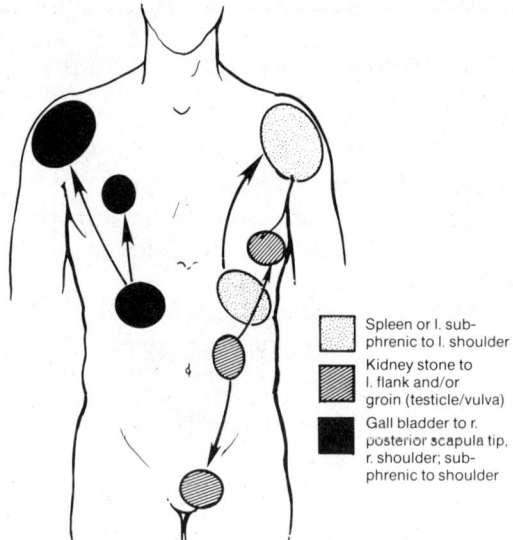

Spleen or l. subphrenic to l. shoulder

Kidney stone to l. flank and/or groin (testicle/vulva)

Gall bladder to r. posterior scapula tip, r. shoulder; subphrenic to shoulder

Figure 8.2. Referral patterns of abdominal pain sites.

Tenderness should be verified using one-finger palpation. It is best to start away from the stated area of pain. If pain is decreased with sitting (i.e., contraction of the abdominal muscles), it is likely intra-abdominal, and vice versa.

Rebound tenderness occurs when gentle pressure elicits less pain than the sudden release of that pressure. Keep in mind that the presence of rebound indicates peritoneal irritation. Any maneuver that jars the inflamed peritoneal cavity should result in rebound. These include direct release of palpation pressure, moving the cart sharply, as well as fist percussion of the soles of the feet. These alternative examination techniques may be especially helpful if the patient is hysterical or malingering.

Referred tenderness occurs when pressure at a distance from an inflamed viscus causes pain over that viscus. An *example* of this is Rovsing's sign in acute appendicitis where left lower quadrant palpation leads to right lower quadrant tenderness.

During palpation, the presence of **masses** is noted. During the **genitorectal** exam, the stool is examined for blood. Fullness, obstruction, and hernia are sought. If a hernia is present, it should be determined if it is easily reducible or not. The exam of a patient with acute abdominal pain is *not* complete without this portion of the exam. The **pelvic** exam falls in the same category.

Tenderness on cervical motion ("chandelier sign") suggests pelvic inflammatory disease. A right-sided pelvic mass suggests an appendiceal abscess, and a left-sided one, tubo-ovarian abscess. Eight-five percent of those patients with an ectopic pregnancy have tenderness on direct cervical palpation.

Some **special signs** may also be present, adding to refinement of the diagnosis:

1. *Iliopsoas sign*—Patients are first instructed to extend (straighten) their knee. They are then asked to attempt to flex (lift upwards from a lying position) the thigh, keeping the knee straight, against the examiner's resistance. Alternatively, the examiner may extend the straightened leg backwards with the patient on his side. If either maneuver causes pain, irritation of the underlying iliopsoas muscle is present, suggesting appendicitis or abscess.

2. *Obturator sign*—The thigh is passively flexed to a 90-degree angle with the knee bent. The examiner first internally, then externally, rotates the leg. Pain with this maneuver suggests pelvic appendicitis (right side) or diverticulitis (left side). These signs are illustrated in Figures 8.3 and 8.4.

The **pulmonary and cardiovascular** examination is crucial as abdominal pain may be due to disease above the diaphragm. Rales in the lungs suggest pneumonia, heart failure, or MI. A left pleural effusion is common with pancreatitis. The presence of atrial fibrillation or a prosthetic (artificial) heart valve suggests the possibility of emboli to the mesentery. Remember, diabetic ketoacidosis can be accompanied by abdominal pain.

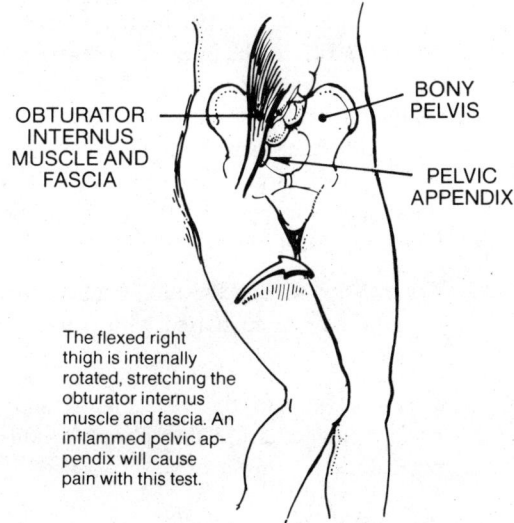

OBTURATOR INTERNUS MUSCLE AND FASCIA

BONY PELVIS

PELVIC APPENDIX

The flexed right thigh is internally rotated, stretching the obturator internus muscle and fascia. An inflammed pelvic appendix will cause pain with this test.

Figure 8.4. The obturator test in acute appendicitus.

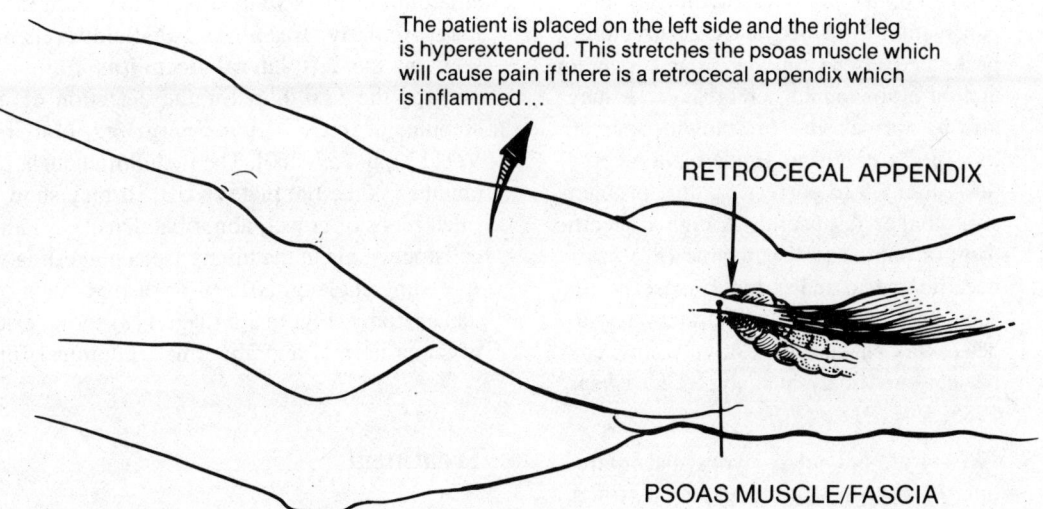

The patient is placed on the left side and the right leg is hyperextended. This stretches the psoas muscle which will cause pain if there is a retrocecal appendix which is inflammed...

RETROCECAL APPENDIX

PSOAS MUSCLE/FASCIA

Figure 8.3. The iliopsoas sign in acute appendicitus.

Laboratory tests

Laboratory results are variable, depending upon the condition involved:

1. *CBC*—The hematocrit may be elevated, indicating dehydration. If there has been concomitant blood loss, several hours will be required for this to be reflected. The white blood cell count (WBC) may be normal or elevated. It is important to note that a viscus may be perforated with a normal WBC. If the WBC is markedly decreased, think of a viral infection or sepsis! The differential may actually be more important than the total white blood cell count. A large percentage [> 75%] of polys and/or many band forms should be noted if present.

2. *Electrolytes*—Check the blood sugar; the calcium may be decreased with pancreatitis.

3. *Urinalysis*—Check for WBC, RBC, and bacteria suggesting pyelonephritis or kidney stones.

4. *Serum and/or urine amylase*—This is the most widely used today. Unfortunately, its discriminatory value is fairly low. Unless isozymes are used, an elevated amylase can be compatible with anything from pancreatitis to cholecystitis, obstruction, perforated viscus, salivary gland irritation, and intra-abdominal hemorrhage. It may also be normal with full-blown pancreatitis. The serum/urine amylase ratio, previously thought to correct for this problem, is no longer felt useful. A highly specific form of pancreatic isoenzyme (P3) has been described and is highly specific for acute pancreatitis. The laboratory test to detect this enzyme is relatively simple, but not yet widely available [*Clin Chem,* 1985, Vol. 31, p. 70].

5. *EKG*—Rule out acute myocardial infarction; of course, if your suspicion is high, a normal EKG should not dissuade you from undertaking the standard workup anyway.

6. Paracentesis (draining ascitic fluid from the abdominal cavity)—This is rarely indicated on an acute basis. This technique is only of use if spontaneous bacterial peritonitis (infection of ascitic fluid without bowel perforation or other obvious source) is suspected.

There are many possible X-ray studies that can be obtained. Remember *not* to leave the potentially gravely ill patient in the X-Ray Department without constant attendance by a trained person! A diagnosis *should not* be excluded by a negative X-ray alone. Films useful in the diagnosis of abdominal pain include the flat plate, upright, left lateral decubitus abdominal films, and the upright chest X-ray. Some experts feel that the upright abdominal film may be eliminated without sacrificing diagnostic accuracy [*AJR,* September 1986, Vol. 147, p. 501]. A barium enema may be helpful acutely, but this should be decided by the consultant surgeon.

The **upright chest X-ray** may show evidence of pulmonary disease, free air under the diaphragm (suggesting perforation of a hollow viscus), or the presence of air-filled viscera in the chest (suggesting a diaphragmatic hernia). The **upright abdomen film** may demonstrate air-fluid levels (suggesting obstruction) or massive dilation of the colon (megacolon). Similarly, free air and air-fluid levels may be seen on the **left lateral decubitus film.** This is perhaps the *best* film for the detection of minute amounts of free air [*Ann Emerg Med,* March 1986, Vol. 15, pp. 257–260]. The first film, though, usually obtained is the flat plate (KUB). It may show fluid-filled loops of bowel, abnormal densities (kidney or gallstones), air in the biliary tree (suggesting severe ascending cholangitis), and/or displacement of normal anatomy. Figure 8.5 (page 118) shows examples of some normal and abnormal abdominal films.

Treatment

Principles of treatment are fairly straightforward:

1. Position of comfort.

2. Nothing by mouth (NPO).

3. O_2 at 4 LPM via NP.

4. IV NS or RL TKO; faster if blood pressure < 90 mm HG. Again, remember to avoid the left arm (if possible) when endoscopy may be indicated.

5. Consider MAST garment if blood pressure < 90 mm Hg.

6. NG TUBE if there is any suggestion of obstruction or at physician's discretion.

7. *Prompt surgical consultation!* In some institutions, culdocentesis (aspiration of the vaginal cul-de-sac with a needle) is performed without gynecological consultation, though generally this is recommended.

8. *Hold* analgesics. They will mask the validity of serial exams, one of the surgeon's most valuable tools. A mild sedative (hydroxyzine 25 mg IM) may help in the evaluation of a hysterical or totally noncooperative patient.

Pearls to Remember

1. Abdominal pain may be the first warning of catastrophic internal bleeding such as a ruptured aneurysm, liver, spleen, or ectopic pregnancy. The bleeding is often not apparent. It is up to you to think of volume depletion and monitor the patient closely to recognize shock. Between 30 and 40% of patients for whom the definitive diagnosis is ectopic pregnancy have previously been seen and discharged by another physician.

2. Regardless of signs or symptoms (or lack thereof), *any* incarcerated (nonreducible) hernia is strangulated (i.e., the blood supply is cut off to it) until proven otherwise.

3. Some have found a diagnostic score for the diagnosis of appendicitis helpful [*Ann Emerg Med,* May 1986, Vol. 15, pp. 557–564]. The mnemonic is "MANTRELS" and a score is given for the presence of each particular item:

M—**M**igration	1
A—**A**norexia-acetone (urine)	1
N—**N**ausea/vomiting	1
T—**T**enderness of right lower quadrant	2
R—**R**ebound pain	1
E—**E**levation of temperature	1
L—**L**eukocytosis	2
S—**S**hift to the left	1
	10

    Proponents of this type of scale feel that patients can often be observed with a score of 5 or 6. Surgery is often required when the score is higher. Though this type of scoring system can be helpful, it is difficult to replace the skilled judgement of an experienced surgeon. It is *not* recommended that the decision to operate (or consult) or not be made solely on the score obtained from a "scoring table."

4. In approximately 20% of all cases, the appendix is ruptured by the time surgery is performed.

5. As many as 30% of the patients with a definitive diagnosis of appendicitis have been previously seen and discharged by another physician. Ten percent of the patients have chronic, recurrent appendicitis (based on pathological findings) diagnosed following surgery. This should be considered in patients presenting with recurrent right lower quadrant abdominal pain [*Surg, Gyn & Obst,* 1986, Vol. 163, p. 11].

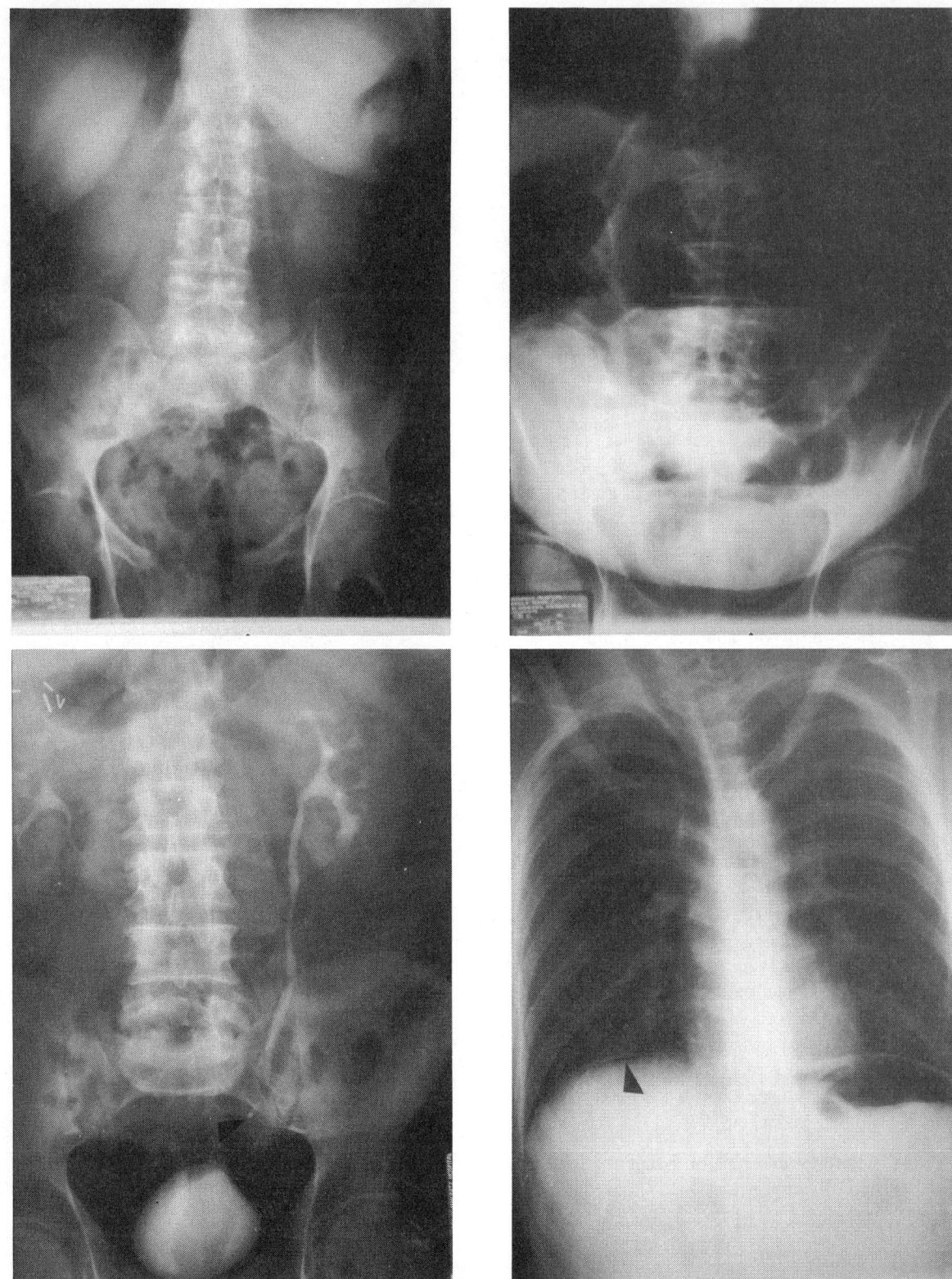

Figure 8.5. Normal and abnormal abdominal films.

Electrolyte Emergencies

The subject of fluids and electrolytes could be the focus of an entire textbook. Many of these problems occur in the hospital. Occasionally, electrolyte problems, other than the acidosis accompanying cardiac or respiratory arrest, present as field situations and in the Emergency Department. Only the most common of these entities will be described in this section:

- Hyperkalemia
- Hypokalemia
- Hyponatremia
- Hypercalcemia.

HYPERKALEMIA

Hyperkalemia is defined as an increased serum potassium (K+) level. In most labs, this is technically a value above 5.1 mEq/L (normal values vary from area to area). Problems do not usually occur, though, unless the serum K+ is in excess of 6.0 mEq/L.

There are numerous **causes** of hyperkalemia. **Decreased excretion/decreased cellular uptake** are common and may be due to:

1. *Renal failure* (acute and chronic)—the most common cause next to a hemolyzed specimen.

2. *Adrenal insufficiency* (Addison's disease)—isolated hypoaldosteronism.

3. *Aldosterone-antagonist drugs*—spironolactone, triamterene, amiloride.

4. *Beta blockers* (propranolol, atenolol, etc.)—may block cellular K+ uptake. This is thought to occur primarily on receptor sites of skeletal muscle cell membranes. A 5–10% elevation in serum potassium is commonly observed in patients taking beta blockers [*Hosp Prac*, 1986, p. 99].

   Angiotensin converting enzyme inhibitors (captopril, and enalapril) lead to decreased concentrations of angiotensin II and aldosterone. This may also result in hyperkalemia. In patients without renal failure, this is usually *not* significant.

5. *Digitalis overdose*—digitalis drugs inhibit the membrane Na-K ATPase which transports sodium and potassium. This blocks both renal tubular K+ excretion and generalized cellular uptake of K+. Thus, the serum level increases.

6. *Heparin*—low-dose heparin, especially in patients with diabetes or chronic renal insufficiency, can lead to hyperkalemia. This is felt to be due to inhibition of aldosterone synthesis. It develops within seven days after starting heparin and resolves within five days of stopping the drug [*Arch Int Med*, 1985, Vol. 145, pp. 1070–1072].

7. Nonsteroidal anti-inflammatory agents—

decrease the glomerular filtration rate and inhibit the renin-angiotensin system, both of which may lead to hyerkalemia [*N Engl J Med,* 1984, Vol. 310, p. 563]. This is likely due to reduced biosynthesis of renal prostaglandins.

8. Hyperglycemia *without* ketoacidosis (in diabetics with even moderately impaired renal function) can lead to hyperkalemia. This is likely related to a concomitant deficiency in aldosterone synthesis but can occur in its absence. It occurs most commonly in the face of glucose loading. Thus, the potassium level must be monitored carefully after giving glucose to an unconscious diabetic [*Med,* 1985, Vol. 64, pp. 357–370]. Hypertonic infusions of other substances, such as mannitol, have also been reported to cause hyperkalemia.

9. Nifedipine—one report has documented serum potassium elevation in a small number of nondiabetic, nonuremic patients treated simultaneously with propranolol. The significance of this is unknown [*Proc Am Soc Nephrol,* 1984, Vol. 17, p. 44A].

10. Neuromuscular blocking agents, such as succinylcholine, often lead to a transient rise in serum K+ of approximately 0.5 mEq/L. This is caused by changes in the membrane permeability for sodium and potassium brought on by these agents. Patients with burns, massive trauma, denervation and spinal cord injuries, CNS disease, brain damage, severe abdominal infections, and tetanus are at an increased risk for the development of life-threatening hyperkalemia with the administration of these agents.

Increased oral load is another significant way a patient may become hyperkalemic. In the presence of normal renal function, the oral route of potassium intake cannot usually increase the serum K+ to dangerous levels. Well over 500 mEq are required. Other processes that *can* include:

1. *Crush injury, rhabdomyolysis*—release of K+ from muscle tissue.

2. *Massive hemolysis*—release of K+ from red blood cells.

3. *Salt substitutes in the face of decreased renal function*—these usually consist of potassium chloride (KCl) salts.

4. *Blood transfusion*—there are 30 mEq/L of K+ in banked blood stored for 10 days. This is due to ongoing hemolysis of red blood cells.

5. *High-dose penicillin*—1.7 mEq K+/million units penicillin.

Acidosis will increase the serum K+ because of redistribution of K+ from the intracellular to the extracellular pool. A final form is **factitious hyperkalemia** which implies that the K+ of the obtained serum is higher than the true K+ of the patient. This includes:

1. *Hemolyzed sample*—The *most common* cause of hyperkalemia. The blood cells are disrupted via the needle when the blood is drawn from the patient.

2. *Prolonged tourniquet placement on the patient's arm*—will cause lysis of red blood cells, with resultant hyperkalemia while still in the blood vessel.

3. *Elevated WBC or platelet counts*—may contribute to an increased potassium load if the elevations are marked. These cells tend to release their potassium during clotting in the collection tube.

Table 9-1 summarizes the causes of hyperkalemia.

Diagnosis

History
The diagnosis of hyperkalemia may be suspected on the basis of a history of renal disease, muscle injury, or ingestion of the above-named drugs.

Symptoms include rapidly ascending muscle weakness and perhaps flaccid quadriplegia. Paresthesias, numbness, and tingling without objective sensory deficits may be present. If dysrhythmias exist, the patient may note palpitations.

Table 9-1. Causes of Hyperkalemia

Decreased Excretion
Renal failure
Adrenal insufficiency
Isolated hypoaldosteronism
Aldosterone-antagonist drugs
Beta blockers
Catopril, enalapril
Digitalis overdose

Increased Load
Oral
Crush injury, rhabdomyolysis
Massive hemolysis
Salt substitutes with renal insufficiency
Blood transfusions (30 mEq/L K+ in
    banked blood)
High-dose penicillin

Redistribution
Acidosis

Factitious
Hemolysis
Prolonged tourniquet time
Elevated WBC/platelet count

Physical Examination

The physical findings are those of the underlying disease. They may also include: decreased reflexes and hypotension if significant dysrhythmias are present.

Laboratory tests

Laboratory examination will reveal a reproducibly elevated serum K+ level.

EKG findings of hyperkalemia are the most specific way to suspect the diagnosis. Symmetric peaking of the T waves occurs in the ranges of 5.5–6.0 mEq/L. At levels of greater than 6.0 mEq/L, there is QRS prolongation, decreased P wave amplitude, and increased PR intervals (6.5–7.5 mEq/L)—eventually, there is atrial standstill and merging of the QRS complex with the T waves. QT prolonga-

tion, ST elevation or depression may be noted (7.0–8.0 mEq/L). Atrial fibrillation may be noted. As the K+ increases further (> 8.0 mEq/L), the QRS may take on a "sine wave" configuration with PVCs, ventricular fibrillation, and, eventually, asystole [*J Emerg Med,* 1986, Vol. 4, p. 449]. These changes are illustrated in Figure 9.1.

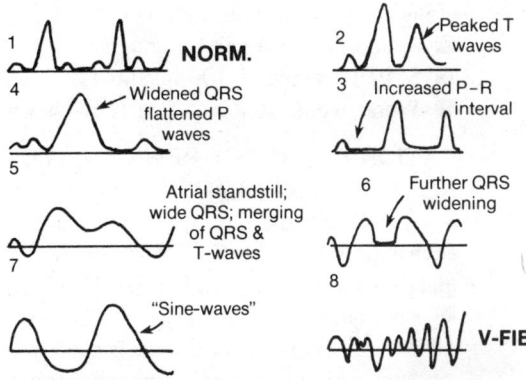

Figure 9.1. Serial EKG changes of hyperkalemia.

Treatment

Treatment is emergent if the measured serum K+ is greater than 7.5 mEq/L OR if EKG changes are present (suggesting cardiac membrane toxicity). A threefold approach is used. If present, membrane toxicity needs to be reversed promptly. Then, agents are used which cause potassium shifts within the body, leading to a decrease in the measured serum K+. Finally, attempts are made to actually eliminate the electrolyte from the body.

1. CALCIUM GLUCONATE directly antagonizes the cardiac toxicity (membrane-effect) of elevated K+ via a membrane-stabilizing effect:
   - 5–10 cc of a 10% solution are given IV over 2 minutes.
   - If EKG changes persist, this may be repeated × 1 in 5 minutes.
   - This works within minutes; lasts 30–60 minutes.

2. SODIUM BICARBONATE causes rapid movement of K+ into cells *regardless* of

the baseline pH (i.e., the patient does *not* have to be acidotic for it to work):
- 1 amp (44 mEq) IV over 5 min; may repeat × 1 in 10–15 minutes.
- Works within minutes, lasts 1–2 hours.

3. GLUCOSE AND INSULIN cause an intracellular shift of glucose which "draws along" K+ with it into the cells:
- 1 amp D_{50} IV over 5 minutes.
- 5–10 U regular U100 insulin IV.
- Works within 30 minutes; lasts 2–4 hours.

4. CATION EXCHANGE RESINS (KAYEXALATE) and SORBITOL actually remove K+ from the body (1 mEq/gram of resin) by exchanging Na+ for K+. Sorbitol leads to diarrhea which decreases K+ levels as well:
- Kayexalate 20–50 grams in 100–200 cc of 20% sorbitol—the oral route is preferred. This should be given every 4 hours to a maximum of 5 doses per day.
- The Na+ load is 1.3–1.7 mEq Na+ for each mEq K+ removed—thus, use this agent with care in patients susceptible to cardiovascular overload.
- Works in 1–2 hours; lasts 4–6 hours.

5. HEMODIALYSIS should be reserved for those with refractory life-threatening hyperkalemia and renal insufficiency.

6. FUROSEMIDE (Lasix) will gradually decrease the serum K+ via its diuretic effect in milder cases.

Table 9-2 summarizes the treatment of hyperkalemia.

Pearls to Remember

When dealing with hyperkalemia, keep in mind that:

1. Under the proper clinical circumstances, if hyperkalemia is suspected (i.e., highly suspicious EKG changes), one should treat before lab work is available (draw blood first).

2. Calcium given to a patient on digitalis may precipitate acute digitalis toxicity. Watch the rhythm carefully and use only if necessary.

Table 9-2. Summary of Treatment for Hyperkalemia

1. Stabilize the cardiac membrane—calcium

2. Shift potassium into cells:
   - $NaHCO_3$
   - Glucose
   - Insulin

3. Deplete potassium stores:
   - Kayexalate with sorbitol
   - Furosemide
   - Dialysis

HYPOKALEMIA

Hypokalemia may be defined as a serum potassium (K+) level < 3.5 mEq/L.

There are numerous causes of this electrolyte disturbance. **GI causes** include diarrhea, vomiting, and loss of K+ via a nasogastric suction (very common in the ICU). **Urinary loss** may occur via many types of kidney disease, through osmotic diuresis (such as in diabetes or with mannitol), use of diuretics, and steroids. Inadequate intake is an uncommon cause of hypokalemia, though it can occur. **Intracellular shifts** of K+ can also lead to abnormalities. These most commonly occur during alkalosis or with the concomitant administration of glucose and insulin (see above). Administration of beta-agonist drugs such as isoproterenol, epinephrine, and terbutaline have been shown to cause intracellular shifts of K+, resulting in sometimes severe hypokalemia [*New England Journal of Medicine,* 1983, Vol. 309, pp. 1414–1419].

An interesting entity known as hypokalemic periodic paralysis is a rare inherited disease which causes intermittent generalized muscle weakness due to severe hypokalemia. Carbohydrates, cold, and rest may all provoke an attack. Symptoms begin proximally and spread distally, with the bulbar muscles and diaphragm spared. Complete recovery usually follows attacks. Acetazolamide seems to have a prophylactic effect for unknown reasons [*J Emerg Med*, 1986, Vol. 4, p. 287].

Clinical manifestations of hypokalemia usually only occur when the serum potassium is below 3.0 mEq/L.

Neuromuscular disturbances may include weakness, hyporeflexia, and paresthesias. Quadriparesis due to potassium depletion has been reported [*Crit Care Med*, 1986, Vol. 14, p. 750].

Cardiac abnormalities such as dysrhythmias and increased sensitivity to digoxin may occur. The literature suggests that hypokalemia in many different settings commonly precipitates dysrhythmias. This is especially true in patients on digitalis and in those with acute myocardial infarction but occurs in others as well.

EKG changes include flat to inverted T waves, prominent U waves and ST-segment depression.

Renal abnormalities, including the inability to concentrate the urine, have been reported.

CNS problems range from irritability to stupor.

Finally, **GI disturbances** may occur such as nausea, vomiting, and other signs/symptoms of decreased gastrointestinal motility.

Treatment

In considering treatment, it is important to remember that only 2% of body $K+$ is extracellular. Thus, the measured serum $K+$ is only a reflection of the total body stores. If this value is markedly decreased, so must be the total body $K+$. Oral replacement therapy is usually adequate unless the $K+$ is < 3.0, and the patient is on digitalis. IV replacement is also recommended if dysrhythmias are present. Most commonly noted are APCs and PVCs:

1. *IV boluses* consist of 10 mEq KCL mixed in 50–100 cc D_5W. This is dripped in IV over one hour per bolus. If the patient complains of pain or burning in the vein, the rate may be slowed. Alternatively, a small amount of 1% lidocaine injected into the IV line will often stop the pain. As a rule, 3–4 boluses are given and the potassium rechecked.

2. *Oral therapy*—numerous preparations are available. The enteric-coated preparations (Slo-K) or microencapsulated versions (Micro-K) are far better tolerated than any of the powders or "fizzy" forms (K-lyte, Kaon, etc.).

Pearls to Remember

When considering hypokalemia, keep in mind the following:

1. Consider the diagnosis when a patient, especially who is on digitalis, has lots of ectopy.

2. Don't forget that pH changes cause shifts in the potassium—acidosis leads to movement of $K+$ from the cells, increasing the measured value; alkalosis results in the opposite.

3. Epinephrine and terbutaline given for asthma may cause hypokalemia. This should be watched carefully, especially in individuals already on diuretics.

HYPONATREMIA

Hyponatremia is technically defined as a serum sodium $(Na+)$ value below 135 mEq/L in most laboratories. However, problems do not usually occur until this value has dropped below 120–125 mEq/L. As we shall see, the rate of fall may also have some effect.

Hyponatremia is often classified based on the status of the extracellular fluid (ECF). The causes include:

1. **ECF volume depletion**—there is usually a loss of both water and salt. Replacement has occurred with salt-deficient solutions.
   a. *Renal losses*
      - Diuretics (use and abuse); the elderly, especially if female and underweight, are especially at risk [*Arch Intern Med,* 1986, Vol. 146, p. 1355].
      - Adrenal insufficiency—due to a deficiency of mineralocorticoid (aldosterone) secretion.
      - Salt-losing nephropathy—impairment of the kidney's ability to retain salt.
      - Renal tubular acidosis Type II—the kidney is unable to reclaim HCO_3, there is loss in the urine, along with obligate $Na+$ loss.
      - Osmotic diuresis (glucose, mannitol, urea).
   b. *Extra-renal losses*—vomiting, diarrhea, "third spacing" (loss of fluid into body spaces or from venodilation, such as in inflammation, sepsis, etc.). Marathon runners who supplement themselves with only dilute fluids (combined with excessive sweat sodium loss) have been noted to develop clinically significant hyponatremia as well [*JAMA,* 1986, Vol. 255, pp. 772–774].

2. **ECF normal or slightly increased**
   a. *Hypothyroidism*—the response to steroids is thought to be blunted; there may also be inappropriate secretion of antidiuretic hormone (SIADH).
   b. *Syndrome of inappropriate antidiuretic hormone (SIADH)*—abnormal production of antidiuretic hormone (ADH) which causes the kidneys to retain water. This usually occurs with tumors. Lung, duodenal, and pancreatic cancers are common causes. Pulmonary and central nervous system infections may also lead to SIADH. Central nervous system trauma is a final consideration.
   c. *Emotional problems* (water intoxication) can cause hyponatremia. Massive amounts (**>** 20 gallons per day) of water must be imbibed. A syndrome resembling this has occurred in otherwise healthy females following surgery. It is felt secondary to a combination of free water intoxication superimposed on increased antidiuretic hormone secretion which is known to occur following surgery [*N Engl J Med,* 1986, Vol. 314, pp. 1529–1535].
   d. *Drugs that may lead to water retention* with hyponatremia include: nicotine, tolbutamide, morphine, barbiturates, carbamazapine, epinephrine, acetaminophen, indomethacin, isoproterenol, and some antitumor drugs.
   e. *Glucocorticoid deficiency.*

3. **ECF—profound excess with edema**—both total body water and sodium are increased with relatively more water than sodium. This implies impaired renal excretion of water—nephrotic syndrome, cirrhosis, congestive heart failure, and renal failure.

4. **Artifact**
   a. *Lab error*—low sodium values can be obtained because the blood was drawn above a running IV line which diluted the sample. A dangerously low $Na+$ value should always be rechecked immediately.
   b. *Hyperglycemia*—the elevated blood sugar causes an increase in local osmolality; fluid is drawn in, leading to an increase in the amount of ECF, and a subsequent decrease in the $Na+$ concentration.
   c. *Hypertriglyceridemia, hyperproteinemia*—patients with a large proportion of lipid or protein substances in their blood have a large percentage of their plasma occupied by these.

Thus, the measured [Na+] appears low. If the lipid/protein is removed by ultracentrifugation, the [ ] is normal. Plasma osmolality will also be within normal limits with this artifact versus the hypo-osmolality usually found with most hyponatremic entities.

Table 9-3 summarizes the causes of hyponatremia in outline form.

Table 9-3. Causes of Hyponatremia

ECF—Volume Depleted
Renal causes
- Diuretics
- Adrenal insufficiency
- Salt-losing nephropathy
- RTA type II
- Osmotic diuresis

Extra-renal causes
- Vomiting
- Diarrhea
- "Third space"

ECF—Normal or Modestly Increased
Hypothyroidism
SIADH
Emotion
Drugs—nicotine, tolbutamide, morphine, barbiturates, carbamazapine, epinephrine, acetaminophen, indomethacin, isoproterenol, antitumor agents
Glucocorticoid deficiency

ECF—Profound Excess with Edema
Nephrotic syndrome
Cirrhosis
Congestive heart failure
Renal failure

Artifact
Lab error
Hyperglycemia
Hypertriglyceridemia
Hyperproteinemia

Clinical Presentation

The clinical presentation of hyponatremia results from the fact that brain swelling accompanies an acute dilution of the total body water (TBW). Severe symptoms are usually present when the Na+ is less than 120 mEq/L. If the patient has been chronically hyponatremic, they may have no symptoms with a Na+ as low as 110 mEq/L. Conversely, a rapid decrease in the [ ] may lead to symptoms with Na+'s in the range of 125–130 mEq/L. Early symptoms can rapidly proceed to seizures and death. Acute hyponatremia is a true medical emergency!

One reason chronic hyponatremia may not be as symptomatic is the fact that brain cells extrude sodium and water after being exposed to 24–48 hours of low serum sodium concentrations. This loss of more solute than water leads to an equalization of hypotonicity between brain cells and extracellular fluid. It also results in decreased cellular swelling. During restoration of osmolality (i.e., treatment of hyponatremia) with saline, brain cells may shrink unless adequate time is provided for them to replenish lost electrolytes. Thus, chronic hyponatremia should never be reversed rapidly. Most literature has suggested a safe rate of correction of 2 mEq per liter per hour [*N Engl J Med*, 1986, Vol. 314, pp. 1573–1574]. A few studies have noted that unusual neurological symptoms may develop unless one-half this rate is used [*N Engl J Med*, 1986, Vol. 314, pp. 1535–1542].

Symptoms of hyponatremia include lethargy and apathy. The patient may be anorexic (no desire to eat) and nauseated. Disorientation, agitation, and muscle cramps may be present.

Diagnosis

The diagnosis is made first by the presence of a reproducibly decreased serum Na+ concentration. The patient should be checked for features of associated conditions (endocrine disease, etc.). It is important to determine if the individual is volume-contracted or not. If so, the urine Na+ concentration is usually < 10–15 mEq/L, indicating an attempt by the kidneys to conserve Na+. Additionally, the BUN, creatinine, and serum uric acid will be elevated in states of volume depletion. Patients with SIADH will usually *not* exhibit these features. If measured, the serum osmolality will be decreased (normal = 290 mOsm/L).

Physical examination

The physical examination will often reveal an abnormal sensorium with depressed deep tendon reflexes. Cheyne-Stokes breathing (see "Synthesis" section in Chapter 13 for explanation) may be present, including severe central nervous system effects. Hypothermia can occur as well as seizures and facial nerve palsies.

Treatment

Treatment of hyponatremia secondary to mineralocorticoid, glucocorticoid, or thyroid hormone deficiencies are best treated by hormone replacement. Acute symptomatic hyponatremia associated with serum Na+ concentrations less than 120–125 mEq/L *and* central nervous system symptoms (stupor, coma, seizures) requires rapid treatment to decrease brain swelling.

1. Hypertonic 3% saline (512 mEq/L) should be given at a rate that raises the serum sodium concentration no faster than 1–2 mEq/L/hour.

2. Furosemide-induced diuresis—to prevent fluid overload from the saline. Use 1 mg/kg IV.

3. DO NOT correct the [Na+] to greater than 125 mEq/L as the brain may acutely sense this as hypertonicity and brain shrinkage could occur.

Chronic or only mildly symptomatic hyponatremia (i.e., lack of significant central nervous system symptoms) can be treated by water restriction alone. If this fails, demeclocycline, a drug which interferes with the renal tubular action of ADH, may be used. This is very helpful in patients with chronic SIADH.

HYPERCALCEMIA

The normal serum calcium (Ca++) concentra-

tion is usually between 9 and 10.3 mg/dl. Theoretically, hypercalcemia is any value above this. For purposes of this discussion, we will be referring to markedly elevated values and so-called "hypercalcemic crises" when Ca+ +is often > 15 mg/dl and significant symptoms (to be discussed) are present.

There are many **causes** of hypercalcemia. **Malignancy** with and without metastases is that most commonly associated with a crisis. Tumors are usually of the breast, lung, head, or neck region. Elevated Ca++ values are thought to occur via direct invasion of bone as well as secondarily to substances produced by the tumors.

Hyperparathyroidism is the second most common cause of a crisis after malignancy. Hypercalcemia results from the overproduction of serum parathyroid hormone (PTH) from a benign adenoma of the parathyroid gland 85% of the time. Theophylline toxicity has been associated with elevated serum calcium levels. This phenomenon may be reversed with beta blockade, suggesting a beta-adrenergic mechanism of regulation [*Ann Int Med,* 1986, Vol. 105, p. 52].

Other causes of hypercalcemia *not* likely to be associated with a crisis are:

- Vitamin D intoxication
- Hyperthyroidism (decreased bone turnover)
- Milk-alkali syndrome (large intake of milk and calcium-containing antiacids)
- Sarcoidosis (abnormal vitamin D metabolism)
- Addison's disease—decreased inhibition of the action of PTH.

Signs and symptoms of hypercalcemia depend upon the severity of the elevation and the rapidity of its development. Four main systems of the body are affected:

1. *Neuromuscular*
   - Apathy, depression, fatigue
   - Muscle weakness
   - Mental obtundation and coma.

2. *Cardiovascular*
   - Hypertension (? secondary to an effect of Ca++ on vascular smooth muscle)

■ Shortened QT interval (with a moderately increased [Ca++])

■ Prolonged QT interval (due to widening of the T wave with a marked elevation).

3. *Renal*
■ Polyuria, nocturia, polydipsia
■ Dehydration, nephrolithiasis (kidney stones)
■ Azotemia, acute renal failure.

4. *Gastrointestinal*
■ Anorexia, nausea, abdominal pain
■ Constipation
■ Peptic ulcer disease.

These are easily remembered by the mnemonic "abdominal moans, muscle groans, and fatigue overtones." Other symptoms may include bone pain and itching (pruritis). With a crisis, stupor, coma, and acute renal insufficiency are common.

Laboratory tests

Laboratory findings consist of a repeatedly elevated Ca++. Electrolytes, BUN, and creatinine should also be checked acutely. There are numerous interesting studies to be performed when one eventually works up the patient for the underlying cause of their hypercalcemia. In the acutely ill patient, most of them are irrelevant.

Treatment

Treatment of very symptomatic hypercalcemia or of a hypercalcemic crisis should proceed as follows:

1. Volume expansion—Give 1–2 liters of NS over one hour. Volume expansion decreases renal reabsorption of calcium and leads to calciuria. Several liters of fluid may be required [*J Kansas Med Soc*, 1983, Vol. 16, p. 17].

2. FUROSEMIDE—Give 40–80 mg IV every 2–3 hours to maintain urine flow; watch the K+ and volume carefully. This drug inhibits sodium and calcium reabsorption in the kidney. Extracellular fluid

volume should be restored to assure an optimal effect. If this fails then give:

3. CALCITONIN—This substance increases the renal clearance of Ca++ as well as inhibits bone reabsorption. Give 4 U/kg IV initially, followed by a repeat of the same dose at 12–24 hours. This is one of the fastest acting drugs (2–3 hours) in terms of lowering serum [Ca++] but fails in 25% of patients. Others who initially respond may develop resistance later (which can be prevented by concomitant steroid administration). Most recommend giving concomitant steroids (hydrocortisone, 100 mg IV every 6 hours). 80% of patients respond to hydration, calcitonin, and steroids. If these fail then give:

4. MITHRAMYCIN 25 µg/kg IV—This is an antitumor agent that works acutely to decrease an elevated serum Ca++ level from malignancy by either inhibiting bone reabsorption or altering the metabolism of vitamin D. Repeated infusions may lead to renal toxicity and thrombocytopenia, but a one-time infusion should not. This works within 24–48 hours.

5. If the above fail, consider either HEMODIALYSIS or EDTA, a chelating agent that binds Ca++ in the blood. Over four hours, give 15–20 mg/kg. This is the *most* effective immediate therapy but is plagued by a high incidence of nephrotoxicity. Therefore, EDTA therapy is warranted only in life-threatening crises when the other therapies have failed!

6. Some experts recommend the administration of 50–100 mEq of phosphate in saline over 4–6 hours. This works, but may only be tried once due to the high risk of calcium deposition in soft tissues. Generally, this is reserved for situations where other modalities have failed and treatment is emergent [*J Intensive Care Med*, 1986, Vol. 1, p. 319].

The treatment of severe hypercalcemia is summarized in Table 9-4.

Table 9-4. Treatment of Symptomatic Hypercalcemia

Volume Expansion
 1–2 liters normal saline under one hour

Furosemide
 40–80 mg IV every 2–3 hours

If these fail:

Calcitonin
 4 units/kg IV initially; repeat same
  dose at 12–24 hours

Mithramycin
 25 μg/kg IV; one-time infusion only

If these fail:

Hemodialysis or EDTA Chelation

Hematological Emergencies

The most common emergency problems related to bleeding are secondary to hemorrhage, be it internal or external. The obvious first consideration is stopping the bleeding by standard means. Persistent or recurrent hemorrhage may be indicative of an underlying chronic or acute hematological problem. We will discuss the following topics:

- The bleeding patient
- Anticoagulant and antiplatelet drugs
- Medical aspects of transfusion therapy.

THE BLEEDING PATIENT

The **physiology of hemostasis** is best understood by examining the four component systems involved—blood vessels, platelets, clotting, and fibrinolysis.

Abnormalities of *blood vessel walls* can lead to bleeding, usually from small vessels. These walls are also rich in compounds involved in clotting such as tissue plasminogen activator and prostacyclin. Defects lead to "purpuric lesions." This is a general term for lesions consisting of petechiae and/or ecchymoses. Petechiae are small, reddish to salmon-colored patches no greater than .5–1 mm in diameter. Ecchymoses are reddish-purple areas that are larger than petechiae; we often refer to these as "bruises."

Platelets form plugs at vessel tears as well as releasing platelet factor 3 which accelerates the clot-ting cascade. Defects in this system also lead to purpuric lesions, most commonly petechiae.

The *clotting system* involves numerous sequential steps that culminate in the formation of thrombin. Two pathways are involved: the intrinsic and extrinsic. Both lead to thrombin generation which then acts as an enzyme in the conversion of fibrogen to fibrin. Fibrin then polymerizes and forms, along with red blood cells and platelets, the final clot. Defects in this system lead to larger vessel bleeding. The clotting system is summarized in Figure 10.1.

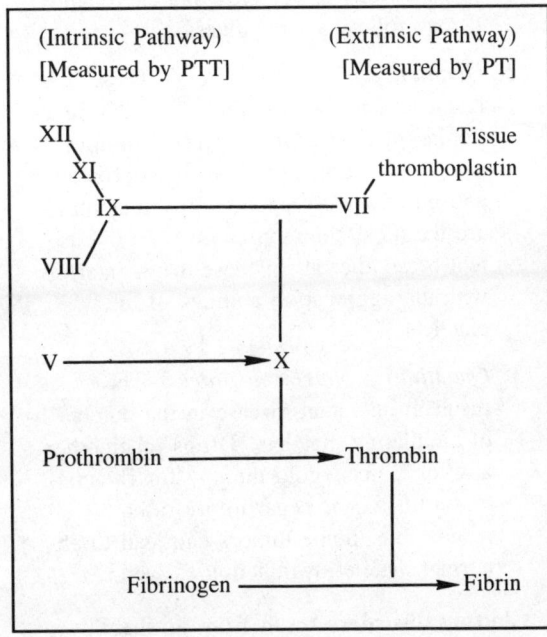

Figure 10.1. The coagulation cascade simplified.

Fibrinolysis is a normal process that dissolves clots formed in the body. Plasminogen is converted to plasmin which leads to the lysis of fibrin clots. When fibrin clots are lysed, small "pieces" are released which are called "fibrin-split products." These are generally of no significance in healthy individuals, though they may cause severe problems during disease states.

Classification of Bleeding Disorders

Three categories of bleeding disorders exist: purpuric disorders, clotting disorders, and hybrid disorders.

Purpuric disorders come about because of small blood vessel or platelet problems with the resultant formation of purpuric lesions. Bleeding in these diseases is more commonly in the form of bruising or oozing from mucosal surfaces (gums, rectum, etc.).

1. *Idiopathic thrombocytopenic purpura* (ITP)—This acquired disorder is thought, perhaps, to be on an immunological basis which results in very low platelet counts. It may follow a viral illness.

2. *Qualitative platelet disorders*—These result in a normal number of poorly functioning platelets. Uremia (renal failure) and various drugs (aspirin, nonsteroidal anti-inflammatory agents, dipyrimadole) are the most common causes. To one extent or another all of these drugs interfere with the aggregation abilities of the platelets.

3. *Quantitative platelet disorders*—These result in an actual disease in the number of circulating platelets. Drugs (chemotherapy for cancer, gold therapy for rheumatoid arthritis, or heparin) are often responsible. Some tumors can lead to abnormal platelet dysfunction as well.

Clotting disorders result from an inability of either the extrinsic, intrinsic, or both clotting pathways to properly result in the formation of thrombin (and thus a clot). Hemorrhage resulting from these defects occurs in large blood vessels. Thus, major bleeding is likely to occur.

1. *Hemophilia*—Due to a hereditary deficiency of clotting factor VIII ("classic" or hemophilia A) or factor IX ("Christmas Disease" or hemophilia B), this disease usually affects males only (due to a sex-linked pattern of inheritance). Spontaneous joint bleeding (into the joint cavity) and massive bleeding following surgery or trauma are common symptoms. This should be suspected with an isolated increase in the partial thromboplastin time (PTT) which measures the integrity of the intrinsic clotting pathway.

2. *Primary fibrinolysis*—For uncertain reasons, the fibrinolytic system may be inappropriately activated. This will result in bleeding from any area where a clot has previously formed. This is actually a rather unusual occurrence, with secondary fibrinolysis accompanying disseminated intravascular coagulation (see below) being much more common. Sepsis and transurethral resections of the prostate gland (TURP) are frequent accompanying disorders when this problem is present (the urinary tract is high in urokinase—much is released during a "TURP").

3. *Heparin and coumadin toxicity*— Coumadin anticoagulation leads to inhibition of the synthesis of vitamin K dependent clotting factors II, VII, IX, and X. Usually an increase in only the protime (PT) occurs, though the PTT may also be elevated due to thrombin inhibition (factor II). Heparin binds to antithrombin III leading to a prolongation of the PTT. The PT is increased with large doses (see section on "Anticoagulation" on page 134. With too large a dose of either, there may be hemorrhage at a single or many sites. Large soft tissue bruises are common with only minor or no preceding trauma.

4. *Circulating "spontaneous" anticoagulants*—These are often present in connective tissue disease (systemic lupus erythematosus), in the elderly, and as a result of various drugs (chlorpromazine, penicillin). They may also occur following normal delivery and, in hemophiliacs, as a result of many transfusions.

5. *Vitamin K deficiency*—Generally, this results in the same effect as coumadin therapy/overdose. This may occur via malabsorption of fat (and thus vitamin K) and in liver disease (where the ability of the organ to synthesize clotting factors despite normal amounts of vitamin K is impaired).

Hybrid disorders involve a combination of platelet-factor and clotting-factor deficiencies:

1. Von Willebrand's disease—a congenital disorder with both platelet dysfunction (poor absorption) and a clotting abnormality (factor VIII is hypofunctional).

2. *Disseminated intravascular coagulation* (DIC)—an acquired disorder. There is abnormal coagulation leading to depletion of the essential clotting factors. As the clots are lysed, fibrin-split products are released. These have an anticoagulant property and further add to the bleeding. DIC should be suspected in any patient with decreased platelets, a clotting disorder, and the presence of fibrinolysis. DIC accompanies other serious diseases such as sepsis, ARDS, abruptio placentae, etc. It is rarely a primary entity. Trauma, as well as suicidal ingestion of glacial acetic acid, have been noted to result in DIC [*Crit Care Med*, 1986, Vol. 14, p. 990]. A chronic form (which will not be discussed) may accompany malignancies. The chronic form of DIC is of much lower virulence than the acute type.

3. *Dilution coagulopathy*—dilution in clotting

factors and platelets from massive blood transfusion. This will be discussed under "Medical Aspects of Transfusion Therapy" on page 137.

Table 10-1 summarizes the classification of bleeding disorders.

Table 10-1. Classification of Bleeding Disorders

Purpuric Disorders—Bruising, Oozing from Mucosal Surfaces
Idiopathic thrombocytompenic purpura (ITP)
Qualitative platelet disorders
- Aspirin
- Sulfinpyrazone
- Persantin
- Uremia
- Nonsteroidal anti-inflammatory agents

Clotting Disorders—Major Bleeding
Hemophilia A (factor VIII deficiency)
Hemophilia B (factor IX deficiency)
Primary fibrinolysis
Heparin and coumadin toxicity
Circulating anticoagulants
- Connective tissue disease
- Elderly patient
- Drugs—chlorpromazine, penicillin
- Hemophilia (after large numbers of transfusions)
- Postpartum
Vitamin K deficiency
- Gastrointestinal malabsorption
- Liver disease

Hybrid Disorders—Major Bleeding
Von Willebrand's disease (factor VIII + platelet problem)
Disseminated intravascular coagulation (DIC)
Dilution coagulopathy

Several factors should lead the health care provider to suspect a bleeding problem:

1. Bleeding at multiple sites or in several body systems concurrently.

2. "Spontaneous" deep hematomas or hemarthroses (joint cavity bleeding).

3. Unusually prolonged bleeding after local injury.

4. Disproportionately large hemorrhage following a minor insult.

5. Late bleeding after a period of apparently normal hemostasis following surgery or trauma.

Diagnosis

History

Many factors need to be noted in taking the history. Is the problem from greater than one site? Bleeding at one site only (unless it is a joint cavity) is unlikely to be secondary to a bleeding diathesis. Is there a family history of bleeding problems? Has the problem been lifelong or just recent in onset. Hereditary bleeding problems usually are lifelong though they may present for the first time following a first operation at an older age. Along the same lines, one must ascertain if there was ever any untoward postoperative bleeding especially if a transfusion was required. Bleeding requiring hospitalization or return to the dentist for control of delayed hemorrhage is significant.

It is important to determine if the pattern suggests a clotting problem or a hemostatic (i.e., platelet plug) defect. **Clotting problems** (e.g., hemophilia) result in large vessel bleeding, not capillary oozing. Hemarthrosis, large hematomas and ecchymoses, as well as excess bleeding following trauma are common. **Hemostatic plug** problems lead to small vessel (capillary) bleeding (oozing). Thus, petechiae, mucous membrane bleeding (nose, gums, gastrointestinal tract) or an "oozing" nature rather than a "gush" are common. Some hematological problems, of course, are associated with both types of bleeding.

Physical examination

Physical examination of the skin and mucous membranes should be carefully performed looking for evidence of hemorrhage. The fundi, large muscle groups, and joints should also be checked. Bleeding into joints is, as mentioned previously, seen almost exclusively in clotting problems.

Laboratory tests

The majority of problems can be detected by simple laboratory tests. A CBC, electrolytes, BUN/creatinine, type and crossmatch, PT, PTT, bleeding time, platelet count, and fibrinogen level should be obtained. The PT/PTT measure the integrity of the intrinsic and extrinsic clotting pathways respectively. The **bleeding time** tests hemostatic plug formation and is increased with significant thrombocytopenia (decreased platelet count) or platelet dysfunction disorders.

The **platelet** count can be either too high or too low (either will result in problems). The normal adult count is usually between 150,000 and 400,000 platelets per cubic mm. Minor bleeding problems will usually be seen with counts < 50,000 or > 500,000. If the platelet count is < 10,000, there is a possibility of spontaneous intracranial hemorrhage. The **fibrinogen level** is decreased in consumption coagulopathy.

The following is a list of laboratory patterns observed with common bleeding problems:

1. *ITP*—decreased (dec) platelets or decreased platelets and increased (inc) bleeding time (BT).

2. *Platelet dysfunction*—increased BT, platelet count WNL.

3. *Hemophilia, heparin*—increased PTT.

4. *Vitamin K deficiency, coumadin, liver disease, massive heparin doses*—increased PT (PTT also increased with heparin).

5. *Primary fibrinolysis*—decreased fibrinogen, increased PT, occasionally increased PTT, platelets *WNL*.

6. *DIC*—decreased fibrinogen, increased PT/PTT, *decreased* platelets.

7. *If all clotting parameters are normal in an abnormally bleeding patient*—suspect autoimmune vasculitis (connective tissue disease directed against blood vessel walls), some other type of blood vessel disorder, or a factor XI deficiency (special factor assays are then required).

Emergency Treatment of Bleeding Disorders

Treatment first involves attention to some **general principles:**

1. A, B, C's

2. Fluid replacement—start IV D$_5$LR and titrate in response to patient's blood pressure.

3. Avoid intramuscular and subcutaneous injections.

4. Apply prolonged pressure to arterial blood gas and venipuncture sites.

Treatment of platelet disorders

Bleeding in the face of **quantitative platelet disorders** may require treatment with platelet concentrates. Each 25 cc unit should raise the platelet count by 6–12,000 platelets per cubic mm. The goal is to try and increase the count by 40–50,000. This should be doubled if surgery is imminent. Prophylactic transfusions are NOT warranted unless the count is < 10,000 in an asymptomatic patient—this is still not felt to be an indication by some. The reason is due to the rapid development of antiplatelet antibodies.

Unless there is massive bleeding or a large number of transfusions given, platelet transfusion (tx) therapy is not usually an Emergency Department consideration. If the cause of the problem is not obvious, prompt hematological consultation is recommended. Bleeding in **qualitative platelet disorders** is usually minor. It is best treated by stopping any offending drugs and observing the patient. Platelet transfusions may be used if necessary.

It has been established that platelet transfusions can raise the platelet count in many patients with immune-based thrombocytopenia and should be used if indicated [*Am J Med,* 1986, Vol. 80, p. 1051]. Bleeding problems in patients with renal failure may be due to platelet survival/aggregation problems. The administration of conjugated estrogens may reduce acute bleeding in these individuals [*N Engl J Med,* 1986, Vol. 315, p. 731].

A relatively uncommon disease, thrombotic thrombocytopenic purpura (TTP), results in a pentad of features: fever, hemolytic anemia, thrombocytopenic purpura, transient or permanent central nervous system signs, and renal failure. It should be suspected in any patient with neurological deficits, renal abnormalities, anemia, and a low platelet count. If diagnosed early, treatment with steroids and plasmapheresis may be lifesaving [*J Intensive Care Med,* 1986, Vol. 1, p. 341].

Treatment of clotting problems

1. *Hemophilia—cryoprecipitate* (see ''Medical Aspects of Transfusion Therapy'' on page 137) is given to raise the missing factor level to at least 40% of normal activity. Commercial concentrates are also available (and may be required in factor IX deficiency). These carry a high risk of transmitting hepatitis. The dose of cryoprecipitate is 2 bags/12 kg body weight followed by one-half this dose every 12 hours as necessary. Von Willebrand's disease may be treated in this fashion as well.

2. *Coumadin or nonspecific problems— vitamin K* administration orally takes 12–24 hours to work. It may be given intravenously with a *high* risk of anaphylaxis but still takes several hours to have any noticeable effect. The *treatment of choice is fresh frozen plasma* (FFP). Give 2 units and observe the effect clinically and on clotting parameters. Remember, once thawed, this component should be used within 2 hours, or it must be thrown out.

3. HEPARIN OVERDOSE—If the administration of the drug is stopped, heparin levels will rapidly decline due to its short half-life (1.5 hours) in the blood. If there is severe bleeding requiring more rapid reversal, then PROTAMINE SULFATE, 50 mg should be given IV over 10 minutes. Protamine has some intrinsic anticoagulant activity of its own and may worsen a situation. Use only when absolutely required!

When reversing any anticoagulant, it is important to keep in mind that this may lead to a rebound hypercoagulable state. In other words, the thrombotic problem for which the medicine was originally given may recur. In patients with small amounts of bleeding, the anticoagulant effect does *not* have to be completely reversed. For example, if the protime is elevated to 40 seconds (therapeutic range = 18–25 seconds), and only a little bit of bruising is present, fresh frozen plasma can be given until the value is within the therapeutic, *not* the control (i.e., "normal"), range.

On the other hand, keep in mind that an individual can bleed 2–3 units into a thigh without noticeable change in size. This is a common location for "coumadin" bleeds. When this occurs, it may be necessary to completely reverse the anticoagulant effect, transfuse the patient, and resume anticoagulation a couple of weeks later. Additionally, keep in mind that hematuria (blood in the urine) in a patient on coumadin with a *therapeutic* protime (PT) is due to something other than the anticoagulant (i.e., tumor, infection, etc.) until proven otherwise!

DIC is best treated via intensive therapy of the underlying disease. Heparin is somewhat controversial but can lead to replenishment of depleted clotting factors by interrupting the clotting process. Currently, heparin anticoagulation is reserved for situations in which massive defibrination is accompanied by fibrinogen levels of less than 100 mg/dl *and* replacement therapy is not stopping hemorrhage. IV infusion has been recommended in these selected patients by several investigators. Others have suggested that the bleeding risk from this form of therapy is too great. Thus, they recommend subcutaneous hepa-

rin (5,000 U SQ every 12 hours) in the hope that the naturally occurring anticoagulant antithrombin III will be potentiated. Low-dose intravenous therapy (500 units/h) may be as safe [*J Am Coll Card*, 1986, Vol. 8, p. 159B].

All agree that heparin should *not* be used in patients who have major bleeding from a localized site, possible central nervous system hemorrhage, uncontrolled hypertension (diastolic blood pressure > 110 mm Hg), or who have undergone surgery in the past five days. If successful, one should expect to see the fibrinogen level rise by 24–36 hours following therapy. Replacement therapy (platelets, fresh frozen plasma) may be necessary but unless ongoing coagulation is stopped, these will all be eventually consumed before they can help.

Treatment of fibronolytic disorders

Primary fibrinolysis is rare. Thus, the diagnosis *must* be confirmed with a hematologist or pathologist before starting therapy. Improperly diagnosing and treating secondary fibrinolysis accompanying DIC as if it was primary fibrinolysis can be a fatal mistake! Most fibrinolysis occurs secondary to DIC and will subside if DIC is treated. If there is an established diagnosis of primary fibrinolysis, then EPSILON-AMINOCAPROIC ACID (EACA), which inhibits fibrinolysis, is used. The dose is 4–5 grams IV initially the first hour, then 1 gram IV each hour for eight hours or until the bleeding is controlled. Table 10-2 summarizes the treatment of bleeding problems.

ANTICOAGULANT AND ANTI-PLATELET DRUGS

The agents, coumadin and heparin, have been mentioned previously. Many people are on these drugs as well as the so-called antiplatelet products. Emergencies related to these compounds are discussed in the previous section. This material is intended as background information only. Formal hematology texts should be sought for more detailed information.

Table 10-2. Summary: Treatment of Bleeding Problems

General Principles
  A, B, C's
  Fluid replacment—IV D$_5$LR
  Avoid IM/SQ injection
  Prolonged pressure for ABG/venipuncture sities

Thrombocytopenia
  Each platelet unit should increase count by 6–12,000/mm³
  Consider indications carefully—antibody formation common
  Stop offending medications in qualitative problems

Clotting Problems
  Cryoprecipitate for hemophilia A, Von Willebrand's
  FFP for hemophilia B (or commercial concentrate)
  FFP for coumadin or nonspecific problem
  Stop heparin—use protamine if situation urgent

Remember: Reversing anticoagulation can lead to a rebound hypercoagulable state!

Disseminated Intravascular Coagulation
  Intensive therapy of underlying disease
  Heparin—hematological consult first
  Replacement therapy—use judiciously

Primary Fibrinolysis
  Most important thing is to confirm diagnosis!
  If confirmed with pathologist or hematologist:

  Epsilon-Aminocaproic acid

An **anticoagulant** is any substance which, when added to blood, decreases the ability of that blood to clot. **Heparin** is given either subcutaneously or intravenously. It works by binding to antithrombin III (ATT). Heparin causes a change in the configuration of antithrombin III. The newly shaped complex is then able to inhibit thrombin as well as activated factors IX-XII in the intrinsic pathway. In very high doses, heparin also affects factor VII (extrinsic pathway). Used therapeutically, heparin leads to elevations in only the PTT. In excess, it may also increase the PT.

A naturally occurring substance which has anticoagulant properties, protein C, has recently been described. This compound interferes with the procoagulant properties of activated factors V and VIII. The net effect is a decrease in thrombin formation, with decreased activation of fibrinogen. Deficiency of protein C can lead to a propensity for thrombotic disease. This is a vitamin K-dependent factor, and its level is reduced in the presence of malabsorption as well as other conditions that decrease the level of vitamin K. Protein C is activated by thrombin. The activated form has a potent anticoagulant effect which inactivates activated factors V and VIII and stimulates fibrinolysis.

Protein S is a recently discovered vitamin K-dependent protein which is a cofactor for activated protein C. Its presence is required for expression of the anticoagulant effects of protein C. Deficiencies have been reported, with recurrent venous thrombosis being noted, as would be expected [*J Am Coll Card*, 1986, Vol. 8, p. 104B].

The side effects of heparin include bleeding and thrombocytopenia. The decrease in platelet counts is thought to be secondary to an immunological phenomenon. Generally, it is related to the duration of therapy. Severe thrombocytopenia usually occurs in the face of full-dose IV therapy but has also been reported with "mini-dose" subcutaneous (SQ) treatment as well. With massive depressions in the platelet count, several days may be required for return to normal following cessation of therapy. The depression recurs if heparin is resumed. Steroids are NOT helpful in this situation. Mild platelet count depressions (80,000–150,000 counts) also occur commonly with heparin therapy. One study noted this in up to

25% of all CCU patients [*Arch Int Med,* April 1978, p. 549]. This may resolve despite continuance of therapy, though not recommended. Heparin has also been reported to increase aggregation of platelets and, rarely, can actually lead to thrombosis.

The following recommendations should be followed to avoid problems in any patient on heparin therapy:

1. Obtain platelet counts daily or every other day.

2. If new thrombosis occurs in a heparinized patient, consider both under-heparinization and the possibility that heparin could have caused the problem.

3. If hemorrhage occurs on heparin, rule out thrombocytopenia.

4. Use heparin with caution, if at all, in patients who have thrombocytopenia.

5. The best treatment for heparin-induced thrombocytopenia is cessation of therapy.

6. An increased protime (PT) in a patient on heparin therapy with therapeutic PTTs is unusual. Rule out DIC as a cause.

7. Subcutaneous heparin is not effective for the treatment of established proximal-vein thrombosis [*N Engl J Med,* 1986, Vol. 315, p. 1109]. Intravenous therapy must be used.

When discontinued, heparin should be gradually weaned. Sudden cessation of heparin (or coumadin) therapy, as mentioned previously, may lead to rebound hypercoagulability. In an emergent situation, heparin may be reversed with protamine sulfate, 25–30 mg IV over 10 minutes. Remember, excess protamine can act as an anticoagulant.

Coumadin (warfarin) inhibits the formation of clotting factors II, VII, IX, and X ("vitamin K-dependent factors") by the liver. It is given orally and takes about five days to have a full effect. Factor VII levels decrease rapidly and the measured PT may be elevated with 24–48 hours of instituting therapy. Coumadin decreases the production of not only the vitamin K-dependent factors, but protein C as well. Protein C inhibits coagulation by inactivating clotting factors V and VIII. This may lead to a false sense of security because the administration of coumadin will decrease protein C levels more rapidly than those of factors II and X. Thus, there is a transient relative deficiency of protein C and a hypercoagulable state. This is perhaps the most important reason to overlap heparin and coumadin therapy by at least five days. Patients with liver and heart failure are more sensitive to the effects of coumadin.

The most common complication of coumadin is bleeding. The longer the duration of therapy, the higher is the risk of medically important bleeding [*Am J Med,* 1986, Vol. 81, p. 255]. As mentioned previously, most hematuria with a therapeutic PT is *not* due to anticoagulant and other causes must be ruled out. Again, vitamin K orally takes 12–24 hours to work. The IV form is more rapid but carries a high risk of anaphylaxis. Fresh frozen plasma works rapidly and is the *treatment of choice* for severe bleeding problems associated with coumadin. Some experts feel that simple transfusion of blood, plasma, or plasma concentrates rich in vitamin K-dependent clotting factors will work and do not necessarily need to be fresh, as the involved factors are relatively stable in banked blood [*J Am Coll Cardiol,* 1986, Vol. 8, p. 10B].

Necrosis of the skin in patients on coumadin can occur and is thought to be related to microvascular hemorrhage. It is more common in patients with protein C deficiency. A final problem that can be noted, often in male patients, is purple toes; this is a transitory phenomenon, and the reason is unknown. It is not from bleeding.

The **antiplatelet agents** include aspirin, dipyridamole, sulfinpyrazone, and the nonsteroidal anti-inflammatory agents (NSAIAs). The various drugs act to inhibit different steps in the biochemical pathway of platelet aggregation. Aspirin (ASA), NSAIAs, and sulfinpyrazone block cyclooxygenase which prevents the formation of prostaglandin endoperoxides by platelets. This is a permanent effect and a single dose of ASA affects all circulating platelets. This effect is *unique* to aspirin (i.e., the one-dose effect). Dipyridamole blocks the platelet phosphodiesterase and simultaneously stimulates adenyl cyclase. This leads to the increased formation of cyclic AMP (cAMP) which leads to inhibition of platelet aggregation.

These drugs are used in many areas including coronary artery disease (to keep bypass grafts patent), cerebrovascular disease (prevention of transient ischemic attacks), and peripheral vascular disease. Some studies have shown a decrease in prosthetic heart valve thrombosis as well. These drugs do not usually affect the platelet count, just the bleeding time. If there has been excessive platelet inhibition, a petechial rash or mucous membrane oozing may be noted. These are usually minor problems and often respond to stopping the offending agent. The stomach lining may be irritated (gastritis) leading to GI bleeding. This may be significant. Additionally, some feel these agents are ulcerogenic.

MEDICAL ASPECTS OF TRANS-FUSION THERAPY

Transfusion therapy (TX) is generally used in the emergency setting for blood loss secondary to trauma. Nonetheless, there are numerous medical aspects of blood transfusions that must be kept in mind, whether transfusion is done in the Emergency Department, ICU, operating suite, or on the ward.

Whole blood is rarely used for active bleeding any more. Too many components are inactivated during the banking process. Fresh whole blood may be indicated in a patient with severe volume loss. One unit = 500 cc. More commonly, whole blood is broken down into components. Current use of transfusion mandates proper understanding of **component therapy:**

1. *Packed red blood cells* (PRBCs)—the hematocrit of this preparation is about 70%, with 250 cc volume; much plasma and platelets are removed from whole blood (WB) to form a unit of packed red blood cells. A 1 U transfusion should raise the hematocrit about three percentage points.

2. *Washed red blood cells*—The WBC have been removed to prevent leukoagglutinin reactions (see below) in multiply transfused patients.

3. *Fresh blood*—This is, by definition, less than six hours old, often from recruited donors during an emergency. It is best used in the patient with large acute transfusion requirements who has received much banked blood (greater than 10 units within 24 hours). The general rule is to give 1 U of fresh blood for every 4 U of banked blood (after the initial 10 U of banked blood have been given). This practice is designed to prevent dilution of coagulation factors and platelets (see discussion on Dilutional Coagulopathy below). One unit of fresh frozen plasma plus one unit of platelets plus one unit of packed red blood cells has the equivalent effect of one unit of fresh blood.

4. *Frozen RBCs*—These allow for long storage times.

5. *Random single-donor platelets*—Platelets are harvested from a single unit of fresh blood and resuspended in 30–50 cc of plasma. They have a relatively short storage time. One U should increase the platelet count 6–12,000 as measured 1 hour following transfusion. These may need to be repeated every 24–72 hours depending on the situation.

6. *Fresh frozen plasma* (FFP)—This consists of plasma that is separated from fresh blood and stored at temperatures less than 20°C or less. It is generally active in clotting factors II, VII, IX, and X as well as the relatively labile components V and VIII. Note that heat-prepared "plasma protein fractions" (Plasmanate) have NO active coagulation factors. One unit fresh frozen plasma = about 150 cc volume. Fresh frozen plasma is used to prevent dilutional coagulopathy, correct coumadin overdose, congenital defects, and Von Willebrand's disease. Fresh frozen plasma has an osmolality of 375 mosm/L and the following electrolyte concentrations:
   - Glucose—535 mEq/L
   - Sodium—172 mEq/L
   - Chloride—73 mEq/L
   - Potassium—15 mEq/L

■ Albumin—60% (5.5 g/dl protein)

It may be a less effective volume expander than other albumin-containing solutions because of the lowered albumin content [*Crit Care Med*, 1986, Vol. 14, p. 145].

7. *Cryoprecipitate*—This is a gelatinous precipitate of a few cc volume containing mostly factor VIII and fibrinogen. It is used in hemophilia, Von Willebrand's disease, and in hypofibrinogenemia.

8. *White blood cells* (WBC)—These may be transfused for severe bone marrow depression and accompanying severe infections. Their discussion is not relevant here for our purposes.

Table 10-3 summarizes the various blood components available.

Problems occurring secondary to massive transfusion (defined as > 10 U banked blood within a 24-hour period) include dilution coagulopathy, hypothermia, citrate intoxication, acidosis, and hyperammonemia. **Dilution coagulopathy** (DC) usually occurs in trauma or surgical patients who receive a massive transfusion of banked blood. This stems from the fact that banked blood is from ten days to three weeks old. Blood becomes rapidly depleted of some active factors with time. Functioning platelets are gone in one day. Other labile components include factors V and VIII. Thus, by giving large numbers of banked units of blood, thrombocytopenia, increases in the PTT (due to loss of factor VIII), PT (loss of factor V), and associated clinical bleeding can occur.

Dilution coagulopathy is the most common cause of "nonsurgical bleeding" associated with massive transfusion. Many experts recommend monitoring the PT, PTT, fibrinogen level, and platelet count with at least every 10 units transfused. Generally, 2 U fresh frozen plasma are given with every 5–6 U packed red blood cells as a prophylactic measure though the standard (as mentioned previously) has been 1 U fresh frozen plasma for every 4 U transfusion following the initial 10 units of banked blood. If dilution coagulopathy occurs, the following is recommended:

Table 10-3. Summary: Blood Components

Whole Blood
  500 cc/U
  Infrequently used

Packed Red Blood Cells
  HCT = 70%
  250 cc/U
  1 U should increase HCT by 3%

Washed Red Blood Cells
  WBCs removed to prevent leukoagglutinin reactions

Fresh Blood
  Less than 6 hours old
  Best used in massively transfused
  1 U for every 4 U of banked blood after an initial 10 U of banked blood
  1 U FFP + 1 U platelets + 1 U PRBC = 1 U fresh blood

Frozen RBC
  Allows for long storage times

Random Single-Donor Platelets
  25 cc/U
  Short storage time
  1 U should increase count 6–12,000/mm³
  Count should be measured 1 hour after transfusion

Fresh Frozen Plasma
  Active in factors II, VII, IX, X, V, and VIII
  Approximately 150 cc volume per U
  Heat-treated products ("plasmanate") not identical

Cryoprecipitate
  Gelatinous precipitate
  Concentrated factor VIII and fibrinogen

White Blood Cells
  Harvest difficult
  Given in severe neutropenia with infection

1. Fresh frozen plasma + packed red blood cells in a 1:1 or 1:2 ratio. Often 6-10 U of fresh frozen plasma are required to make a difference.

2. If the fibrinogen level is < 100 mg/dl and not increased with fresh frozen plasma, cryoprecipitate should be given in a dose of 4 U/10 kg of body weight (should raise fibrinogen level by 150 mg/dl).

3. Expeditious control of surgical bleeding.

4. If excess bleeding is occurring with a platelet count < 50,000, consideration should be given to platelet transfusion. It is rare that a platelet problem is responsible for bleeding until > 10 units of banked blood have been given. The American College of Surgeons (ACS) recommends giving 6-10 bags of platelet concentrate per 20 units of banked blood.

Hypothermia during transfusion is common. This is proportional to the rapidity of and the amount transfused. Blood warmers should be used and the patient's core temperature followed carefully. **Acidosis** could theoretically occur during transfusion because banked WB is acidotic. This could contribute to the acidosis already present in a shocky patient. This has *not* been found to be a clinically significant problem. Prophylactic $NaHCO_3$ is NOT recommended! **Hyperammonemia** is also a theoretical problem as ammonia (NH_4) is present in stored blood. Although this could possibly cause problems during transfusion of a patient with severe liver disease, no clinical significance of this finding has ever been demonstrated.

Citrate intoxication can occur by virtue of the fact that citrate is used as an anticoagulant during blood storage. This works by binding Ca++, which is essential to blood clotting. By giving large amounts of citrate, the patient's own calcium could possibly be bound as well. Most patients DO NOT develop clinically significant hypocalcemia (with bradycardia and hypotension). Regardless of the volume of blood given, if the transfusion rate is less than 50-75 cc/minute, the patient's Ca++ mobilization rate should be sufficient. If blood is given at a rate > 100 cc/min, Ca++ should be given.

The ACS recommends giving .2 gram $CaCl_2$ (2 cc of a 10% solution) in a *separate* line for every 500 cc blood given. This applies only to transfusions given at a rapid rate. The total dose of Ca++ should not exceed 2 grams (2 amps). The patient's QT interval should be followed. It increases with hypocalcemia, decreases with mild hypercalcemia, and again increases with large elevations in Ca++ (due to widening of the T wave by massive hypercalcemia).

Transfusion Reactions

Transfusion reactions are a final area of concern. An **acute hemolytic reaction** occurs when incompatible donor cells are agglutinated by the recipient's antibodies. This is often secondary to a "clerical" error whereby the wrong blood is given to a patient. These are best *prevented* by double-checking all blood orders. Table 10.4 summarizes the potential problems associated with transfusion therapy.

Signs and symptoms begin following transfusion of 50 cc of blood or less. They include jaundice (may develop over days), flushing, chills, fever, tachypnea, tachycardia, and flank, back, or extremity pain. The patient may bleed from wounds, develop hemoglobinuria, or acute renal failure.

Laboratory evaluation will show free hemoglobin in the blood and urine. A repeat crossmatch is indicated. A direct Coomb's test should be obtained as well as a haptoglobin level. Haptoglobin binds free hemoglobin and will be acutely depressed following hemolysis.

Treatment of the patient is as follows:

1. STOP the transfusion immediately.

2. If further blood is required after re-crossmatching, use washed cells.

3. Forced alkaline diuresis with mannitol and HCO_3.

4. Watch for DIC.

Leukoagglutinin reactions occur secondary to the presence of white blood cell antibodies. They are far more common than hemolytic reactions.

The **symptoms** are chills and fevers which occur later on in the transfusion. These may be effectively prevented by premedicating the patient with diphenhydramine (Benadryl—give 25 mg po, IM, or IV one-half hour before the transfusion begins, then every four hours as needed). Leukoagglutinin reactions are rare in a patient premedicated in this fashion.

If chills and fever do occur during transfusion and the workup as outlined below is negative for a hemolytic reaction, you may be able to continue the transfusion (after giving Benadryl). Most chills and fevers that occur during transfusion are due to leukoagglutinin reactions.

Volume overload reactions are still the most common serious hazard of blood transfusion. Be careful with elderly patients, those with congestive heart failure, and individuals requiring transfusion acutely on top of an already existent chronic anemia. Individuals with chronic anemia have "reset" their body's thermostat, so to speak, and are used to lower hematocrits (circulating blood volumes). Suddenly increasing these parameters could have devastating consequences. If rapid transfusion is required in a hemodynamically unstable patient, the placement of a Swan-Ganz catheter is mandatory.

Pearls to Remember

In summary, the evaluation of any suspected transfusion reaction (except, of course, volume overload) should proceed as follows:

1. **STOP** the transfusion immediately!

2. Perform a careful clerical check of the identity of the recipient and the accuracy of blood bank and clerical records.

3. Draw a blood sample into an anticoagulant-containing tube, centrifuge, and examine the supernatant for hemoglobin (will appear pink if positive).

4. Draw blood for repeat cross-match, direct Coombs' test, and haptoglobin.

5. Check the urine for free hemoglobin.

6. Consider sepsis. Culture the patient's blood as well as the bag of blood. Rarely, chronic blood donors can develop bacterial colonization at the venipuncture site, which can then be transmitted to the donated blood [*Am J Med,* 1986, Vol. 81, p. 405].

Table 10-4. Problems with Massive Transfusions

Dilution Coagulopathy
  Banked blood usually devoid of platelets, factors V and VIII
  Thrombocytopenia, increased PT and PTT with associated bleeding can occur
  Give 1 Unit fresh frozen plasma/4 Units of blood transfused after the first 10 blood Units
  Give 6-10 bags of platelet concentrate for every 20 Units of banked blood
  Consider cryoprecipitate in difficult cases

Hypothermia
  Proportional to the amount and rapidity of the transfusion given
  Use a blood warmer
  Monitor patient's core temperature carefully

Acidosis
  Usually not clinically significant
  Prophylactic bicarbonate *not* recommended

Hyperammonemia
  Ammonia present in banked blood
  Theoretically a problem in patients with liver disease
  No clinical significance has ever been demonstrated

Citrate Intoxication
  Citrate binds calcium
  Does *not* occur with transfusion rates less than 50–75 cc/minute
  With rapid transfusion, give 2 cc of a 10% solution of calcium chloride in a separate line for every 500 cc of blood given

Transfusion Reactions
  Acute hemolytic reaction
  Leukoagglutinin reaction
  Volume overload reaction

Infectious Disease Emergencies

11

Patients with infectious diseases commonly present to emergency care providers. Many of these diseases consist of colds, pneumonia, and urinary tract infections, none of which are particularly difficult to handle. There are several life-threatening conditions that every emergent care provider should be aware of. In this chapter, we will discuss the following:

- Toxic shock syndrome
- Bacterial meningitis
- Septic arthritis
- Bacterial infections of skeletal muscle and contiguous structures.

TOXIC SHOCK SYNDROME

Though initially described in young children, the presence of a life-threatening illness in menstruating females using tampons was noted only a few years ago. This disease process became known as the toxic shock syndrome (TSS). At first, toxic shock syndrome seemed to be associated with the use of one particular brand of feminine tampon. Soon, though, it became obvious that any type could be responsible. In fact, (see below) nonmenstruating females, as well as male victims, have been reported.

TSS is due to the production of a toxin at the site of what is often a relatively localized, and often asymptomatic, infection by any one of several strains of the bacteria *Staphylococcus aureus*. The most common site of primary infection is the vagina, and this is virtually always associated with tampon use. Other sites have been described with males also being affected. Generally, these have involved foreign bodies, most often sutures in surgical wounds. A case of TSS developing in a male child with a large burn has been reported [*Jrnl of Trauma,* 1985, Vol. 25, p. 1004]. The clinical manifestations of the syndrome are produced when the toxin is absorbed into the body.

Diagnosis

History

Generally, the patient is not aware of the localized infection until TSS "strikes." TSS is heralded by the dramatic and sudden onset of high fever, muscle aches, profuse nausea, vomiting, and watery diarrhea. An early rash may or may not be present.

The patient will complain of the above symptoms. They will have usually been well immediately before. If asked, a history of tampon use or recent surgery can usually be obtained.

Physical examination

The examination will reveal an extremely sick-looking patient. The blood pressure is usually low, though (as in other types of shock) it may initially remain "within normal limits." If old records are available, however, the obtained BP is usually significantly less than the patient's current reading. A high temperature is noted. The abdominal examination is relatively unimpressive in terms of tenderness, rebound, and guarding. Pelvic may reveal mild cervical tenderness, but the the primary purpose of performing this exam is to obtain a cervical culture for *Staph.*

Within the first few days an erythematous (red) rash appears over the entire body. This is followed by the "classic" rash of TSS—desquamation (loss of skin) of the hands and feet. This is noted within 7–10 days. It is unlikely that the patient has TSS without this rash being present sometime in the disease course. Diffuse injection (redness) of the conjunctivae, mouth, or vaginal wall may also be noted. Signs and symptoms of TSS are summarized in Table 11-1.

Table 11-1. Signs and Symptoms of Toxic Shock Syndrome

Symptoms	% With Symptoms
Fever	100
Rash with desquamation	100
Myalgia	97
Vomiting	89
Diarrhea	88
Abdominal tenderness	75
Pharyngeal hyperemia	73
Sore throat	71
Conjunctivitis/conjunctival hyperemia	60
Decreased sensorium	59
Rigors/chills	55
Vaginal hyperemia	40
Pelvic tenderness	26

Laboratory tests

Findings are nonspecific. Blood cultures are often negative, though cervical culture may reveal the presence of the offending organism. Serum albumin is often low. Multisystem organ dysfunction is noted by the presence of abnormal liver, muscle, and sometimes kidney function tests. Low platelets may also be noted.

The clinical course of TSS consists of progressive deterioration with increasing levels of shock. A diffuse capillary leak syndrome often develops with adult respiratory distress syndrome, renal failure, and multisystem organ failure as defined above. Despite this, the prognosis is usually favorable. Five to ten

percent of patients die from TSS.

Treatment

The treatment of TSS consists of massive fluid therapy. A CVP or Swan-Ganz line may be helpful in monitoring the situation. Antibiotics are given to eradicate the *Staph*, but there is no conclusive evidence that these shorten the course of TSS. An effective antistaphylococcal penicillin should be used such as nafcillin or oxacillin. Patients thus treated appear to have a decreased incidence of recurrent disease. All vaginal tampons or sponges must be removed. Recurrences may occur, it is thus recommended that women who have had TSS avoid the use of tampons for at least six subsequent menstrual cycles.

BACTERIAL MENINGITIS

Bacterial meningitis is defined as inflammation of the arachnoid, pia mater, and intervening cerebrospinal fluid (CSF) from bacterial infection. It extends via the subarachnoid space about the brain, spinal cord, and ventricles (open areas in the brain that collect CSF).

The most **common cause** for each individual depends upon their age. Adults are arbitrarily defined as individuals > 15 years old. In this group, *Streptococcus pneumoniae* is responsible for 30–50% of cases with *N. meningitidis* the cause of 10–25%. In sicker individuals, other organisms such as staphylococci and *Listeria monocytogenes* may be prevalent. Note that the causes of bacterial meningitis in patients less than 15 years old are often markedly different than in the adult. This younger age group will not be discussed further here. The common causes of bacterial meningitis are summarized in Table 11-2.

There are often **predisposing factors** noted in individuals who contract bacterial meningitis. Meningococcal meningitis may occur in outbreaks especially in military recruits. Pneumococcal disease has several interesting associations. Acute otitis media (middle ear infection) is noted to be present in 30%

Table 11-2. Common Causes of Meningitis

Neonates
- Gram-negative rods—50–60% (40% are *E. coli*)
- Group B *Streptococci*—20–40%

Children
- Hemophilus influenza type B—40–60%
- *Neisseria Meningitidis*—25–40%

Adults (> 15 years old)
- *Streptococcus pneumoniae*—30–50%
- *Neisseria meningitidis*—10–25%
- Others:
  - *Staphylococci*
  - *Listeria monocytogenes*

tive hydrocephalus (blockage to the drainage of CSF) can occur. Once infection is established in any part of the meninges, it spreads rapidly throughout the entire subarachnoid space.

Table 11-3. Predisposing Factors in Bacterial Meningitis

Meningococcal
- Outbreaks common
- Military recruits, institutions

Pneumococcal
- Acute otitis media—30%
- Pneumonia—25%
- Sinusitis
- Previous head injury—10%
- CSF rhinorrhea—5%
- Sickle cell anemia, asplenia
- Alcoholism—10–25% of cases

Staph Aureus
- Complication of neurosurgery
- Penetrating skull trauma
- *Staph* bacteremia (endocarditis)

Gram-negative Rods
- Post-trauma/surgery
- Spontaneous in diabetics
- Immunosuppression

of the patients and pneumonia in 25%. A pneumococcal sinusitis may be the initial focus in some patients. A previous head injury (recent or remote) is noted in 10% with CSF rhinorrhea (leakage) in 5%. Sickle cell anemia and asplenia make individuals more susceptible to pneumococcal infections in general, including meningitis. Alcoholism is present in 10–25% of adults with pneumococcal meningitis.

Staph aureus meningitis is usually a complication of a neurosurgical procedure, penetrating skull trauma, or secondary to a bacteremia (usually from endocarditis). Gram-negative rod-caused meningitis occurs following trauma, surgery, and spontaneously in immunosuppressed individuals, particularly diabetics. *Klebsiella* are responsible for 40% and *E. coli* for 30% of cases. If there is underlying malignant disease, organisms such as *Pseudomonas aeruginosa* may be more commonly seen. Table 11-3 summarizes the predisposing factors to meningitis.

In terms of **pathophysiology,** no direct invasion of brain tissue occurs by either the organism or inflammatory exudate. This is due to the effectiveness of the pial barrier. This is why cerebral abscess does NOT complicate bacterial meningitis. *If* the two do coexist, it is because the abscess has ruptured leaking into the ventricular cavity with resultant meningitis. The brain may also become congested and edematous. Ventriculitis is common; rarely, obstruc-

Diagnosis

History

The history is that of acute onset of fever, generalized headaches, vomiting, and a stiff neck. There is often antecedent or accompanying upper respiratory infection, otitis media, or pneumonia. Myalgias, backache, and general weakness are common. The patient may be confused, obtunded, or comatose. The history may be atypical with the patient merely presenting with a change in mental status.

General physical findings

These will include signs of the predisposing factors mentioned above. Signs of meningeal irritation are also present. Drowsiness, decreased mentation, and a stiff neck are common. Positive Kernig's (pain and resistance on extending the leg at the knee after flexing the thigh on the body) and Brudzinski's signs (reflex flexion of the lower limbs with passive flexion of the head on the chest) are highly suggestive of meningeal irritation. These are illustrated in Figures 11.1 and 11.2.

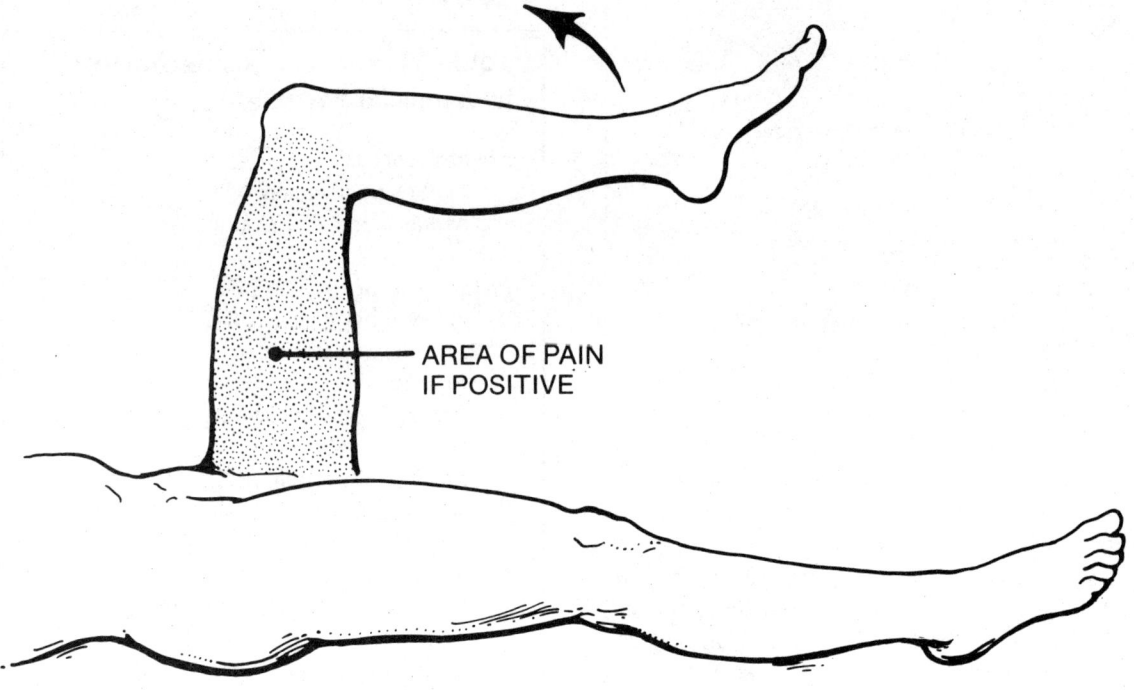

AREA OF PAIN
IF POSITIVE

The hip and knee are flexed to 90 degrees. The hip is held immobile and the knee extended. Pain in the hamstring region suggests meningeal irritation.

Figure 11.1. Kernig's sign in acute meningitis.

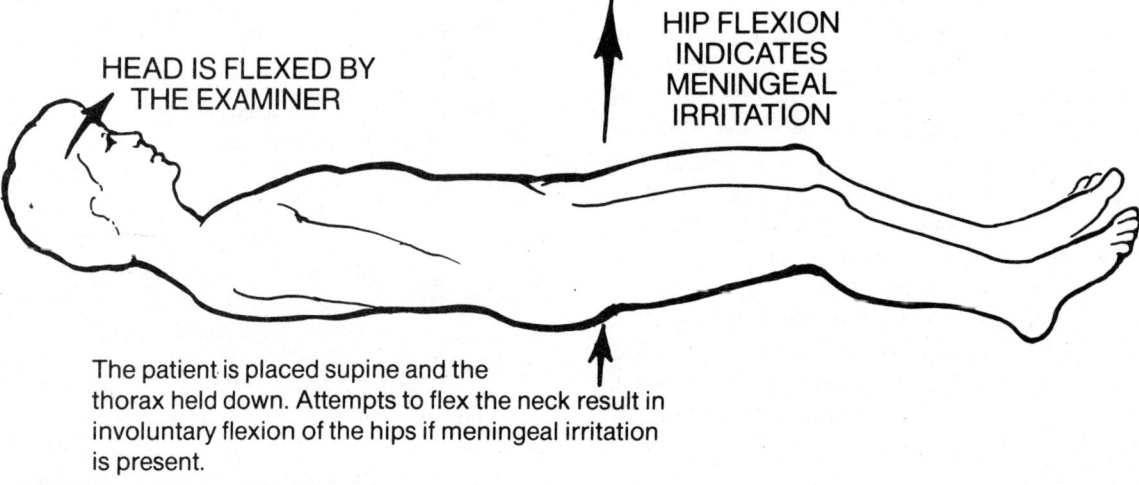

HEAD IS FLEXED BY
THE EXAMINER

HIP FLEXION
INDICATES
MENINGEAL
IRRITATION

The patient is placed supine and the thorax held down. Attempts to flex the neck result in involuntary flexion of the hips if meningeal irritation is present.

Figure 11.2. Brudzinski's sign in acute meningitis.

It is important to note that these findings can be minimal or absent in an obtunded or elderly patient. The skin should also be examined carefully for any type of petechial, purpuric, or ecchymotic rash. This is common with meningococcal infection.

Neurological findings

Neurological findings are common. Abnormalities of the cranial nerves (3, 4, 6, or 7) occur in 10–20% of patients, disappearing with treatment. Seizures are present in 20–30%. Brain swelling with increased CSF pressure can lead to abnormal reflexes, coma, hypertension, and bradycardia. Despite this, papilledema is *rare* even with increased CSF pressure. If this finding is present, you MUST rule out concomitant or other CNS infectious processes (brain abscess, subdural empyema). Focal cerebral signs (hemiparesis, dysphasia, visual field defects) are present in 15% of patients. Residual neurological damage occurs in 10–20% of victims. Table 11-4 summarizes the clinical presentation of bacterial meningitis.

Laboratory tests

Laboratory diagnosis is best made by examination of CSF obtained during lumbar puncture. The absence of papilledema should first be verified before performing this procedure. The spinal tap should be done promptly in the emergency department. The following tests should be done with the fluid:

1. CSF pressure—usually moderately increased (normal = less than 20 cm H_2O).

2. Gram stain of CSF—will demonstrate the etiologic organism in 70–80% of cases.

3. CSF culture—(+) in 80–90% of cases. Special immunological techniques are available (but not widely) that can aid in rapid identification of many organisms.

4. CSF cell count—usually 100–10,000 WBC/cubic mm with the differential showing > 80% polys. Later on, more lymphocytes are seen. Counts > 50,000 are *rare* and suggest intraventricular rupture of a cerebral abscess. Initially, WBC count may be low or close to normal, resembling the findings in the more benign viral meningitis.

Table 11-4. Clinical Presentation of Bacterial Meningitis

History
> Fever, generalized headache, vomiting, stiff neck
> Antecedent or accompanying URI, otitis, pneumonia
> Myalgias, backache, generalized weakness
> Confusion, obtundation, coma

General Physical Findings
> Signs of meningeal irritation:
> - Drowsiness, decreased mentation
> - Stiff neck
> - Positive Kernig sign (pain with leg extended and flexed on thigh)
> - Positive Brudzinski's sign (reflex leg flexion occurring with head and flexion)

Note: These may be absent or minimal in the elderly or obtunded patient.

Skin rash—petechial, purpuric, ecchymotic

Neurological Findings
> Cranial nerve abnormalities—10–20%
> Seizures—20–30%
> Abnormal reflexes, coma, HBP, bradycardia
> Papilledema *rare*
> Focal cerebral signs—15%
> Residual neurological damage in adults—10–20%

---

5. CSF glucose—generally < 40 mg% (or < 50–60% of a blood sugar drawn 15–30 minutes earlier—this time is required for equilibration to occur between the blood and CSF sugar contents). There should *always* be a comparison of the CSF glucose to the blood value as some patients (such as diabetics) may have high serum levels of blood sugar which may result in increased absolute CSF

values—the percentages will still be abnormal when compared.

6. CSF protein—usually > 100 mg/dl.
Other lab tests that should be obtained include:

a. Blood cultures may be positive, depending on the organism as follows:
■ H. influenza—80%
■ S. pneumoniae—50%
■ N. meningitidis—30–40%

b. Upper respiratory tract cultures are NOT helpful.

c. Electrolytes, BUN/creatinine

d. If extensive skin lesions are present, you should obtain clotting parameters to rule out a coagulopathy.

e. X-rays—bacterial meningitis is a life-threatening emergency requiring immediate diagnosis and rapid institution of therapy. Delay for X-rays or CT scans is generally unwarranted. Later on, after treatment has been started, a chest X-ray, sinus, and mastoid films may be appropriate.

Table 11-5 summarizes the laboratory findings in bacterial meningitis.

Treatment

General field treatment of the patient with suspected meningitis involves giving high-flow oxygen (10 LPM via mask), starting an IV of NS at a TKO rate, and transporting the patient as soon as possible to the emergency department. Again, this is a life-threatening problem and no delays are warranted.

Antibiotic treatment of meningitis is based upon the most likely bacterial cause. If an organism is seen on the CSF gram stain, appropriate therapy should be directed against it. Otherwise, treat for the most likely organism based on the clinical circumstances. The following are the adult doses for the most common causes of bacterial meningitis in this age group.

1. *Pneumococcus*—PENICILLIN G, 24 million units IV/24 hours in divided doses every 2 hours. CEFTRIAXONE (8 gm/day in 2 divided doses), CEFOTAXIME (16 gm/day in 6 divided doses), or CEFUROXIME (9 gm/day in 3 divided doses) are alternative possibilities. If a major penicillin allergy is present, use instead CHLORAMPHENICOL (CAP) 4–6 gm/day IV in 4 divided doses.

2. *Meningococcus*—PENICILLIN G is the first drug of choice. Alternatively, CHLORAMPHENICOL or CEFOTAXIME may be used. The same dosing schedules as mentioned for Pneumococcal meningitis are used.

3. *Staphylococcus*—NAFCILLIN (9 gm/day in 6 divided doses) is the first drug of choice. Either VANCOMYCIN (2 gm/day in 6 divided doses) or CEFUROXIME (9 gm/day in 3 divided doses) are acceptable alternatives.

Table 11-5. Laboratory Features of Bacterial Meningitis

CSF Examination
Pressure—moderately elevated
Gram stain—(+) 70–80% of the time
Culture—80–90% (+)
Cell count—usually 100–10,000
    WBC/cu mm; > 80% polys
Glucose—< 40 mg% or < 50–60% of
    blood sugar
Protein—usually > 100 mg/dl

Other Lab Tests
Blood cultures positive:
• Hemophilus influenzae—80%
• *Streptococcus pneumonae*—50%
• *Neisseria meningitidis*—30–40%
Upper respiratory cultures—not helpful
Electrolytes/creatinine
Clotting parameters if extensive skin
    lesions
X-ray—defer until later!

4. *Gram-negative rods* (*Pseudomonas, E. coli, Klebsiella,* etc.)—most experts recommend starting with a combination of a third-generation cephalosporin agent (such as Ceftazidime) and an aminoglycoside (such as amikacin) until susceptibilities are determined. It is recommended that the reader consult with appropriate local infectious disease experts to determine specific area sensitivity patterns.

5. *Listeria*—AMPICILLIN 2 gms IV every 4 hours, combined with gentamicin, 1.5 mg/kg IV every 8 hours may be ideal, though many opt to go with ampicillin alone.

Presumptive therapy in adults may be guided as follows:

1. Otherwise healthy, less than 45 years old; SUSPECT *Strep pneumonia*, or *Neisseria meningitidis*. Penicillin G is the first drug of choice.

2. Elderly, cirrhotic, diabetic, or patient with other underlying disease; SUSPECT *Strep pneumoniae*, gram-negative bacilli, *Staphylococcus*, or *Listeria*. Cefotaxime and ampicillin should provide adequate preliminary coverage.

3. Trauma, neurosurgery; SUSPECT gram-negative bacilli, *Staph aureus, Strep pneumoniae*, unusual or resistant gram-negative bacilli (such as *Pseudomonas*). A combination of nafcillin or vancomycin plus cefotaxime is recommended. Some would also add gentamicin.

4. Hospital-acquired infection or immunosuppressed patient; SUSPECT *Listeria*, in addition to those mentioned for trauma, neurosurgery. Amikacin (5 mg/kg IV every 8 hours) IV as well as intrathecally (in the spinal fluid) plus piperacillin or ticarcillin (75 mg/kg every 6 hours) are recommended. Many would also add vancomycin to this high-risk group of patients until culture results are available.

Prognosis is determined by many factors. With treatment, the mortality in meningococcal disease is 10% and in pneumococcal meningitis, 25%. Poor prognostic factors include advanced age, the presence of other foci of infection, underlying disease (leukemia, alcoholism), coma, and a *delay* in instituting therapy.

Chemoprophylaxis for close contacts of a patient with known meningococcal disease (same household, same day-care center, mouth-to-mouth resuscitation) is absolutely necessary. These exposures can lead to infection in the exposed individual within four days so prophylaxis should be begun as soon as the initial case is identified. RIFAMPIN 600 mg twice daily for two days in adults is 80–90% effective in preventing infection.

Pearls to Remember

Keep in mind that:

1. Obtunded or elderly patients with congestive heart failure or pneumonia can develop meningitis without prominent meningeal signs. Lethargy should be investigated carefully.

2. The presence of a petechial, purpuric, or ecchymotic rash in a patient with meningeal findings almost always implies the presence of meningococcal infection requiring prompt therapy.

3. If bacterial meningitis is suspected and the initial spinal tap is negative or nonspecific AND the patient does not improve, consider repeating the tap in 24 hours. Bacterial meningitis can initially present with benign appearing CSF (unusual but it does occur).

SEPTIC ARTHRITIS

Septic arthritis is defined as an acute infection in a joint space with resultant accumulation of excess joint fluid (effusion), white blood cells (WBCs), and microorganisms. Usually, only one isolated joint is involved with the exception of gonococcal arthritis (see below). The consequences of failure to treat septic arthritis may be devastating—joint destruction, disseminated infection, and death.

Sources of infection include spread from contiguous abrasions and lacerations (such as from a "fight bite"). Most commonly, though, the joint is "seeded" from hematogenous spread of a microorganism. The **commonest organism** in adult age 15–40 is *Neisseria gonorrhoeae*. Following this are *Staph aureus* (35%), *Streptococci* (10%), and GNR (5%).

Predisposing factors are often present in cases of septic arthritis:

- Extra-articular infection [49%]
- Previous joint damage (rheumatoid, etc) [27%]
- Serious underlying disease (CA, liver) [19%]
- Previous antibiotic therapy [20%]
- Immunosuppressive or steroid Rx [50%].

Diagnosis

History

The history is that of pain, redness, and swelling usually occurring over 2–3 days. There is decreased joint mobility. Most commonly, only one joint is involved. The knee or hip is most likely. A multiarticular presentation is more common in *N. gonorrhoeae* (GC) infection. Systemic symptoms may include weakness, malaise, and fever. There may be complaints referable to concomitant infections—skin, sinus, ear, lung, or venereal diseases.

Physical examination

The physical examination reveals mono or polyarticular arthritis with warmth, swelling, and joint effusion. The temperature is elevated over 100°F in 90% of victims. The skin should be checked carefully for vesicular lesions with dark (necrotic) centers suggesting gonorrhea.

Laboratory tests

General laboratory evaluation will show WBC elevation in 70% of patients. All possible foci of infection should be cultured, as in 49% of cases the organism

will be recovered. An X-ray of the involved joint(s) should be done but not on an acute basis. **Synovial fluid aspiration** using sterile technique and a large-bore (#18) needle is the next step. Hip joint aspiration should be performed by an orthopedic surgeon. Aspiration is done as soon as possible in the emergency department. The following parameters are evaluated in the fluid:

1. *Culture*—inoculate as soon as possible. Be sure to include anaerobic and GC cultures.

2. *Gram stain*—the type of initial therapy is made based on this.

3. *Glucose*—usually < 50% of the serum level. It may be WNL in GC arthritis.

4. *Cell count/differential*—ranges widely; 40% of patients have a WBC > 100,000 (mostly polys). There is an overlap between infectious arthritis and acute inflammatory arthritis (gout, rheumatoid). Infection is *highly* unlikely if the joint fluid WBC is < 2500 WBC/cu mm.

If the patient is seen by the prehospital care provider, the joint should be gently supported and the patient brought to the emergency department as soon as possible. **Initial antibiotic therapy** is based upon the gram stain results. Therapy should be begun within two hours of initial presentation and is given intravenously. Culture results may lead to later modification of antibiotic schedules. For all patients greater than 15 years old, the following are recommended as initial treatments of choice (the second antibiotic listed is the choice in a patient who is allergic to the first one):

1. *Gram-positive cocci (Staph/Strep)*—Nafcillin 150 mg/kg/24 h in divided doses every 6 hours; Cephalothin 100 mg/kg/24 h in divided doses every 6 hours.

2. *Gram-negative cocci (GC)*—Penicillin G, 10 million units IV every 6 hours; Erythromycin 1 gm IV every 6 hours.

3. *Gram-negative rods (E. Coli, Klebsiella)*—Gentamicin 5 mg/kg/24 h IV every 8 hours. It is imperative to obtain serum lev-

els (peak and trough) when aminoglycoside antibiotics are used.

In all patients with a negative gram stain but the clinical picture of a septic joint, penicillin is given if the patient is less than 40 (to cover GC) in the dose outlined above (erythromycin if the patient is allergic to PCN). If the individual is over 40, then nafcillin or cephalothin are given to cover the most likely organism, *Staph aureus*. Analgesics that don't affect the fever curve (codeine, propoxyphene) should also be given. Nonsteroidal anti-inflammatory agents will alter the fever and should be avoided.

Gonococcal (GC) arthritis is very common and may have severe associated systemic toxicity. Polyarthritis and monoarthritis appear in this entity with almost equal frequency. Pustulovesicular lesions that develop a necrotic (black) central eschar are present in 44% of cases. Tenosynovitis (inflammation of tendon and joint membranes) is noted in about 68% of persons. Cultures of all possible sources should be obtained. Positive results may be expected as follows:

- Synovial fluid—60%
- Urethra—81%
- Blood—24%
- Rectum—13%
- Pharynx—17%.

BACTERIAL INFECTIONS OF SKELETAL MUSCLE AND CONTIGUOUS STRUCTURES

These infections represent a continuum with different degrees of severity. The exact terminology employed depends on the extent of tissue involvement and damage. Included under this general category are bacterial myositis (muscle infection), cellulitis (infection of the skin and subcutaneous tissues), fasciitis (infection of the fascia), and clostridial myonecrosis (gas gangrene).

These infections are often preceded by a penetrating wound or local trauma. There is an increased predisposition in patients with poor arterial circulation (diabetics, peripheral arterial disease). The **cause of the infection** in microbiological terms are often gram-positive cocci. There is usually a mixture of aerobic, anerobic, and facultatively aerobic streptococci. *Staph aureus*, gram-positive rods (i.e., *Clostridium*), and gram-negative rods are also responsible at times. The *most frequent cause of gas in the tissues* is one of the gram-negative aerobic bacteria, often *E. coli;* nonetheless, the presence of clostridial infection (gas gangrene) MUST be ruled out.

Diagnosis

History
The history usually relates a penetrating wound or some other type of local trauma. Symptoms of local infection in the extremity (or other area) for less than a week are noted. Pain is progressive and severe. Swelling in the region of the wound is noted along with lethargy, chills, and fever. The patient may be aware of a foul odor to the secretions of the wound or lesion. It is important to determine if the patient has ever been diabetic. There appears to be a strong link between clostridial myonecrosis and malignancy. Thus, a history of neoplastic disease must also be sought.

Physical examination
On physical examination, the patient appears quite ill. Despite this, the fever may be only modestly elevated. Lethargy, toxemia, and dementia may be present and appear to be out of proportion to other physical findings of infection. There is often marked swelling of the involved tissues. They are very tender as a rule—tenderness and pain is often decreased, and sometimes lacking altogether, in diabetics. Progressive discoloration leading to a "sickish" purple-bluish hue is noted. There may be bullae and crepitation of the overlying skin, indicating the presence of gas in the deeper tissues. Secretions often have a rancid odor.

Laboratory tests
Laboratory examination will reveal a markedly increased WBC. The blood sugar should be checked at initial presentation. Previously undiagnosed diabetics commonly can present with this type of an infection.

X-ray may show gas in the tissues. Gas bubbles immediately around the wound or a surgical site are of questionable significance. If visible along fascial planes, you should be very concerned! Material for culture (aerobic and anaerobic) and gram stain should be obtained. Unbroken bullae should be aspirated. Draining areas need to be swabbed, and needle aspiration of deeper tissues done. The gram stain leads to a correct diagnosis in a high percentage of cases. Blood cultures should also be obtained.

Treatment

These infections are MEDICAL AND SURGICAL EMERGENCIES! A fatal outcome can result with great rapidity.

Prehospital treatment consists of high-flow O_2 (10–15 LPM via mask), an IV of D_5W at a TKO rate, and rapid transportation. In the hospital the following should be done:

1. PROMPT SURGICAL CONSULTATION!

2. Immediate antibiotic therapy after viewing the gram stain:

   a. Gram positive or no organisms—Penicillin 10–12 million U IV every 6 hours (use CAP if allergic).

   b. Gram negative (With or without gas in the tissues)—CAP 4 gm/24 h + an aminoglycoside (such as gentamicin 3–5 mg/kg/24 h in divided doses every 8 hours). It is important to obtain serum levels (peak and trough) when aminoglycosides are used.

   c. Some authors recommend the addition of either carbenicillin or ticarcillin to the above regimens.

3. Tetanus prophylaxis.

4. Hyperbaric oxygen may be helpful if conveniently available. Controlled clinical studies do NOT exist that adequately demonstrate the efficacy of this often employed therapy.

5. Polyvalent gas gangrene antitoxin should NOT be used; no clinical studies prove its efficacy and serum sickness is a common result.

Diving Emergencies

Diving is rapidly gaining in popularity throughout the country. Because of the transportation conveniences of our society, it is also possible for individuals to have the rapid mobility necessary for some postdiving problems (such as flying in an airplane shortly after diving) to occur. This chapter is not designed to be an extensive treatise on diving emergencies but, rather, a brief review of potential problems that may be seen by any emergency care provider. The types of problems we will discuss are related to the breathing of compressed air under water. Topics to be discussed include:

- Diving physiology
- General principles
- Air embolism
- Nitrogen narcosis
- Decompression sickness
- The "squeeze"
- Hyperpnea exhaustion syndrome
- Differential diagnosis of diving accidents.

DIVING PHYSIOLOGY

When diving, an individual is exposed to atmospheric pressures greater than those on land. This results in contraction of the gases in the lungs. As a rough estimate, pressure increases about one pound per square inch (psi) with each 2 feet of depth. The exact figures are 0.445 psi per foot in saltwater and 0.432 psi per foot in freshwater.

To compensate, air must be taken in from self-contained underwater breathing apparatus (SCUBA) so that the lungs will not collapse. The events discussed here can also occur with *any* source of compressed air used for breathing—SCUBA gear, a hose from the surface, a bucket, or air trapped in a submerged car.

The term "atmosphere" (ATM) is used as an arbitrary unit of pressure. At sea level, the pressure on the body is 1 ATM. At 33 feet of water depth (34 feet in fresh water), it is 2 ATM, 3 ATM at 66 feet, etc. **Boyle's law** states that the volume of a gas varies inversely with the absolute pressure. In other words, as the pressure increases, the gas volume decreases. If a pair of lungs contains 2,000 cc of air at sea level, this volume will decrease with descent—1,000 cc at 33 feet, 500 cc at 66 feet, etc.

If a SCUBA tank is added to normal lungs at sea level, the volume of air in the lungs stays constant as the diver forcefully inhales supplemental air from the tank. Thus, the volume in the lungs remains constant, regardless of depth (assuming proper breathing techniques).

If the diver ascends, but forgets to exhale on the way up, the pressure will decrease with ascent and the volume of gas "trapped" (due to failure of exhalation) in the lungs will expand. Thus, if a diver at 33 feet with a combined lung volume of 4,000 cc ascends and fails to exhale, the total lung volume at sea level will be 8,000 cc! Figure 12.1 illustrates diving applications of Boyle's law.

Other hazards are also associated with breath-holding during diving. As one descends, more oxygen is made available to the tissue due to the increased pressure. At depth, one's breath-holding ability is thus markedly increased. With ascent, the drop in pressure of the tissue oxygen supply decreases sharply. This may lead to a sudden loss of consciousness, upon surfacing, in a diver who has pushed his limits at depths in terms of improper breathing. This has been called "shallow water blackout." Thus, a cardinal rule of scuba diving is that *a diver must never hold his or her breath while underwater!*

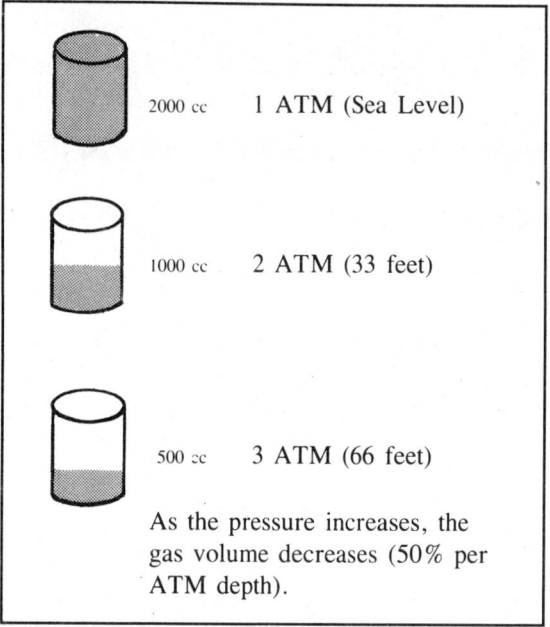

2000 cc   1 ATM (Sea Level)

1000 cc   2 ATM (33 feet)

500 cc   3 ATM (66 feet)

As the pressure increases, the gas volume decreases (50% per ATM depth).

Figure 12.1. Boyle's law of gases as applied to diving.

Henry's law states that a constant temperature, the solubility of any gas in a liquid, is almost directly proportional to the pressure of the liquid. In other words, the deeper one dives, the greater the pressure and the greater the soluble gas (i.e., nitrogen) that becomes dissolved in the blood and tissue fluids. The reverse occurs on ascent. It may take a much longer period of time for the gas to revaporize upon ascent than it did to originally dissolve in the fluid. Thus, a certain time is required for dissolved nitrogen to properly resume the gaseous phase.

GENERAL PRINCIPLES

It is extremely important to take an adequate **his-**

tory on any patient potentially suffering an emergency related to diving. The first question one *must* ask: Did the victim breathe compressed air under water? Remember, this can occur with SCUBA gear, a surface hose, bucket, or within a submerged car. Make *certain* the patient was not just snorkeling and that you are really dealing with a near-drowning victim (see Chapter 3, Respiratory Emergencies)!

A detailed history of the *entire diving day* is necessary in order to give the best possible care. If the patient needs to be sent to a hyperbaric (decompression) chamber, this information will be vital. The number of dives, depth of each, and bottom time are important. The type of equipment used as well as the diver's activities should be noted (hard work increases the risk of certain problems). Environmental factors, such as type of water and the conditions as well as the type of water entry, may be significant. It is useful to know if the diver was with a companion (who should then also be questioned) and exactly what type of gas mixture was being breathed. You also need to ask if in-water recompression was attempted. Finally, the examiner should note if the diver flew in an airplane or jogged before developing symptoms (either can precipitate "the bends").

AIR EMBOLISM

Air embolism is defined as the presence of air bubbles in the central circulation. It is the most serious of diving-related emergencies. The **cause** is breath-holding on ascent with resultant expansion of air in the lungs. As the lung tissue expands, alveoli eventually rupture, resulting in the escape of air.

Though it may certainly occur, pneumothorax is not a necessary consequence of alveolar rupture. Interstitial air occurs first which can track anywhere in the body including the pleural space (pneumothorax), pericardial space (pneumomediastinum), and distant sites via the bloodstream (air embolus). Since divers most commmonly ascend in a vertical position, bubbles of air in the bloodstream often travel to the brain. This can occur during an ascent from as little as four feet of water!

Air embolism may also occur in divers with lung conditions that result in local air trapping—any lung infection, lung cysts, tumors, scar tissue, mucous plugs (asthma), and obstructive lung disease. Smokers, for unknown reasons, have an increased risk as well. Table 12.1 illustrates the pathophysiology of air embolism.

Signs and symptoms of air embolism include chest tightness and shortness of breath. Pink frothy sputum may be noted coming from the nose and mouth. Vertigo, paresthesias, paralysis, seizures, and loss of consciousness may be noted in cerebral emboli. Findings tend to appear suddenly during or immediately after surfacing and may resemble a stroke. Signs and symptoms of tension pneumothorax may also be present.

Table 12-1. Pathophysiology of Air Emboli

Breath-holding on ascent leads to:
- Overexpansion of air in the lungs
- Air trapping, localized or generalized
- Rupture of lung tissue
- Escape of air into the bronchial circulation which then passes through the heart, entering the central circulation
- Pneumothorax may or may not occur

Treatment

The treatment of suspected air embolism is as follows:

1. High-flow O_2 (mask 10–15 LPM; 100% if possible); beware of using positive pressure devices with the possibility of an untreated pneumothorax.

2. Emergency needle thoracostomy if a tension pneumothorax is present—use the second intercostal space (ICS-2) in the midclavicular line. A chest tube may be placed when the situation is stabilized.

3. Trendelenberg position (feet elevated) with the patient on his left side (left lateral decubitus position) is used to attempt to trap air within the heart and prevent it from traveling to the brain, causing cerebral embolism.

4. Recompression should be attempted as soon as possible. The National Diving Accident Network (DAN) provides a 24-hour number (919-684-8111). The network phone is answered by the Duke University Hospital operator who then refers the caller to the DAN on-call person. Physicians who specialize in diving medicine are available for consultation if necessary as well.

   Alternatively, one can call the U.S. Navy Experimental Diving Unit (US-NEDU) [1-202-433-2790] at any hour of the day or night and ask for the duty officer. DO NOT attempt recompression in the water! This may lead to incomplete recompression and increased loading of dissolved nitrogen.

NITROGEN NARCOSIS

Nitrogen narcosis, often referred to as "rapture of the depths," is the development of an apathetic, slightly euphoric mental state due to the narcotic effect of dissolved nitrogen (N_2). This effect is analagous to excessive ethanol levels. The **cause** of this is a result of Henry's law.

As the pressure increases (i.e., the depth of descent), so does the amount of dissolved N_2 (which is normally 79% of room air). The greater the depth, the greater the amount of N_2 dissolved and the "high" achieved. Mild effects may be noted at as low as 50 feet of water depth. This problem has been referred to as "martini's law": the mental effects of each 50 feet of descent, while breathing compressed air, are approximately equivalent to those of one dry martini. As depth increases, so does the severity of the **signs and symptoms.**

At 125–150 feet, narcosis usually begins. At 150–200 feet, the diver exhibits drowsiness and decreased mental functioning. At 200–250 feet, there is decreased strength and coordination, and at 300 feet, the diver is essentially "useless." At depths between 250–400 feet, unconsciousness and death can occur. Generally speaking, recreational divers should descend no deeper than 100–150 feet.

Treatment

The treatment of this problem involves gradual ascent to shallower water. Assistance from one's diving companion (NEVER DIVE ALONE!) is usually necessary. This problem may be prevented by avoiding dives to excess depths.

DECOMPRESSION SICKNESS

Decompression sickness is an illness occurring during or after ascent secondary to rapid release of nitrogen bubbles. The **cause** is a sudden decrease in environmental pressure from a too-rapid ascent. This releases previously absorbed excess N_2 from the tissues into the bloodstream in the form of bubbles.

The "cola-bottle" analogy is helpful in understanding what is thought to occur. An undisturbed bottle of cola can have the cap slowly removed without any fizzing or bubbling. If allowed to sit, the carbon dioxide within it will gradually equilibrate with the atmosphere, and the soda will go "flat." If, on the other hand, the bottle is shaken before opening it, or the cap rapidly removed, bubbles form. This is similar to what occurs in the bends. One can imagine the diver somehow "shaken" with resultant nitrogen bubble formation. Multiple factors appear to be responsible for the development of decompression sickness in one diver and not in another who had had equal bottom time.

Many feel that the bends occur when the tissues become "supersaturated" with inert gas, such as nitrogen. As pressure is reduced, these gases will leave via the lungs. This takes a while, though, and if the pressure changes too rapidly, the "unloading process" will fall behind. Thus, the partial pressure of gas in the tissue far exceeds that of the ambient pressure and supersaturation exists. Rapid pressure changes favor the formation of bubbles as tissue supersaturated with gas attempts to release it and equilibrate the pressure. Only small degrees of this can be tolerated.

The "coke-bottle" analogy has also been applied to explain supersaturation. Before the cap is removed, gases are dissolved quietly in solution. Removing the cap leads to a sudden drop in pressure, and a state of supersaturation with resultant bubbling.

Current research suggests that more may actually be involved than the physical occlusive effects of gas bubbles. Hemoconcentration in the microcirculation occurs even in asymptomatic divers, as do venous gas emboli. This commonly clears within a few minutes of surfacing. Platelet aggregation may also play a role.

The microcirculation of the spinal cord venous plexus is especially favorable for the formation of gas bubbles. This may explain why patients with the bends tend to have spinal cord symptoms that resolve with time—venous occlusion has a far better prognosis than does arterial blockage [*Phys & Sport Med*, 1986, Vol. 14, p. 196].

Most cases of decompression sickness are due to repetitive diving, i.e., greater than one dive in a 12-hour period. It takes about 12 hours for a liquid to become completely desaturated of a gas. Thus, cumulative effects occur when a diver enters the water more than one time within this period.

Within the first hour of ascent, 85% of the **signs and symptoms** occur. Very few people develop new symptoms or initial symptoms greater than 3 hours following ascent. Up to 1% of patients may present later than 24 hours.

There are a variety of symptoms that may be noted affecting many organ systems. These result both from the physical effects of N_2 bubbles in the lung tissues and the activation of numerous body systems, including the intrinsic clotting, kinin, and complement systems. These responses lead to platelet activation, cellular clumping, lipid emboli, increased vascular permeability, interstitial edema, and microvascular sludging. The net effect is a decrease in tissue perfusion and ischemia. A vicious cycle can result with decreased perfusion leading to tissue hypoxia and interstitial edema, which further decreases perfusion.

1. Skin—a blotchy red rash on the torso may be present. The patient may complain of burning, prickly, or mottled skin (the "itches"). This is due to subcutaneous air bubbles.

2. Pain in the legs or joints is present in 90% of cases (the "bends"). The most commonly involved joint is the shoulder, though multiple joints may be involved in serious cases. Recurrent pains are common.

3. Dizziness (the "staggers"), vertigo, visual, or hearing abnormalities may be noted in up to 5% of patients.

4. Paralysis occurs in 2% of victims; permanent sequelae are possible though uncommon. The development of spinal cord manifestations may be preceded by abdominal pain.

5. Shortness of breath (the "chokes") may occur in up to 2% of patients. A firey red pharynx (back of throat) is noted, and there may be pleuritic chest pain and a nonproductive cough. Spinal cord symptoms commonly accompany this, warranting careful neurologic evaluation as well.

6. Collapse is present in .5–1% of victims. Death, if it occurs, is usually from a cardiovascular cause. A delayed shock syndrome with pulmonary edema (adult respiratory distress syndrome) can occur 1–3 hours later.

Factors which increase the severity of the signs and symptoms include: extremes of water temperature, increasing age, and obesity. Fatigue, poor conditioning, alcohol ingestion, and heavy work during diving may also play a role. A previous case of decompression sickness may increase one's susceptibility to recurrence.

Diagnosis

Laboratory and X-ray findings may include right heart enlargement on the chest X-ray. Blood gases reveal hypoxia, and hypocarbia (low pCO_2) with a metabolic acidosis, suggesting a metabolic component (see Appendix C).

Treatment

To treat decompression sickness:

1. Contact either DAN or the USNEDU to arrange for *immediate* transportation to a decompression chamber.

2. *Total* bed rest in the combined Trendelenberg and left lateral decubitus position—transport and KEEP the patient in this position at all times!

3. 100% O_2 via mask.

4. IV D_5 NS at a TKO rate—increase as necessary for hypotension (which is common if the condition is severe). In serious cases, judicious fluid administration may help hemoconcentration. Low molecular weight dextran has been shown to improve flow in the microcirculation and minimize platelet aggregation but cannot be universally advised at this time. DON'T use D_5W alone (due to the possibility of increased intracranial pressure).

5. Cardiac monitor.

6. IV $NaHCO_3$ if the pH is less than 7.10.

7. Steroids may be advised to treat cerebral swelling if central nervous system signs are present. Work demonstrating definitive efficacy is lacking, though.

8. If a chamber is not available, the patient can be closely monitored, following the steps outlined above. This is NOT recommended.

9. Some experts recommend giving 2 aspirin (325 mg each) as an antiplatelet agent to conscious patients. There is not uniform consensus on this matter.

Pearls to Remember

Keep in mind that:

1. Any complaint of joint soreness (in the absence of obvious injury) 24–48 hours after a dive should be considered for decompression therapy. At the minimum, a diving medicine consultation should be obtained.

2. Decompression sickness can occur at depths less than 33 feet. They are more likely if the diver has been below that depth with sufficient bottom time to permit supersaturation of the body tissues with inert N_2 gas. One should suspect air embolism in symptomatic divers who have been at depths < 33 feet and whose dive times are well within the U.S. Navy Dive Tables.

3. Common errors include a victim's failure to report signs and symptoms, failure to treat a patient in questionable cases, and failure to identify severe symptoms as resulting from a diving accident.

4. Prevention of diving accidents may be achieved by not diving too deeply or staying down too long. As a minimum, the U.S. Navy Repetitive Dive and Decompression Tables should be followed.

   Unfortunately, most sport divers do not take into consideration the fact that the Navy tables were designed for young, male military personnel. Additionally, these were intended to be used in ocean diving only. They do not apply for freshwater, and at any altitude above sea level. Thus, the Navy tables DO NOT provide an adequate margin of safety for the average sport diver. Divers should ALWAYS carry a SCUBA ID card for at least 48 hours after a dive.

   Finally, it is unwise to fly in an unpressurized aircraft for at least 24 hours following a dive. It is worth keeping in mind that correctly functioning commercial aircraft pressurize their cabins to about 8,000 feet. Thus, exact waiting times vary, depending on the bottom time.

5. If the patient needs to be air evacuated, the pilot should be instructed to fly as close to the ground as possible (1,000 feet are recommended). If the aircraft is pressurized, the cabin pressure should be kept as near to sea level as possible. It is best to use an airplane (either helicopter or fixed-wing) that is capable of cabin pressurization to 1 ATM (Lear Jet or Hercules C130). Be sure to bring the patient's equipment along and give to the hyperbaric medical experts.

6. If paralysis involves both sides of the body (i.e., both hands, legs, etc.—it transverses ACROSS the body), suspect decompression trauma with a spinal cord syndrome. If loss of sensation or motion is unilateral, the odds favor an air embolus to the brain.

7. Late recompression (even 10 days or greater) or decompression sickness problems can be accomplished with relief of symptoms and morbidity. Long delays are common in the lay diving population because of the lack of recognition of symptoms and "wishful thinking" that symptoms will "go away." [*Ann Emerg Med,* March 1985, Vol. 14, pp. 254–257].

"THE SQUEEZE"

This is defined as "severe pain" caused by compression of air trapped in hollow "chambers." The **cause** is breath-holding on descent or air getting trapped in a hollow cavity. These symptoms occur when the outside pressure is greater than that inside the body. Though not the most severe potential adverse effects of diving, these are the most common. They may occur in these areas:

1. *Ears, sinuses*—secondary to blocked eustachian tubes, sinus ostia (openings), or external ear canals. The trapped air is then compressed with resultant painful bulging of the tympanic membrane (eardrum). This usually occurs early in the dive.

   Rupture of the eardrum can occur. If the diver is bareheaded, cold water can rush in, markedly effecting one's balance leading to vertigo and nausea. Devastating circumstances may result.

2. *Lungs, airways, and thoracic cavity—* usually occurs during "free diving" (diving without a compressed air source). It is rare nowadays because this practice is not common. If symptoms develop (crushing chest pain), they are often at great depths.

3. *Teeth* (cavities, dental abscesses).

4. *Added air spaces*—face mask, wet suit—at times, severe bruising of the skin can occur. The eyes and eyelid linings are the most susceptible to damage, especially if only goggles, which have no method of pressure equalization, are used for anything but very shallow diving. A tight diving suit covering the external ear canal can result in "squeeze" of the canal with possible tympanic membrane rupture.

5. "Gut" squeeze does not occur commonly due to the fact that the structures of the gastrointestinal tract have supple walls which are easily compressed. Expansion within the GI tract with ascent may lead to discomfort, though. Significant flatulence or diarrhea can occur at this time. This usually occurs in novice divers who swallow a lot of air or those who ate heartily before diving.

Signs and symptoms include pain, edema, rupture, and bleeding, depending on the area involved. The **treatment** is gradual ascent to shallower depths, reassurance, and analgesics as needed. Decongestant medications may be helpful. Antibiotics should be administered if infection or eardrum rupture are present or if the diver was swimming in polluted water.

HYPERPNEA-EXHAUSTION SYNDROME

This is a syndrome of exhaustion and fear secondary to diver fatigue. The **signs and symptoms** include tachypnea, anxiety, feelings of impending doom, difficulty floating, and exhaustion. The **treatment** consists of ascent to the surface and rest aboard a flotation device or boat.

DIFFERENTIAL DIAGNOSIS OF DIVING ACCIDENTS

It is helpful to think of a dive as being divided into five stages, each of which is associated with particular potential problems:

1. *The predive surface phase*—This may include considerable surface swimming to the site. Motion sickness, hyperventilation, physical trauma, near-drowning, and marine animal encounters may occur.

2. *Descent phase*—Squeeze syndromes (especially involving the ears) and gas-associated problems (such as carbon monoxide poisoning or hypoxia due to faulty equipment) commonly occur at this point.

3. *At-depth or bottom phase*—Either physical trauma or encounters with dangerous marine life may occur. If nitrogen narcosis ensues, it is at this phase in the dive. It should also be remembered that divers are highly susceptible to the dangers of hypothermia.

4. *Ascent phase*—Barotrauma ("squeeze") syndromes occur here but less commonly than with descent. Decompression sickness may begin to occur during ascent. If it does, it is usually very serious in nature.

5. *Postdive surface phase*—This is divided into two subphases:
   a. *Immediate* (within 10 minutes of surfacing)—Air embolism is the cause of problems at this time until proven otherwise. Other potential problems may include: pneumothorax or related entities, motion sickness, exhaustion, or irritant reactions to marine flora/fauna.

b. *Delayed* (after 10 minutes)—Decompression sickness is the "culprit" of any problems at this time until proven otherwise. More than 50% of patients will be symptomatic within the first hour following ascent, though 1–2% may note their first symptoms at 24–48 hours.

SUMMARY OF TREATMENT FOR DIVING EMERGENCIES

It is worth keeping in mind some basic tenets for *all* diving-related problems:

1. 100% oxygen by nonrebreather mask.

2. Always rule out pneumothorax.

3. Left lateral decubitus-Trendelenberg position.

4. Communication with DAN (919-684-8111) and appropriate transport to a treatment facility.

5. Cardiac monitor, IV fluids, etc. as needed.

A few selected references should be mentioned that will be of particular help to the interested reader, in addition to those noted in the bibliography:

1. *Field Guide for the Diver Medic,* Daugherty, C. G.; National Association of Diver Medical Technicians, 1983. This book is the official field guide for this organization and contains much on prehospital care and diving emergencies that is very helpful.

2. *The Skin Diver's Bible,* Lee, O.; Doubleday & Company, 1986. Well-written and up to date with many illustrations.

3. *The New Science of Skin and Scuba Diving,* Council for National Cooperation in Aquatics, Smith, R. W., editor; New Century Publishers, Inc., 1985. Has some excellent illustrations of diving physiology and underwater wildlife.

Synthesis: A Generalized Approach

It is the goal of this final section to "put together" some of the previous material as well as the general approach to the patient. A systematic and general approach to three common emergency care situations will be presented:

- The breathless patient
- Nontraumatic coma
- The "shocky" patient.

THE BREATHLESS PATIENT

The breathless patient is defined, for our purposes, as a person having either difficulty breathing or shortness of breath from a nontraumatic cause. Potential **causes** of this problem are:

1. *Obstruction*—either complete (as in the "cafe coronary") or incomplete.

2. *Hyperventilation*—remember that pulmonary and cardiac disease can lead to hyperventilation. Central nervous system problems, anxiety, drugs (aspirin, amphetamines), septic shock, fever, anemia, and acidosis can also cause hyperventilation.

3. *Cardiac*—chest pain, myocardial infarction, pulmonary edema, congestive heart failure, arrhythmias.

4. *Respiratory*—asthma, COPD, pneumothorax, pneumonia, pulmonary embolism, pleurisy, allergy, anaphylaxis.

Diagnosis

History
The diagnostic approach to the breathless patient first involves obtaining a brief history. Are the symptoms acute or chronic? Is there a history of heart or lung problems? Is the patient on any medicines? Has there been any past allergic reactions? Is home oxygen in use?

It is also important to ascertain if patients have had recent surgery which would make them more susceptible to either pulmonary embolism or infection. Associated symptoms, such as chest pain and paresthesias of the mouth and hands, should be sought.

Physical examination
The general physical examination involves checking the vital signs, evaluating the level of consciousness, and observing for cyanosis, drooling, coughing, inspiratory stridor, irrational behavior, and poor cooperation (a sign of hypoxia). One should note unusual sounds of respiration:

- *Stridor* is a high-pitched musical inspiratory noise representing the presence of partial obstruction of the upper airway.
- *Hoarseness* is caused by any process leading to inflammation and edema of the larynx.
- *Gurgling noises* are produced by liquids in the airway, regardless of type.
- *Snoring* signifies upper airway obstruction.

159

■ *Cough* just indicates any inflammatory, chemical, mechanical, or thermal stimulation of the cough receptors [Rosen, et al., *Emergency Medicine—Concepts and Clinical Practice*, 1985].

The examiner should be on the lookout for signs of congestive heart failure (CHF) such as distended neck veins when the patient is upright, wet lung sounds, and peripheral edema. Signs of trauma are noted if present. The presence of hives, airway edema, and sputum production is ascertained.

Respirations are then evaluated on the basis of **respiratory pattern.** Different types of patterns suggest various etiologies:

■ *Agonal respirations* are slow, weak, shallow, and gasping with a rapid inspiratory component. These indicate terminal respiratory distress and usually mean that immediate airway control is required.
■ *Cheyne-Stokes respirations* are phasic in nature; they involve rapid, peaking crescendo-decrescendo patterns followed by pauses. These usually indicate a metabolic derangement though they may also occur with neurologic or cardiac disease.
■ *Chaotic (or ataxic) respirations* are irregular with varying volumes and indicate anatomic or metabolic disturbance of the central nervous system respiratory center (pons, medulla).
■ *Kussmaul respirations* are deep, regular, and rapid. These represent an attempt to compensate any severe metabolic acidosis with deep respirations. These patterns are summarized in Figure 13.1.

Auscultation of the lungs is straightforward. There are three major types of breath sounds.

■ *Wheezes* are high-pitched, squeaky sounds which may be heard on either inspiration or expiration. In asthmatics, wheezing may be audible without a stethoscope.
■ *Rhonchi* are course, groaning sounds originating from larger airways. Wheezes

as a rule, on the other hand, are from smaller airways.
■ *Rales* are bubbly or crackling sounds that emanate from the alveoli.

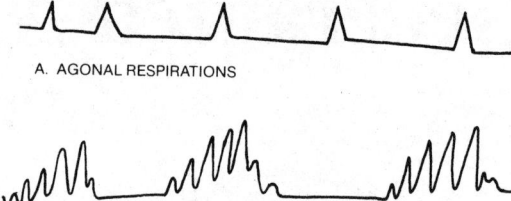

A. AGONAL RESPIRATIONS

B. CHEYNE-STOKES RESPIRATIONS

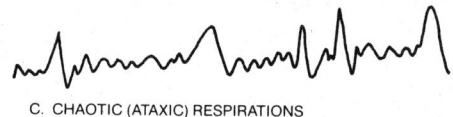

C. CHAOTIC (ATAXIC) RESPIRATIONS

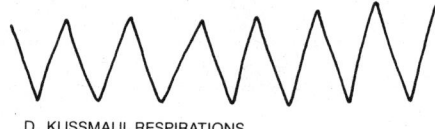

D. KUSSMAUL RESPIRATIONS

Figure 13.1. Respiratory patterns.

A *summary of the physical examination* and important findings to look for follow:

1. **Inspection**
   ■ Rate—increased, normal, decreased?
   ■ Depth—shallow, deep?
   ■ Effort—use of accessory muscles, abdominal breathing, panting, pursed-lip exhalation?
   ■ Rhythm—pattern of inhalation and exhalation
   ■ Chest—absent, shallow, unequal, or unilateral expansion? Paradoxical respirations, sternal retractions?
   ■ Sputum—thick, purulent, drooling, bloody, frothy?

2. **Palpation**
   ■ Tracheal shift

- Flail chest
- Pain

3. **Percussion**
   - Hollow
   - Dull

4. **Auscultation**
   - Upper airways—inspiratory/expiratory stridor, wheezes
   - Lower airways—crackling, moist, bubbling rales

Laboratory tests

In making the diagnosis of the cause of respiratory distress, laboratory work should include arterial blood gases, a chest X-ray, and an EKG. S-T segment elevation in hyperventilation has been reported in the absence of enzymatic evidence of MI. The mechanism is uncertain but may include respiratory alkalosis, transient changes in extracellular potassium, excess vagal activity, endogenous catecholamine release, and altered position of the heart secondary to diaphragmatic motion [*Ann Emerg Med*, November 1985, Vol. 14, p. 1122]. Other studies should be obtained depending upon the suspicions of the health care provider at the time.

Treatment

The general treatment for the breathless patient is as follows:

1. Place in a position of comfort.

2. Be prepared to assist ventilations.

3. Identify and treat an obstructed airway if present.

4. O_2—low flow if a history of COPD and not emergent; otherwise, 4–6 LPM via NP or higher by nonrebreather mask.

Specific therapy should be initiated for any particular problem suggested by the history and physical. Some clues from breath sounds of patients in respiratory distress may be obtained:

1. *Clear symmetric sounds*—hyperventilation, MI, pulmonary embolism, metabolic.

2. *Wet (rales), symmetric*—pulmonary edema, extensive pneumonia.

3. *Wheezing, symmetric*—asthma, pulmonary edema, COPD.

4. *Clear, asymmetric, or absent*—pneumothorax, pulmonary embolism, or COPD.

5. *Wet, asymmetric*—pneumonia, pulmonary edema (uncommon)

6. *Wheezing, asymmetric*—foreign body, pulmonary embolism, COPD.

Practically speaking, under most cases, *symmetrical wet lung sounds* should be treated as pulmonary edema, assuming other factors are compatible with the diagnosis (age, history, etc.). *Symmetrical, expiratory wheezes* in the patient under 40 years old strongly suggest asthma. The asthmatic may also have inspiratory wheezing, *but* the presence of inspiratory wheezing alone, *especially* if it is localized, should STRONGLY suggest foreign body airway obstruction!

Pearls to Remember

An IV of D_5W at a TKO rate and cardiac monitoring are appropriate. Some helpful "PEARLS" to keep in mind are:

1. If unable to differentiate the cause of respiratory distress, administer oxygen and transport (or get consultation if in the hospital).

2. Wheezing in older persons is frequently due to pulmonary edema, not asthma. Pulmonary embolism is also a possibility. Aminophylline will cover both of the first two possibilities and should not hurt in embolism (and may help as reflex bronchospasms sometimes exists).

3. Don't overdiagnose "anxiety-type" hyperventilation in the field. It is best to give

the patient the benefit of the doubt. Treatment with oxygen will not harm them.

4. When the patient's breathing becomes so labored that he can no longer ventilate himself, intubation should be considered.

NONTRAUMATIC COMA

Coma is defined as the absence of any understandable response to stimulus or inner need. There are numerous causes. Common **intracranial causes** of coma are: bleeding, infarction, neoplasm, infection (meningitis, encephalitis, abscess), and postconvulsive. Some common **extracranial causes** of coma are: electrolyte disorders (acidosis, hypernatremia, hyponatremia, hyperglycemia, hypoglycemia), high and low blood pressure, hepatic/uremic coma, myxedema, thyrotoxicosis, Addison's disease, Wernicke's encephalopathy, and drugs. Involved drugs can include sedatives, barbiturates, tranquilizers, opiates, ethanol, methanol, and salicylates.

Catatonia may present as coma or stupor. This is defined as a marked decrease in one's reactivity to their environment and/or a reduction in spontaneous movements or activity. These patients often appear semistuporous rather than comatose, are often unresponsive, and may lie with their eyes open. Their pulse, respiratory rate, and blood pressure may all be elevated. Pupillary and optokinetic reflexes (doll's eyes—see page 163) are all normal. They will blink in response to a visual threat. They often demonstrate "waxy flexibility" which is the assumption and maintenance of any position in which their arms or legs are placed. Their eyelids do not drift back into place after being opened.

Though often associated with the manic phase of manic-depressive psychosis, several organic problems can also cause catatonia: encephalitis, biparietal infarcts, glutethimide withdrawal, epileptic seizures, and bilateral subdural hematomas. Brain tumor and hemorrhage, as well as high-potency neuroleptic medication may also lead to catatonia [*Ann Emerg Med*, April 1985, Vol. 14, pp. 359–361].

Table 13-1 summarizes the causes of coma.

Table 13-1. Causes of Coma

Intracranial Causes
Bleeding
Infarction
Neoplasm
Infection
• Meningitis
• Encephalitis
• Abscess
Postconvulsive

Extracranial Causes
Electrolyte disorders
• Acidosis
• Hyponatremia
• Hypernatremia
• Hypokalemia
• Hyperkalemia (rare)
• Hypoglycemia
• Hyperglycemia
High/low blood pressure
Hepatic, uremic coma
Myxedema
Thyrotoxicosis
Addison's disease
Wernicke's encephalopathy
Drugs
• Sedatives
• Barbiturates
• Tranquilizers
• Opiates
• Ethanol
• Methanol
• Salicylates
Catatonia

Diagnosis

History
The history should reveal when the patient was last well, as well as the progression of their symptoms. Any antecedent symptoms, such as seizures, confusion, or trauma should be noted. The past med-

ical history and medication list should be obtained. It is vital to note the patient's surroundings and check for pill bottles, syringes, and strange odors.

Physical examination

The physical examination consists first of the A, B, C's. Lack of a gag reflex may suggest the need for urgent intubation. The level of consciousness is then evaluated using the Glasgow Coma Scale. Note that this scale does NOT evaluate brain stem function, and other tests (such as the doll's eyes maneuver—see below) must be used for this purpose. The respiratory pattern is noted; Cheyne-Stokes or ataxic breathing suggests a neurologic lesion while a Kussmaul pattern is more compatible with a metabolic etiology.

1. *Diaphoresis* is compatible with shock, hypoglycemia, sepsis, salicylate intoxication, organophosphate poisoning.

2. *Dry skin* is compatible with dehydration, hyperglycemia, hyperosmolar states (i.e., hyperosmolar hyperglycemic nonketotic coma), and anticholinergic poisoning.

3. *Hypothermia* is compatible with cold exposure, hypoglycemia, Addisonian crisis, Wernicke's encephalopathy, hypothyroidism, barbiturate, phenothiazine, or alcohol intoxication.

4. *Hyperthermia* is compatible with heat stroke, hyperthyroidism, sepsis, pontine hemorrhage, and anticholinergic poisoning.

The eyes are examined for the presence of contact lenses, which should be removed. The pupils are observed for their size and reactivity. *The pupillary reaction is the single most important diagnostic sign in distinguishing structural from metabolic causes of coma.* Absent pupillary reactions imply structural lesions in the absence of asphyxia, hypothermia, glutethimide, barbiturate, atropine, or scopalamine ingestion. Some commonly observed pupillary changes and their significance are listed below:

1. *Midposition, nonreactive*—midbrain

damage or glutethimide intoxication.

2. *Normoposition, reactive*—suggest drug or metabolic etiology.

3. *Pinpoint, reactive*—suggest pontine bleed or narcotics; pilocarpine eyedrops (used for glaucoma) will also cause this.

4. *Dilated, fixed*—atropine, brain death.

5. *Ocular palsies*—commonly associated with Wernicke's encephalopathy, especially of the sixth cranial nerve (abducens). Skew deviation of the eyes (one eye is turned downward and inward, and the other is deviated upward and outward) may also be associated with this entity, as well as tumors, infections, and trauma [*J Emerg Med,* 1985, Vol. 3, pp. 361–363].

The eyes are then checked for **doll's eyes.** (OMIT THIS MANEUVER IF THERE IS ANY SUSPICION OF CERVICAL SPINE INJURY!) The head is rotated side-to-side rapidly. The eyes should move in the opposite direction normally. If they follow the head, suspect a brain lesion (pons, midbrain) or barbiturate poisoning. This maneuver is illustrated in Figure 13.2

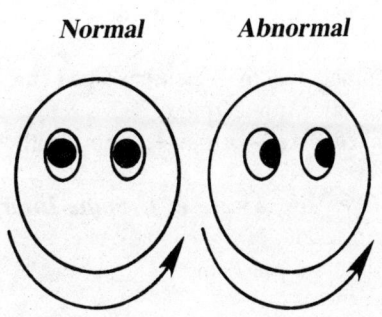

Normally, the eyes remain fixated straight ahead when the head of an unconscious person is turned to the side. If they appear to follow, suspect brain stem damage or barbiturate poisoning.

Figure 13.2. The doll's eye reflex test.

Movements, or lack thereof, are noted. Are there any jerks or seizures? Any obvious paralysis? **Posturing** is noted. **Decorticate posturing** involves flexing the arms toward the cortex (head) and indicates a lesion above the midbrain area. Extension or **decerebrate posturing** is compatible with a lesion further down. Finally, the neck should be checked for stiffness, and the body searched for needle tracks and unusual odors. Table 13-2 presents a summary of the physical findings in nontraumatic coma.

Table 13-2. Summary of Physical Examination in Coma

A, B, C's

Level of Consciousness—Glasgow Coma Scale

Respiratory Pattern
    Cheyne-Stokes/ataxic = neurological lesion
    Kussmaul = metabolic problem

Pupils—Size, Reactivity (Contact Lenses in Eyes?)
    Midposition, nonreactive—midbrain damage, glutethimide
    Normoposition, reactive—drug, metabolic
    Pinpoint, reactive—pontine bleed, narcotics, pilocarpine
    Dilated, fixed—atropine, brain death

Doll's Eyes—Be Aware of C-Spine Injury!
    Brain lesion
    Barbiturate poisoning

Movements—Jerks, Seizures, Paralysis

Posturing
    Decorticate—lesion above the midbrain
    Decerebrate—lesion further down

Nuchal Rigidity

Needle Tracks, Unusual Odors

Laboratory tests

Laboratory tests should include CBC, electrolytes, BUN/creatinine, glucose, toxicology screen (blood and urine), and possibly gastric aspirate for drugs. An EKG should be performed. A lumbar puncture is done if there is a possibility of infection or intracranial bleeding. It is important to check for papilledema first before performing a spinal tap.

CT scan should be done looking for mass lesions, as should the EEG if seizure activity is suspected. A high yield should be expected following CT scanning in comatose patients (46%) [*Ann Emerg Med,* October 1986, Vol. 15, p. 1167]. A normal EEG in a comatose patient rules out metabolic causes, which produce diffuse, symmetric slowing of all brain activity.

Skull X-rays may show a midline shift of the pineal gland (if calcified) but are usually not helpful acutely in nontraumatic coma.

Treatment

Treatment of nontraumatic coma should proceed as follows:

1. A, B, C's.

2. O_2—nasal prongs, nonrebreather mask, or intubation if necessary.

3. IV D_5W TKO—use normal saline if increased intracranial pressure is suspected.

4. Draw 1 red top tube or fingerstick for instant blood sugar determination.

5. Thiamine 100 mg IV; 1 amp (25 grams) of glucose (D_{50}) should then be given IV.

6. Naloxone (Narcan), .8 mg IV if no response to D_{50}.

7. Monitor cardiac rhythm.

Pearls to Remember

Keep in mind:

1. Be particularly attentive to the airway.

Comatose patients tend to have difficulty clearing secretions. Inadequate tidal volumes are also common.

2. Hypoglycemia may present as a focal neurological deficit or coma (stroke-like picture) in elderly persons.

3. Naloxone is useful in any potential overdose situation. It reverses a wide spectrum of agents. Its action is relatively shorter than many narcotics and can be repeated (and often MUST be). To reverse propoxyphene (Darvon) overdose 8–10 ampules may be required. It has also been reported to reverse coma from massive alcohol (ethanol) intoxication [*Am J Emerg Med,* September 1984, p. 444].

4. Patients less than 20 years old who survive greater than 48 hours after the onset of coma have a good prognosis for mental and neurological recovery. Less than one-half of adults over 50 years old return to normal lives if their coma lasts greater than 24 hours.

THE "SHOCKY" PATIENT

Shock may be defined as a state of inadequate tissue perfusion and oxygenation with abnormal tissue metabolism at the cellular level. Shock has been classified in many ways. The currently accepted **classification of shock** involves four types:

- Hypovolemic
- Cardiogenic
- Obstructive
- Distributive.

Hypovolemic shock occurs when the volume within the intravascular compartment is inadequate for tissue perfusion. It may be the result of exogenous causes such as hemorrhage, plasma loss from burns or inflammation, or electrolyte loss from diarrhea or dehydration. Endogenous causes include extravasation ("third spacing") due to inflammation, trauma,

anaphylaxis, and envenomation.

Cardiogenic shock occurs when the cardiac pump is impaired to the extent that it cannot adequately circulate the available volume. Myocardial infarction is the most common cause, though acute mitral insufficiency, ventricular septal defect, heart failure, and hemodynamically significant dysrhythmias may also be responsible. Fifty percent of the patients who develop this syndrome do so within 24 hours following their myocardial infarction.

Anterior infarcts more commonly lead to cardiogenic shock than do inferior ones. If greater than 40% of the left ventricular muscle is lost, shock will result. Without appropriate treatment, there is a 55–85% mortality within 24 hours. Patients with a cardiac index (cardiac output/body surface area) less than 2.0 L/minute/m² (normal = 3.2–5.2 L/min/m²) and a pulmonary artery wedge pressure (a measure of left ventricular filling) greater than 15 mm Hg (normal = 7–10) have a very high mortality. Ventricular fibrillation can be viewed as the "ultimate" form of cardiogenic shock.

Obstructive shock results from obstruction in the great veins, heart, pulmonary arteries, or aorta to a degree which physically impedes the main stream of blood flow. This may occur in the various parts of the circulatory system as follows:

1. *Vena cava*—compression.

2. *Pericardium*—tamponade.

3. *Cardiac chambers*—ball-valve thrombus.

4. *Pulmonary circuit*—pulmonary embolus.

5. *Aorta*—dissecting aneurysm.

Distributive shock is due to a major defect in the arterial resistance, venous capacitance, or both. In other words, there is a loss of vascular tone. Sepsis, drug overdose, anaphylaxis, and spinal cord injury can all result in distributive shock.

Profound myocardial depression is described in the late stages of almost all types of shock. Elevation of the CPK-MB fraction has been noted as well, with 31% of patients having EKG evidence of acute myocardial infarction in one study [*Crit Care Med,* 1984, Vol. 12, p. 1024]. Reversible segmental myocardial dysfunction causing EKG changes consistent with myocardial infarction and negative autopsy findings has also been described [*Crit Care Med,* 1986, Vol. 14, p. 587].

Table 13-3 summarizes the causes of shock.

It is instructive to examine the **pathophysiology of shock.** There are many similarities between the different types of shock when one looks at end-organ damage. The basic defect in shock is failure of oxygen delivery at the cell level. The mechanisms presented here are specifically in reference to hypovolemic shock, though.

The body's initial response to hypovolemia is a reflex that results in the release of norepinephrine (NE) and epinephrine (E). These compounds cause tachycardia and increase the contractility of the heart. Additionally, there is venous and arteriolar constriction. In effect there is a decrease in the blood flow to skin, muscle, the gastrointestinal tract, and, to some degree, the kidney, with a relative redistribution to the brain and heart. Capillary hydrostatic pressure decreases in early shock, allowing fluid from the interstitium to flow into the vessels. This "autotransfusion" effect, along with the other mentioned mechanisms, allows the body to adequately compensate for up to a 25% volume loss.

As the patient decompensates, perfusion of the brain and coronary arteries decreases. Cells switch to anaerobic metabolism producing a lactic acidosis. This has the potentially beneficial effect of shifting the oxygen-dissociation curve to the right which increases tissue oxygen delivery but also decreases cardiac function and makes the myocardium more susceptible to catecholamine effects (dysrhythmias).

There is decreased synthesis of the compound adenosine triphosphate (ATP), the major intracellular energy compound. This state of "energy failure" leads to increased intracellular sodium and water, with subsequent intracellular swelling. Calcium increases in the cytosol and mitochondria, further impairing ATP synthesis. The cells' lysosomes then lyse, releasing enzymes which further increase cellular permeability. Other enzymes, including histamine, serotonin, kinins, and prostaglandins are also present which lead to increased vascular permeability with subsequent fluid loss back to the interstitium.

The effects of microscopic energy failure are also evident on a gross level. There is progressive cardiac failure. Some feel this is due to the presence of

---

Table 13-3. Causes of Shock

Hypovolemic Shock

Exogenous Causes
- Hemorrhage
- Plasma loss—burns, inflammation
- Electrolyte loss—diarrhea, dehydration

Endogenous Causes—extravasation due to:
- Inflammation
- Trauma
- Anaphylaxis
- Envenomation

Cardiogenic Shock

Myocardial infarction
Acute mitral insufficiency
Ventricular septal defect
Heart failure
Hemodynamically significant dysrhythmias

Obstructive Shock

Vena cava—compression
Pericardium—tamponade
Cardiac chambers—ball-valve thrombus
Pulmonary circuit—pulmonary embolism
Aorta—dissecting aneurysm

Distributive Shock

Low resistance—normal or high cardiac output; vasodilation with arteriovenous shunting
- Cervical spine transection
- Inflammation
- Peritonitis
- Gram-negative shock (early)

High or normal resistance—cardiac output normal/low; increased venous capacitance
- Gram-negative shock (late phase)
- Barbiturate intoxication
- Ganglionic blockade

a circulating "myocardial depressant factor." This is compatible with the fact that coronary flow is preserved, and global ischemia does NOT appear to be the cause of myocardial depression [*Circulation,* 1986, Vol. 73, No. 4, pp. 637–644]. Lung water increases, as does disruption of the epithelial integrity. Atelectasis (collapse) and hemorrhage occur, leading to ventilation-perfusion mismatching, progressive shunting, and eventually ARDS.

Hepatobiliary and pancreatic function are hampered, including impaired insulin release. Thus, the "diabetic-like" state that is so often seen in most kinds of shock. Gastrointestinal motility is decreased, and stress ulcers may form. Urine production tends to decrease and frank renal failure may ensue. Free radical formation in the kidneys may contribute to this [*Ann Emerg Med,* December 1986, Vol. 15, p. 1397].

Finally, function of the white blood cells and blood clotting system is impaired. There is decreased resistance to infection and frank disseminated intravascular coagulation (see Chapter 10, Hematological Emergencies) is possible. Thus, the full-blown shock syndrome is a state of multiple system organ failure with metabolic acidosis, leaky capillaries, and widespread cellular dysfunction. Figure 13.3 summarizes the pathophysiology of hypovolemic shock.

Diagnosis

History

Factors that should be determined in the history include the onset of the shock state and associated symptoms. Was it sudden or gradual? Can anyone identify a precipitating cause or event? Is there any itching, peripheral or facial edema, thirst, weakness, hives, shortness of breath, chest pain, or dizziness on standing? Does the patient have allergies? Is he on medications? Has there been bloody vomitus or stools (suggests internal bleeding)? Does this person have any other significant medical diseases? In one study, a history of anterior thigh pain or tenderness without generalized muscle aches or CPK elevation was highly suggestive of bacteremia [*Arch Int Med,* 1985, Vol. 145, p. 657–658].

Physical examination

Physical findings vary with the severity of shock. Deterioration in vital signs, especially blood pressure,

is only one sign of shock. This actually occurs relatively late in the course of events. Pulse, pulse pressure, capillary refill, respiratory rate, skin tone, and sensorium can all be assessed to make a diagnosis of shock with a relatively *normal* blood pressure (in the vicinity of 90–100 mg Hg systolic). Evidence of pump failure (increased venous pressure, rales edema) should also be sought.

Bradycardia may be present. If this occurs in the face of severe shock, it is usually indicative of a preterminal condition due to myocardial ischemia and impending cardiac arrest. Otherwise, it is often due to a vagal response to fear, pain, and stress. This same reflex may also decrease the cardiac output and total peripheral vascular resistance, leading to orthostatic hypotension. Despite this, hypovolemia may still be present and should be aggressively treated. Hypothermia occurs initially in 13% of patients with septic shock. Failure to mount a febrile response within 24 hours is associated with increased mortality [*Surgery,* 1979, Vol. 86, p. 409].

Table 13-4 illustrates findings on the physical examination with different levels of shock.

Laboratory tests

Laboratory tests in the shocky patient should include: CBC, blood cultures, electrolytes, cardiac enzymes, and blood gases. Arterial catheter blood cultures do not appear to be reliable sampling sites for obtaining blood cultures—standard venous cultures are recommended [*Crit Care Med,* 1985, Vol. 13, p. 664].

Arterial blood lactate levels are considered by many to be the best single indicator of shock but are not widely available on a STAT basis. Values exceeding 2 mmol/L are considered a poor prognostic sign. A simple bedside instrument has been developed that works well and allows this important parameter to be easily measured [*Crit Care Med,* 1985, Vol. 13, p. 323 (abstract)]. There is excellent correlation between blood lactate levels and oxygen delivery in critically ill patients [*Chest, 1985, Vol. 85, pp. 580–584*]. Trends in the blood lactate level may be even more helpful in the monitoring of critically ill patients [*Intensive & Critical Care Digest,* 1986, Vol. 5, p. 15].

Disseminated intravascular coagulation (DIC) may occur (see Chapter 10, Hematologic Emergencies) during shock. Interestingly, 97% of patients who die of traumatic (hemorrhagic) shock have evidence of coagulation defects *prior* to fluid or blood administration. The most frequent abnormality was elevated protime (97%), followed by depressed platelet counts (72%) and elevated partial thromboplastin time (70%). Patients with head trauma seemed to have the greatest incidence. DIC was felt to be responsible for this [*Ann Emerg Med,* July 1985, Vol. 14, pp. 650–655]. DIC commonly complicates the course of septic shock as well.

Hypovolemia → Release of norepinephrine/epinephrine
|
Tachycardia, increased cardiac contractility, venous and arteriolar constriction, and decreased capillary hydrostatic pressure
|
Decreased blood flow → skin, muscle, GI tract, and kidney +
Increased blood flow → brain and heart + flow of fluid from interstitium to blood vessels

The Autotransfusion Effect

Further decompensation→ Decreased perfusion of brain, coronary arteries → anaerobic metabolism
|
Lactic acidosis, decreased cardiac function, dysrhythmias

Subsequently → Decreased ATP synthesis with intracellular energy failure
|
Increased intracellular sodium and water → swelling
+
Release of lysozomal enzymes → increased cell permeability
+
Enzyme release (histamine, serotonin, kinins, prostaglandins) → increased vascular permeability
|

Multiple system organ failure:
Progressive cardiac failure—myocardial depressant factor
+
Increased lung water with atelectasis and hemorrhage → Adult respiratory distress syndrome
+
Hepatobiliary and pancreatic failure → Hyperglycemia
+
Decreased gastrointestinal motility → Stress ulcers
+
Decreased urine output and renal failure
+
Impaired white blood cell and clotting function → Infection, Disseminated intravascular coagulation

---

Figure 13.3. Pathophysiology of hypovolemic shock.

Table 13-4. Findings in Shock

Test	Normal	Mild Shock	Moderate Shock	Severe Shock
Sensorium	Oriented	Slightly anxious but oriented	Anxious, confused	Lethargic Confused Incoherent
Pulse	60–100	100–120	120–150	> 140; rapid, thready
Pupils	Equal, 2–4 mm	Normal	Normal	May be dilated Slow to react
Blood pressure	120/80	110/80	70–90/50–60	< 50–60 systolic
Pulse pressure	40	30	20–30	10–20
Capillary blanch	Normal	Normal	Slow	Slow
Respiratory rate	12–16	14–20	20–30	> 35
Urine output cc/H	40–50	30–35	15–30	Negligible
Skin	Dry	Slightly moist	Sweaty	Cool, clammy

In some patients, thrombosis, rather than hemorrhage, may be present. This is because the liver is unable to remove activated clotting factors from the circulation. These persist, and thrombosis occurs. There are two naturally occurring "anticoagulants," Protein C and antithrombin III. These are rapidly depleted during DIC, thus promoting a thrombogenic tendency in some patients. Symptoms seen in a patient whose primary problem from DIC is thrombosis include skin necrosis, gangrene of distal parts, and renal failure. Low-dose heparinization potentiates antithrombin III activity and may limit the extent of intravascular coagulation. Doses of 5,000 U SQ every 12 hours seem to work well without causing any significant bleeding problems. As mentioned earlier in this text, some experts favor full-dose intravenous heparinization. Of course, this is only indicated in the face of an overwhelming thrombogenic tendency (see Chapter 10, Hematologic Emergencies).

An EKG should be obtained in all patients. Progressive changes may be noted. These are commonly described in hypovolemic shock but may be seen in other types as well. Initially, and through many of the stages of shock, sinus tachycardia is seen. Preterminally, there is a decrease in the sinus rate with widening of the PR interval. A nodal rhythm often ensues. There is gradual slowing of conduction in the His-Purkinje system (widening of the H-V interval) to the point where eventually an idioventricular rhythm takes over. Asystole is usually the terminal event, though it may at times be ventricular fibrillation.

Treatment

The generalized therapeutic approach to the patient in shock is as follows:

1. Stop exsanguinating hemorrhage if present. Preliminary reports of the "Percluder" occluding aortic balloon in humans are promising. This device is placed via a femoral cutdown or percutaneously.

It essentially occludes the aorta, functioning similarly to aortic cross-clamping, but without the requisite thoracotomy. Further data are needed before this promising technique can be widely applied [*Ann Emerg Med*, December 1986, Vol. 15, p. 466].

2. Apply the MAST suit to the patient—inflate as necessary.

3. Lay the patient down with the legs elevated 10–12 inches, unless respiratory symptoms predominate or are aggravated by this—then utilize the position of comfort.

4. High flow O_2 (10–15 LPM via non-rebreather mask) with ventilatory assistance as required.

5. IV Ringer's Lactate at a wide open rate. Either 2 large-bore (16 gauge) lines should be started or an 8.5 French catheter placed to allow for maximum fluid flow in the shortest time. There are some animal data suggesting that warmed fluids may be more effective, especially in hemorrhagic shock [*J of Trauma*, 1984, Vol. 24, p. 957].

6. Cover the patient to avoid heat loss. DO NOT overbundle, or excessive vasodilation may worsen shock (the afterdrop phenomenon).

7. Consider MAST suit inflation if vital signs do not improve rapidly or you are unable to start an IV.

8. Cardiac monitor.

9. Attempt to define the type of shock present and treat specifically if possible.

10. If there are no signs of pump failure, a fluid challenge is reasonable. Though it is possible to follow the results with either central venous or pulmonary artery wedge pressure monitoring, the easiest way is to rapidly (over 15–30 minutes) infuse 250–500 cc of a volume-expanding fluid.

Observe for changes and improvements in the patient's status. This can be repeated if it appears to have helped and the patient later deteriorates (or if improvement is only transient).

Debate continues over whether colloid or crystalloid should be used. Many favor Ringer's Lactate. For hemorrhagic shock, some experts prefer to use uncrossmatched Group O blood [*Ann Emerg Med*, November 1986, Vol. 15, p. 1282]. Small-volume infusion of 7.5% NaCl in 6% Dextran 70 has been used for hemorrhagic shock in a swine model [*Ann Emerg Med*, October 1986, Vol. 15, p. 1132]. One study has demonstrated human efficacy of this treatment [*Ann Emerg Med*, December 1986, Vol. 15, p. 1411].

Several red blood cell substitute solutions have been developed for use in acute hemorrhagic shock. The earliest of these, Fluosol-DA is a perfluorochemical emulsion which has been shown to be ineffective in severe acute anemia [*N Engl J Med*, 1986, Vol. 314, p. 1653]. A polymerized hemoglobin solution has yielded more promising results [*Ann Emerg Med*, December 1986, Vol. 15, p. 1416].

Careful measurement of hemodynamic parameters in patients with shock have shown that increases in the pulmonary artery wedge pressure (PAWP—a measure of left ventricular filling) and blood pressure may not correlate with changes in the cardiac output (the amount of blood, in L/minute pumped by the heart). Despite increases in mean arterial pressure (and PAWP), cardiac output decreased in some patients. Thus, it is recommended to monitor cardiac output as well if hemodynamic parameters are to be followed [*Heart & Lung*, November 1984, p. 649].

11. There is much research literature suggesting that naloxone and/or massive doses of steroids may be helpful in shock. Much of the data is in septic shock models, but animal data for neurogenic and hemorrhagic shock exist as well. At this time,

no firm recommendations can be made for the use of either drug [*Arch Surg,* May 1984, p. 537; see also previously referenced article in the *Am J Emerg Med]*.

In fact, current evidence suggests that naloxone does not reliably improve mean arterial pressure or other physiological variables and may cause severe adverse reactions including pulmonary edema, seizures, and severe hypotension when given in septic shock [*Crit Care Med,* 1985, Vol. 13, p. 28]. The opinion of most experts at this time is that this agent should be avoided [*Crit Care Med,* 1986, Vol. 14, pp. 170–171].

One study suggested that massive doses of steroids (methylprednisolone, 30 mg/kg IV over 10–15 minutes) resulted in reversal of shock. The improvement was only transient, lasting up to 150 hours. Patients treated within four hours after the onset of septic shock had a higher incidence of shock reversal than those not. Long-term survival was not improved though [*NEJM,* 1984, Vol. 311, pp. 1137–1143]. Thus, many experts suggest that pharmacological doses of steroids should be given within 4 hours of the development of the shock syndrome and repeated 4 hours later if a failing blood pressure is unresponsive to fluid challenge [*Crit Care Med,* 1985, Vol. 13, p. 864].

12. Antisera to endotoxin has been shown to reduce mortality in patients with gram-negative shock. It had no effect on infection prophylaxis though. This is a promising area, but, currently, no commercial preparations are available [*Lancet,* July 13, 1985, pp. 59–64].

    Administration of low doses of the antibiotic polymyxin B has been shown to reverse postburn immunosuppression. It is felt that this drug binds endotoxin, thus allowing for a return of normal lymphocyte function. As of yet, no effects on

survival have been demonstrated [*J of Trauma,* 1986, Vol. 26, p. 995].

13. Pressor agents may be tried. There is some evidence that dobutamine may be especially helpful in shock associated with pulmonary embolism [*Crit Care Med,* 1985, Vol. 13, p. 1009].

14. Preliminary research has suggested that calcium-blocking agents can improve both short- and long-term outcomes in experimental shock. At this time, though, these results cannot and should not be extrapolated to humans [*Ann Emerg Med,* December 1986, Vol. 15, p. 457].

Pearls to Remember

Keep in mind that:

1. A decreased blood pressure is indicative of severe shock. If the cause is unknown, a trial of IV fluids is warranted. As unrecognized cardiogenic shock may be aggravated by a fluid challenge, MAST suit inflation may be preferable as a rapid but reversible form of fluid challenge. Note: there is currently widespread debate in the literature as to whether or not the MAST garment actually provides a 1–2 unit "autotransfusion" or not. See Appendix D for further information on this.

2. Vital signs in hypovolemic shock (as well as other types) can be misleading. A high index of suspicion is necessary. Don't wait for the blood pressure to drop!

3. DO NOT overwrap the patient; this may cause peripheral vasodilation and aggravation of shock.

4. Cardiogenic shock is difficult to treat both in the field *and* in the hospital. The *most* treatable factor is hypovolemia if present.

Glossary of Terms and Abbreviations

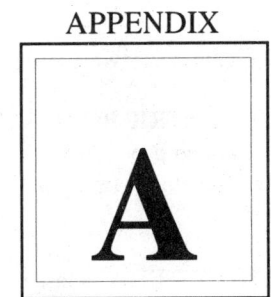

APPENDIX

A

AMYLASE—an enzyme that catalyzes the hydrolysis of starch into smaller molecules. Present primarily in the salivary glands and the pancreas.

ANOREXIA—the loss of appetite and/or the desire to eat.

ANTICHOLINERGIC—a drug that blocks the passage of impulses through the parasympathetic nerves.

AORTIC STENOSIS—narrowing of the orifice of the aortic value usually via calcification and fibrosis. There are many etiologies for this, including rheumatic fever and the calcification of a congenital bicupsid (two- instead of three-cusped) valve. The latter is now the most common cause of aortic stenosis seen.

ARACHNOID—one of the three membranes (meninges) covering the central nervous system. The outside layer is the dura mater. The arachnoid is the middle layer, and the pia mater, which is closely applied to brain and spinal cord tissue, is inside.

ASAP—abbreviation for As Soon As Possible.

AURA—a subjective sensation or motor phenomenon that precedes and marks the onset of a seizure.

BILIRUBIN—a bile pigment that is a breakdown product of hemoglobin.

BLAKEMORE TUBE—a special tube designed for use in bleeding from esophageal varices. There are two balloons—one inflates within the stomach, the other in the esophagus. Additionally, there is a middle channel through which the gastric contents can be aspirated.

BRONCHOSPASM—spasmodic contraction of bronchial muscle.

BUN/CREATININE—kidney function tests.

CARBOXYHEMOGLOBIN LEVEL—(COHb); measured arterial blood level of the complex of carbon monoxide and hemoglobin. Serves to indicate the severity of carbon monoxide poisoning.

CARDIAC ENZYMES—serially measures blood tests, usually consisting of CPK and LDH determinations. If elevated in certain patterns, indicative of myocardial damage (i.e., myocardial infarction).

CARDIAC OUTPUT—the volume of blood pumped by the heart in liters per minute.

CARDIOPULMONARY BYPASS—the heart-lung machine. Designed to bypass the normal circulatory path by circumventing the patient's heart and lungs. Mechanical devices pump the blood and a membrane oxygenator functions like the lungs.

CBC—Complete Blood Count; usually includes the hematocrit, hemoglobin, red and white blood cell count, a differential percentage of different types of WBCs, and sometimes a platelet count.

CEREBROSPINAL FLUID (CSF)—the fluid found in the subarachnoid space which surrounds and bathes the central nervous system at all times.

CHEMSTRIP BG/DEXTROSTIX—chemically impregnated paper strips; by placing blood from a fingerstick on the tip, color changes measure the blood sugar.

CHEST TUBE—a large diameter sterile tube which is surgically inserted into the pleural cavity between the ribs. This is used to drain air and/or blood.

COMPARTMENT SYNDROME—a syndrome whereby pressure builds up in a group of muscles that is surrounded by fascia, forming a compartment. This can lead to ischemic death of the muscle if the tension is not relieved by a fasciotomy.

COOMB'S TEST—a laboratory test for the presence of certain antibodies which may result in the hemolysis of blood cells.

COSTOCHONDRITIS—a nonspecific irritation of the rib cartilage, often caused by a virus. This can result, at times, in severe chest pain which is often aggravated by a deep breath.

CPAP—Continuous Positive Airway Pressure; this is a special respiratory therapy technique whereby the airway always has a small amount of positive pressure applied to it. This prevents smaller airways from collapsing and increases the percentage of alveoli that are effectively ventilated. This is referred to as recruiting alveoli and reducing shunting.

CT—stands for Computerized Tomography (CT scan); this is a special X-ray device that essentially takes serial "cuts" through planes of the body. The resolution is so good that the shadows appear as easily recognizable densities.

D₅LR—5% dextrose solution + Lactated Ringer's in the same bottle.

D₅NS—5% dextrose solution + normal saline solution in the same bottle.

D₅W—5% dextrose solution.

D₅W 1/2 NS—5% dextrose solution + 1/2 normal saline (i.e., half strength) solution in the same bottle.

DIABETES TYPE I/II—the new classification of diabetes mellitus. Type I diabetics were formerly referred to as "juvenile onset" and Type II as "adult-onset." There are many more significant distinguishing features, but they are beyond the scope of this text.

DRUG SCREEN—chemical tests performed on blood, urine, or both for the presence of various legal and illegal medications.

ECCHYMOSIS—a small hemorrhagic spot forming a nonelevated, rounded or irregular blue to purplish patch (a small bruise).

ECLAMPSIA—convulsions and coma occurring in a pregnant woman associated with hypertension, swelling, and/or proteinuria (protein in the urine).

EDEMA—swelling caused by fluid in the subcutaneous tissues.

EEG—electroencephalogram; measures brain wave activity.

ELECTROLYTES—blood test panel usually consisting of sodium ($Na+$), potassium ($K+$), chloride ($Cl-$), and bicarbonate (HCO_3-).

EMPYEMA—accumulation of pus in a cavity in the body.

ENDOSCOPY—visual inspection of the body via an instrument designed to view inside of hollow viscera, often via fiberoptic bundles.

ESCHAR—a blackish, dead area of skin produced by many things, including burns and gangrene.

EWALD TUBE—large-bore rubber or plastic tube used to evacuate the stomach.

FASCIOTOMY—surgical procedure whereby a longitudinal incision is made down to and including fascia that encloses a group of muscles. This is designed to release tension that may have built up in the muscle "compartment" defined by the fascial plane (see also "compartment syndrome").

FEV$_1$—Forced Expiratory Volume in 1 second; the volume, in liters, of air forcefully exhaled in one second.

FIO$_2$—Fraction Inspired Oxygen—the percentage of oxygen in the inspired air (= 21% in room air).

FLOW VOLUME LOOPS—specialized pulmonary function tests that measure the inspiratory and expiratory airflow throughout the entire breathing period.

FUNDUS—the back of the eye as seen when looking through the pupil. The blood vessels, as well as the optic disc where the optic nerve and vessels enter the eye, are seen.

GALLOP—an extra heart sound indicative of cardiac dysfunction.

GASTROPARESIS—neuromuscular dysfunction of the stomach whereby it is unable to empty itself in the normal direction and manner. The stomach then dilates massively, causing severe pain (gastric dilatation) and/or frequent nausea and vomiting.

GLOMERULONEPHRITIS—disease of the small filtering components (glomeruli) of the kidneys. Various entities may be responsible.

GLUCOSE TOLERANCE TEST—a laboratory examination where the patient is given a sugar load (either orally or IV). Blood sugar measurements are then drawn from a vein every 30 to 60 minutes. The duration of the test depends upon the purpose. At times, five hours are required for the diagnosis of hypoglycemia.

H—abbreviation for "hour."

HEMATOCRIT—the percentage by volume of red blood cells in whole blood.

HEMOGLOBIN—the oxygen-carrying protein of red blood cells.

HEMOPTYSIS—coughing up of blood from a pulmonary source.

HYPERPYREXIA—elevated temperature; a fever.

HYPERTROPHIC CARDIOMYOPATHY—a hereditary syndrome with disproportionate enlargement of portions of the heart muscle. The commonest variant is when the interventricular septum is involved (idiopathic hypertrophic subaortic stenosis—IHSS).

HYPERVISCOSITY—excessive "thickness."

IM—abbreviation for intramuscular.

INCONTINENCE—inability to control excretory functions.

INTRADERMAL—within the dermis (layer immediately below the external part of the skin).

JUGULAR VENOUS PRESSURE—the pressure "head" in the internal jugular vein as measured by external visual inspection. When elevated markedly, the patient is noted to have "bulging neck veins."

LACTIC ACID—an end product of anaerobic metabolism. Indicates that the tissue or patient has undergone a lack of oxygen at the tissue level.

LDH—lactate dehydrogenase; a blood enzyme that, when elevated, indicates dysfunction in several body systems. Most commonly obtained for detection of myocardial and liver problems.

LR—Lactated Ringer's solution.

LYMPHOCYTES—white blood cells which partake in immunological functions.

mEq—abbreviation for milliequivalents; a measure of electrical charge and weight.

MITRAL VALVE PROLAPSE—a hereditary syndrome whereby there is infiltration of the mitral valve with a type of connective tissue (myxomatous) that causes it to stretch (prolapse) into the left atrium during systole.

MYXEDEMA—condition used interchangeably with adult hypothyroidism.

NASOGASTRIC TUBE—a long, relatively narrow rubber or plastic tube that is placed via the nose into the back of the throat, the esophagus, and, finally, the stomach.

PEEP—Positive End Expiratory Pressure; the application of positive pressure during the end of the patient's expiratory phase. This is done only with individuals who are intubated and on a ventilator. The purpose is the same as that of CPAP.

PERITONEAL LAVAGE—the flooding of the peritoneal cavity with fluid which is then subsequently drained out.

PHLEBITIS—inflammation of a vein.

PLASMANATE—trade name for the most commonly used variety of heat-purified plasma protein fraction. Used as colloid fluid replacement. It contains NO active clotting factors.

PLEURAL SPACE—a potential space between the visceral pleura (which is closely applied to the lung tissue) and the parietal pleura, which is closely applied to the thoracic wall.

PNEUMOMEDIASTINUM—the presence of air in the mediastinum; often accompanied by a pneumothorax.

PRN—abbreviation; signifies "as needed."

PULMONARY ANGIOGRAM—specialized radiographic test whereby a catheter is placed transvenously into the pulmonary arteries. Dye is then injected visualizing the left then the right branches and their subdivisions.

q—abbreviation for "every"; i.e., every six hours = q 6 H.

RADIONUCLEOTIDE LUNG SCAN—specialized nuclear medicine test in which a radioactive scanner material is injected intravenously (perfusion scan), inhaled (ventilation scan) or both (ventilation-perfusion scan). Used in the detection of pulmonary emboli.

REFLUX ESOPHAGITIS—the "backwash" of stomach acid into the esophagus which leads to irritation—esophagitis.

RETRACTIONS—visible inward movements of portions of the chest wall indicating contraction of the accessory muscles of respiration. These are not seen during normal breathing.

RHABDOMYOLYSIS—disintegration or dissolution of muscle with result release of myoglobin in the urine. Can cause acute renal failure.

SERUM CORTISOL LEVEL—blood test measuring the blood cortisol which is indicative of the functioning of the person's adrenal gland.

SGOT—a liver function test.

SPIROMETRY—a type of pulmonary function test.

SQ—abbreviation for subcutaneous, usually referring to the type of injection.

STAT—abbreviation for "EXTREMELY URGENT!"

STRIDOR—harsh, high-pitched respiratory sound.

SUBARACHNOID SPACE—space between the arachnoid and pia mater. Filled with cerebrospinal fluid.

SUBCLAVIAN STEAL—a vascular syndrome whereby the peripheral circulation is compromised in the subclavian artery. At times of blood need to the arm, blood may be shunted beyond the obstruction from the vertebral artery, leading to syncope.

SWAN-GANZ CATHETER—specialized catheter which is transvenously placed into the pulmonary artery. Measures reflected left atrial pressure which, under most circumstances, indicates left ventricular end diastolic pressure (preload). From the items measured with this catheter, several hemodynamic parameters may be calculated.

THORACOTOMY—surgical procedure involving opening the thoracic cavity, usually through a rib-splitting incision. A midline procedure may also be done by splitting the sternum (midline thoracotomy). This is commonly used for coronary artery bypass procedures.

THYROTOXICOSIS—a syndrome resulting from overactivity of the thyroid gland. The patient is often anxious, hot, sweaty, and tachycardic. Reflexes may be hyperactive.

TKO—abbreviation for "To Keep Open." Refers to an IV rate which should be slow but fast enough to keep the line and intravenous catheter from clotting off. Usually anywhere from 25–50 cc/hour, depending on the equipment.

TORR—a measure of pressure where 1 torr = 1 mm Hg.

TOXEMIA—used by some to refer to eclampsia of pregnancy; also indicates a general condition of a patient looking very sick ("toxic").

TRANSUDATE—fluid substance with a low content of protein and cells.

UA—abbreviation for urinalysis; involves the chemical and microscopic examination of a urine specimen for blood, protein, sugar, and cellular elements. The presence of bacteria and crystals is also sought.

UREMIA—state of chronic kidney failure.

WBC—white blood cell count; done with the CBC.

WERNICKE'S ENCEPHALOPATHY—an organic brain syndrome, primarily in alcoholics, caused by depletion of the vitamin thiamine. Often consists of altered mental status and cranial nerve palsies—especially the abducens (sixth).

Brief Drug Reference

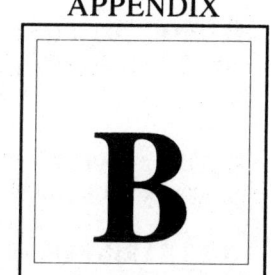

ACTIVATED CHARCOAL—a specialized preparation of granulated charcoal. Used to absorb poisonous substances from the stomach and blood (via the stomach blood vessels).

AMINOPHYLLINE (Theophylline)—a xanthine derivative; functions as a bronchodilator. Also has a mild cardiostimulatory effect.

ATROPINE—drug which blocks the parasympathetic nervous system. Specifically reverses the effects of vagus nerve stimulation.

CALCIUM CHLORIDE/GLUCONATE—salts of calcium ($Ca++$) for intravenous injection.

CHLORPROMAZINE (Thorazine)—a major tranquilizer used in treating shivering during heat stroke therapy and in psychosis.

CIMETIDINE (Tagamet)—blocks the H_2 receptors of stomach tissue leading to a reduction in the secreation of gastric acid.

CLONIDINE (Catapress)—a centrally acting antihypertensive agent whose acute withdrawal can lead to a severe hypertensive crisis.

DEXTROSE (D_{50})—solution of 50% dextrose, commonly referred to as "D_{50}" for intravenous injection.

DIAZEPAM (Valium)—a minor tranquilizer used for seizure control and anxiety.

DIAZOXIDE (Hyperstat)—rapidly acting IV antihypertensive agent; has several significant side effects including hypotension, sweating, chest pain, and hyperglycemia.

DIGOXIN (Lanoxin)—most commonly used preparation of the digitalis leaf drugs.

DIPHENHYDRAMINE (Benadryl)—a moderately strong antihistamine useful in severe allergic reactions and as a mild tranquilizer.

EPINEPHRINE—potent stimulator of adrenergic receptors throughout the body.

FUROSEMIDE (Lasix)—a potent diuretic available in both IV and oral forms.

GLUCAGON—a hormone that stimulates the production of the compound cyclic AMP. This leads to an increase in the blood glucose concentration. It is used intramuscularly in hypoglycemia.

GLUTETHIMIDE (Doriden)—a potent hypnotic/sedative. Not widely used, except illegally and for suicide attempts.

HALOTHANE—colorless, inhalational anesthetic agent.

HYDRALAZINE (Apresoline)—potent antihypertensive agent; available for parenteral or oral use.

HYDROCORTISONE (Solu-Cortef)—an adrenocortical steroid with primarily glucocorticoid effects.

IPECAC—an organic medication that causes vomiting via a central action.

ISOETHARINE (Bronkosol)—an inhaled brochodilator that works by stimulating beta receptors.

ISOPROTERENOL (Isuprel)—a drug available for inhalational, oral, or IV use. Stimulates beta receptors leading to bronchodilation and increased heart rate.

ISOSORBIDE DINITRATE (Sorbitrate)—a member of the nitroglycerin family. Causes both veno- and arteriodilitation. Used for angina and congestive heart failure.

LIDOCAINE (Xylocaine)—the most commonly used IV antidysrhythmic agent.

MAGNESIUM CITRATE—magnesium salt used orally as a cathartic (causes diarrhea).

MEPERIDINE (Demerol)—potent, narcotic analgesic.

METAPROTERENOL (Alupent)—similar to isoethrane.

METHYLPREDNISOLONE (Solu-Medrol)—a potent steroid with predominantly glucocorticoid effects.

MORPHINE SULPHATE—potent narcotic analgesic; also has venodilatory properties which make it an ideal cardiac analgesic.

N-ACETYL CYSTEINE (Mucomyst)—used as an antidote in acetaminophen poisoning; also thought by some to help loosen pulmonary secretions. This is extremely DANGEROUS if used in the acute asthmatic. It will further increase bronchoconstriction!

NALOXONE (Narcan)—specifically reverses narcotic intoxication. Has no narcotic action of its own.

NIFEDIPINE (Procardia)—a calcium channel-blocking agent that has vasodilatory effects on smooth muscle. It has virtually no effect on the cardiac conduction system.

NITROPRUSSIDE (Nipride)—a potent arterial vasodilator, useful IV in heart failure and hypertensive crisis.

NITROGLYCERIN—available in numerous forms (sublingual, IV, oral, transdermal, paste, and lingual spray); for the treatment of ischemia, hypertension, and heart failure.

NOREPINEPHRINE (Levophed)—a sympathomimetic amine used to raise the blood pressure by virtue of vasoconstriction. There is very little direct cardiac stimulation by this agent.

PARALDEHYDE—potent hypnotic agent useful in status epilepticus.

PHENOBARBITAL—potent barbiturate drug used in seizure control.

PHENYTOIN (Dilantin)—used as an antiseizure and antidysrhythmic preparation. Available in IV and oral forms.

PROPRANOLOL (Inderal)—a beta-blocker; blocks adrenergic receptors. Used for hypertension, dysrhythmia control, and in mitral valve prolapse.

PROTAMINE SULFATE—IV drug to immediately reverse the action of heparin. Has some intrinsic anticoagulant activity itself and must be monitored carefully.

QUINIDINE—antidysrhythmic agent available mostly for oral use.

RANITIDINE (Zantac)—newer agent similar to cimetidine.

RESERPINE—an antihypertensive agent useful also as a vasodilator and tranquilizer.

SALBUTAMOL—similar (but longer acting) to isoetharine.

SODIUM BICARBONATE—basic solution usually in 44 mEq ampules.

STREPTOKINASE—derived from the bacteria *Streptococcus*. Used as a thrombolytic agent. May cause severe allergic reactions in some.

TERBUTALINE (Brethine)—injectable and oral agent with similar effects to epinephrine.

THIAMINE (vitamin B_1)—usually lacking in alcoholics. Deficiency can lead to Wernicke's encephalopathy, a severe organic brain syndrome.

TRIMETHAPHAN—an antihypertensive agent that works via ganglionic blockade.

UROKINASE—thrombolytic agent derived from human urogenital tract cells.

Arterial Blood Gases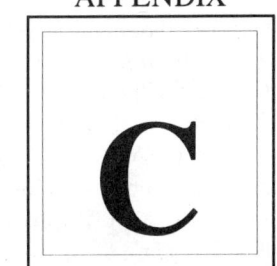

Arterial blood gas (ABG) determinations are frequently used in emergency medicine and referred to often in this text. The following is designed to be a brief discussion of ABGs which will present a simplified approach to reading and understanding them. If you desire further information, refer to the excellent discussion in the AHA *Advanced Cardiac Life Support Textbook.*

ABGs are drawn from an artery, usually percutaneously, into a heparanized syringe. Either the radial or brachial arteries are commonly used. During a CPR situation, the femoral is an easier "target." The blood is then placed into a special machine. The device measures several parameters and calculates a few others. For our purposes, we need only be concerned with the measured parameters.

Measured parameters include pH, pCO_2, and pO_2. The pH is a measure of the acidity or alkalinity of the blood. The "pX" function is mathematically defined as follows:

pX = − Logarithm (Base 10) of the concentration of X

Thus, the pH is defined as the negative logarithm of the hydrogen ion concentration. The $H+$ concentration is directly proportional to the acidity of the blood. More important than the mathematics is the fact that the pH scale is a logarithmic one. In other words, a change of .1 pH units represents a 10-fold change in the hydrogen ion concentration, a change of .2, a 100-fold change, and the like.

The normal pH of arterial blood is 7.40. An acceptable range is usually defined as 7.35–7.45. Values above this indicate the presence of a basic (alkalotic) state. Values below suggest an acidic con-

tent to the blood (acidosis). Technically, an alkalosis or acidosis refers to a *process* which results in the presence of either an alkalemia or an acidemia. This is a semantic point. For purposes of our discussion, we will use the terms interchangeably. Thus, the arterial blood pH indicates whether the blood is acidotic, alkalotic, or normal in terms of acid-base balance. This is illustrated in the examples below:

pH = 7.56 — too high ⟶ alkalosis
pH = 7.23 — too low ⟶ acidosis
pH = 7.38 — just right ⟶ normal

The pO_2 represents the **partial pressure of oxygen** in the arterial blood. It is measured in millimeters of mercury (mm Hg). This is NOT determined by the "pX" scale—only the pH is measured this way. The pO_2 is a direct measurement reflecting the oxygen concentration in the arterial blood. If you are interested, refer to a biochemistry text for a complete discussion of partial pressure determinations. The normal pO_2 depends on the altitude at which the individual is. Generally, on room air, the sea level pO_2 should be 80–100 mm Hg. Values considerably lower than this indicate room air hypoxia (lack of blood oxygen). The pO_2 should, of course, increase with the presence of supplemental O_2. There are formulas to calculate exactly how much, but this is beyond the intended focus of this discussion.

The pCO_2 represents the **partial pressure of carbon dioxide** in arterial blood. The units are the same as those for pO_2. Again, this is NOT determined by the "pX" scale. This number represents the concentration of carbon dioxide in arterial blood. The normal value (at all altitudes) averages 40 mm Hg. An acceptable range is 35–42 or so. As the pCO_2 increases, so does the acidity of the blood (i.e., the pH will *decrease*). As the pCO_2 decreases, the alkalinity (and pH) will *increase*. Changes in the pCO_2 are effected by respiration. Hyperventilation will "blow off" more CO_2, leading to a decreased pCO_2, thus an increased pH. In cases of respiratory failure, CO_2 is not "blown off" properly. It accumulates in the blood, leading to an increased pCO_2 and a decrease in the pH.

Changes in the pCO_2 always occur via the respiratory system. Factors determining how the lungs handle CO_2 may be either intrinsic to the respiratory system or extrinsic. In other words, high or low pCO_2s may be a *primary* response to a respiratory condition or a *secondary* response to some other problem elsewhere in the body. Usually, a secondary response occurs when a metabolic condition has changed the pH significantly. The body attempts to compensate by changing respiration to either increase or decrease by excretion of CO_2. This occurs relatively rapidly. When a primary respiratory problem changes the pCO_2 and, thus, the pH, the body also tries to compensate metabolically. This process takes a while longer and will not be discussed here.

Based on the above responses, we define acid-base deviations as either an alkalosis (basic, pH > 7.45) or acidosis (acid, pH < 7.35). Either condition can be caused by respiratory or metabolic problems. Depending on the time involved, either primary problem may be *partially compensated for* by a secondary process. This is not always the case, though. Generally, the conditions seen by the emergency care provider are either pure acidosis or pure alkalosis. A few significant exceptions are discussed in Chapter 3 on Respiratory Emergencies and will be mentioned again below.

Thus, a **pure respiratory acidosis** involves the retention (usually acutely) of CO_2 due to either hypoventilation (i.e., drug overdose) or intrinsic lung disease (COPD, ARDS). The pCO_2 is increased (> 42) and the pH is decreased below 7.35. The pO_2 is usually decreased but this value is irrelevant in diagnosing the acid-base state. It should be viewed *separately*! A **pure respiratory alkalosis** involves "blowing off" CO_2, usually due to hyperventilation (for any of a number of causes). The pCO_2 is decreased (below 35) and the pH increased above 7.45. Examples of ABGs demonstrating these con-

ditions are shown below:

Case 1—a 21-year-old male with acute respiratory failure from narcotic intoxication. Respiratory rate = 4/minute. pH = 7.20, pCO_2 = 60, pO_2 = 45. This patient is retaining CO_2 due to hypoventilation. The pH is *decreased*, indicating an acidosis. The pCO_2 is *increased*, indicating a **respiratory acidosis.**

Case 2—a 35-year-old female with pleuritic chest pain and a pulmonary embolism. Her respiratory rate is 35/min. pH = 7.60, pCO_2 = 20, pO_2 = 55. This patient is hyperventilating, thus "blowing off" CO_2. This lowers her pCO_2 and increases the blood pH. The increased pH indicates an alkalosis. The decreased pCO_2 defines a **respiratory alkalosis.**

A **pure metabolic acidosis** involves the retention of metabolic acids. The pH is *decreased*, indicating a higher hydrogen ion concentration (the H+ concentration is directly proportional to the acidity of the blood). The pCO_2, at least initially, is unchanged. A **pure metabolic alkalosis** occurs with loss of acid or massive increase in metabolic base. The pH is *increased* indicating a lower H+ ion concentration. Again, initially, the pCO_2 is unchanged. Examples of these processes are shown below:

Case 3—a 60-year-old male who goes into acute renal failure following an intravenous pyelogram (kidney X-ray using IV contrast). pH = 7.25, pCO_2 = 37, pO_2 = 70. The pH is decreased, indicating an **acidosis.** The pCO_2 is normal. This indicates that there is NO respiratory component. This indicates the patient has a **pure metabolic acidosis.**

Case 4—a 45-year-old woman who has received NG suction for the last 36 hours and inappropriate fluid replacement. (NG suction removes stomach acid and commonly leads to an alkalotic state.) pH = 7.56, pCO_2 = 35, pO_2 = 80. The pH is *increased*, indicating an **alkalosis.** The pCO_2 is *normal*, meaning, again, there is NO respiratory component. Thus, the patient has a **pure metabolic alkalosis.**

In many real-life situations, acid-base disturbances are mixed. There are many formulas to determine the contribution of each. These are beyond the intended scope of this discussion. There is a simpler way to get a rough idea of what is happening.:

1. *Look at the pH.* Is it high, low, or normal? A high pH defines an *alkalosis;* a low pH defines an *acidosis.* A normal pH may mean no acid-base disturbance or the result of two or more disturbances which "balance each other out."

2. *Look at the pCO_2.* If it is elevated, there is a component of respiratory acidosis. An *elevated pCO_2* with a *decreased pH =* **pure respiratory acidosis.** An *elevated pCO_2 with a normal* or *increased pH =* primary metabolic process *(alkalosis)* with a **compensatory respiratory acidosis.** If the pCO_2 is decreased, there is a component of respiratory alkalosis present. A *decreased pCO_2* with an *increased pH =* **pure respiratory alkalosis.** A *decreased pCO_2* with a *normal* or *decreased pH =* primary metabolic process (acidosis) with a **compensatory respiratory alkalosis.** In other words, the pCO_2 and pH should deviate in *opposite directions* in primary respiratory processes and in the *same direction* in compensatory respiratory processes. If the pCO_2 is normal, the acidosis/alkalosis is a primary metabolic problem with no significant attempt at respiratory compensation.

3. *Look at the pO_2.* You should also determine, in addition to acid-base status, if the patient is hypoxemic or not.

To the experienced reader, the above will seem a bit oversimplified at times. Nonetheless, this scheme seems to be far more helpful "under heat" than groups of formulas. All you really need to know is:

1. Is the patient acidotic/alkalotic?

2. If so, is it *primarily* a respiratory or a metabolic process?

3. Is the patient hypoxemic?

Using the above scheme will rapidly answer these questions. These principles are summarized below:

If by pH there is an acidosis and the pCO_2 is:
Elevated—pure respiratory acidosis
Decreased—metabolic acidosis with respiratory compensation
Normal—metabolic acidosis without respiratory compensation

If by pH there is an alkalosis and the pCO_2 is:
Decreased—pure respiratory alkalosis
Elevated—metabolic alkalosis with respiratory compensation
Normal—metabolic alkalosis without respiratory compensation

A few *case examples* will help in illustrating the utility of this system:

Case 5—a 35-year-old female with diabetic ketoacidosis. Her respiratory rate is 25. pH = 7.25, pCO_2 = 20, pO_2 = 110. The pH is *low* indicating an **acidosis.** The pCO_2 is also low. Thus, there is also a **respiratory alkalosis.** This suggests a **metabolic acidosis** (lowering the pH) with a **compensatory respiratory alkalosis** (hyperventilating in an attempt to correct the metabolic acidosis by creating a respiratory alkalosis). This is a commonly observed pattern in diabetic ketoacidosis.

Case 6—a 20-year-old male with an acute asthma attack. Despite three shots of epinephrine, he is still very "tight" and short of breath. His respiratory rate is 40. pH = 7.30, pCO_2 = 50, pO_2 = 59. The pH is *low* indicating an **acidosis.** The pCO_2 is *elevated.* Thus, this patient has a **respiratory acidosis.** There is also significant hypoxemia.

Case 7—a 65-year-old male with a "cold." He is coughing up copious amounts of greenish sputum. There is a known history of COPD. Patient's respiratory rate =

35/min. pH = 7.35, pCO_2 = 70, pO_2 = 50. (This is somewhat of a "trick" question but highly relevant). The pH is *normal* (a bit toward the low side). The pCO_2 is *elevated*. This suggests a **respiratory acidosis,** but why is the pH normal? The reason is because this patient is a chronic CO_2 retainer. His body has become used to this condition and fought it by developing a chronic **metabolic alkalosis.** If one measured the patient's serum bicarbonate level, they would find it to be markedly elevated, proving the hypothesis. Thus, this gentleman has a **primary respiratory acidosis with a compensatory metabolic alkalosis.**

Case 8—the same patient as in 7, except that he appears to be more obtunded. ABGs now show pH = 7.15, pCO_2 = 110, and pO_2 = 75. There is now a significant **acidosis.** The pCO_2 is *markedly elevated* indicating a severe **respiratory acidosis.** Thus, there is an **acute respiratory acidosis superimposed** upon a chronic **respiratory acidosis** with a **compensatory metabolic alkalosis.** This is exactly the type of acid-base pattern a chronic CO_2 retainer will develop when they acutely decompensate.

MAST Garment Update

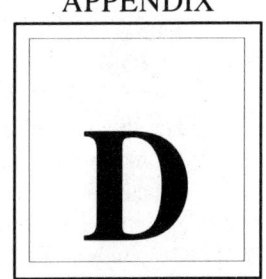

The use of a pressure suit for blood pressure control dates back to 1903 when an inflatable rubber suit was used to combat postural hypotension. Many years passed until the military initiated the use of G-suits (anti-gravity pants) designed to prevent loss of consciousness in pilots undergoing strenuous G-forces. A medical modification was also used on war casualties in Vietnam. Civilian use has caught on rapidly as the MAST garment (MAST suit) has been adopted for bleeding control and numerous other uses. An excellent review by K. R. Kaback et al. [*JAMA*, 1984, Vol. 252, p. 2598] serves as the basis for this discussion, though several other articles will be presented as well.

One of the most hotly debated topics in the emergency medicine literature today is the physiology of the MAST suit. Originally, it was taught that the garment increases blood pressure due to an "autotransfusion" of up to two units of blood (500–1000 cc). Several studies have suggested that the primary action is really by increasing the systemic vascular resistance (constricting blood vessels) as well as by tamponading bleeding vessels. The *JAMA* article cites much evidence to this effect. Other studies, though, have suggested at least a component of "autotransfusion," though the literature must be examined carefully.

A study on baboons [Holcroft, J. W., et al., Venous Return and the Pneumatic Antishock Garment in Hypovolemic Baboons, *Journal of Trauma,* 1984, Vol. 24, p. 928] made hypovolemic and "masted" showed that inflation of the MAST suit increased the driving pressure for venous return in some animals. Unfortunately, at the *same time,* the venous resistance increased so that the net effect was NO increase in

the cardiac preload (i.e., venous return, "autotransfusion effect"). This increased resistance was thought secondary to compression of the vena cava and veins to the abdominal organs. Blood pressure did increase in the animals. The authors suggest increased resistance with diversion of flow to the upper body as a mechanism. They also feel that tamponade of bleeding and stabilization of fractures in an indication for the garment.

In a swine model, the effects of MAST inflation with and without hypovolemia were studied (Bellamy, R. F., et al., Immediate Hemodynamic Consequences of MAST Inflation in Normo- and Hypovolemic Anesthetized Swine, *J of Trauma,* 1984, Vol. 24, p. 889]. Inflation of the suit lead to an increase in the mean aortic pressure (MAP) of 25% in normovolemic and 62% in hemorrhaged animals. Though the cardiac output was unchanged in the control group, it increased 41% following MAST garment inflation in the hemorrhage group. Systemic vascular resistance increased 32% in the control and 16% in the hemorrhage group. The authors noted that MAST inflation translocated about 3 ml/kg of blood in both groups (measured using tracer studies).

There was no change in myocardial, cerebral, hepatic, small intestinal, or renal blood flow in the control group. There was a 50% increase in coronary perfusion and a 33% increase in cerebral perfusion following MAST inflation in the hemorrhage group. The authors caution that their results may not be immediately applicable to human beings for many reasons but nonetheless feel that the MAST suit has its effect at least partially by increasing preload. There appear to be other factors as well, as 3 ml/kg is far less than two units of whole blood!

In humans with adult respiratory distress syndrome (ARDS) ventilated with positive end expiratory pressure (PEEP), the ability of MAST inflation to predict the response of the patient to a fluid challenge has been studied. PEEP tends to cause hypotension by decreasing venous return and perhaps by changing the geometry of the heart muscle itself. It often responds to fluid infusion. It is the better part of valor to keep patients with ARDS on the "dry" side if at all possible. Thus, this was an ideal way to try and see if additional fluid would benefit without potential risks of necessarily giving the fluid first. Thus, this article investigated MAST garment use as a form of "reversible fluid challenge" [Jastremski, M. S., and Beney, K. M., Military Antishock Trouser (MAST): Application as a Reversible Fluid Challenge in Patients on High Peep, *Chest,* 1984, Vol. 85, pp. 595–599].

Patients on high PEEP with a cardiac index less than 4 L/min had the leg compartments then the abdominal compartment of the MAST suit inflated. Aortic pressure was measured and the suit then slowly deflated. Fluid boluses were given to maintain the blood pressure. The volume of fluid necessary to maintain the increase in blood pressure brought about by MAST inflation was determined to average 2,974 cc per patient! When ventricular function curves were plotted, it appeared that the improvement in cardiac output and blood pressure was due to an increased preload. These authors conclude that in this population the MAST garment 1) increases blood pressure and cardiac output by increasing preload (venous return), and 2) predicts the ability of the patient to respond to a fluid challenge. It is unknown why the average amount of fluid required was well above the "two unit autotransfusion" supposedly provided by the MAST suit. Is it possible the device "transfuses" more than two units? Or is there a combination effect of increasing preload and perhaps another factor? The answer is not clear from this study.

After reviewing this data, it is safe to conclude that the MAST garment appears to increase the blood pressure in many models. It is likely that the mechanism by which hypotension is reversed differs depending on the clinical situation. It is possible that several mechanisms may be operative together. It does not appear that the "autotransfusion theory" is completely ruled out nor that the "increased SVR" totally proven at this time.

Let's discuss indications for the MAST garment. Obviously, the most common is hypovolemic shock. This can be from bleeding, trauma, sepsis, a ruptured aneurysm, or ectopic pregnancy. The suit MAY be of help in hypotension secondary to decreased cardiac output (though increased SVR may actually HURT the heart). In cardiac tamponade and tension pneumothorax, MAST inflation may act as a temporizing measure until definitive therapy can be performed, despite the fact that it may elevate an already increased central venous pressure. Human studies are lacking.

One study conducted by Mackersie et al. in San Francisco [The Prehospital Use of External Counterpressure: Does MAST Make a Difference, *J of Trauma,* 1984, Vol. 24, p. 882] suggests that in an urban setting MAST inflation in trauma patients with short transport times had NO demonstrable effect on the trauma score, BP, or mortality. Interestingly, though, the study also showed NO delay in transport time by using the MAST suit. Another study of MAST in an urban setting with hypotensive penetrating trauma victims concluded that the suit offered ". . . no specific advantage in an urban paramedic-regional trauma center system that is closely scrutinized . . . by full-time physician supervision that emphasizes rapid response and evacuation along with aggressive prehospital airway management and immediate in-hospital surgical intervention" [*Ann Emerg, Med,* December 1986, Vol. 15, p. 1407]. The reader should be aware that there is NOT uniform agreement in reference to these investigators' conclusions. The populations studied and geographical restrictions limit widespread conclusions in regards to this device.

Application of the MAST garment was part of one group's standard protocol (along with the prehospital IVs and intubation) in penetrating trauma. Extremely high survival rates were reported, with no evidence to suggest that in this particular urban setting (Denver, Colorado) that paramedic intervention was detrimental (Pons, P. T., et. al, Prehospital Advanced Trauma Life Support for Critical Penetrating Wounds to the Thorax and Abdomen, *J of Trauma,* 1985, Vol. 25, p. 828].

Additional indications include stabilization of fractures. Most amenable are those of the femur, lower leg, and pelvis. The MAST suit may be used to effect hemostasis in ruptured aortic aneurysms, post-renal biopsy bleeding, postoperatively, and in severe pelvic fractures. It may also be used on external bleeding sites if other methods have failed. The suit's use as a "reversible fluid challenge" is somewhat debatable, as mentioned, but many still use it for this purpose.

A final very helpful role is the MAST suit's prophylactic placement in air and ground ambulance transfers. If the patient gets into trouble, the suit only need be inflated. This is especially useful in an aircraft. In most smaller cabins, it is impossible to put the suit on the patient AFTER an emergency has occurred. Thus, prophylactic placement (while still on the ground) is the only viable alternative in a high-risk patient.

Possible contraindications to the use of the MAST garment will now be discussed. Pulmonary edema is an absolute contraindication. Irrespective of how the suit works, both increased venous return (preload) and/or an increase in afterload (arterial resistance) is bad for the failing heart. The inflation of the abdominal compartment is contraindicated in pregnancy, evisceration, and when there is an impaled object in the abdomen.

The optimum inflation pressure is another widely debated point. Many authors feel gauges to be unnecessary. Others feel strongly about not exceeding certain pressures. The ultimate end point is the patient's blood pressure. Most of the literature would suggest that with the exception of fracture stabilization, higher pressures may be better (see below for controversy!). It is very important to keep in mind the environmental effects on the suit pressure. It will increase with increasing altitude (i.e., in an airplane) and temperature (as well as vice-versa).

Many potential complications of the MAST suit are discussed in the literature. Changes in pulmonary function are theoretically possible. The weight of the evidence suggests they are unlikely to occur. There may be slight increases in intracranial pressure, but this appears more than compensated for by increased cerebral perfusion pressure resulting from an increase in the MAP! Some have suggested renal compromise may occur. There is no documented evidence proving this point.

A compartment syndrome results from ischemic necrosis to muscle and nerves with a fascial compartment. This is particularly applicable in the legs, where several separate fascial compartments exist. Although rare overall, several case reports do exist of MAST garment inflation causing this horrible problem. The externally applied pressure from the suit is transmitted all the way to the muscle compartment in at least 90% of cases (Chisholm, C.D., and Clark, D.E.: Effect of the pneumatic antishock garment on intramuscular pressure. *Ann Emerg Med*, August 1984, Vol. 3, pp. 581-583) leading to the recommendation that the lowest pressure possible be used.

Bilateral iliofemoral thrombosis was reported to occur following MAST suit inflation in a critically ill patient with a nifedipine overdose. The inflation time was well over *four hours* [*Ann Emerg Med*, December 1984, Vol. 13, pp. 1155–1157). The authors, M. W. Frampton and colleagues, suggest that further evaluation of the garment's use in nonhemorrhagic shock is needed.

It appears that compartment syndromes and thrombotic events can occur from MAST suit inflation. *Every* case report of this documents inflation time well over two hours! All standard MAST protocols clearly state that the use of the garment over two hours is NOT recommended.

The inflation of the suit may lead to accumulation of some acid waste products in the legs, especially if there is a "shunting" effect of the circulation to the upper body. Some fear that releasing the leg compartments will "flood" the system and create severe problems. There is some basis for this fear in that a slight decrease in pH DOES occur. It is easily managed, though, by monitoring the pH and using $NaHCO_3$ and ventilation as necessary to control it.

A final concern is that MAST garment inflation might eliminate the possibility of using leg veins for venous access. No good human studies are available but some dog studies are reassuring [*Ann Emerg Med*, October 1984, Vol. 13, pp. 885–890]. In this study, MAST suit inflation during CPR had no effect on venous injections into distal hindlimbs.

A couple rather "experimental" uses of the MAST garment include its utility in CPR and in dysrhythmias. There have been reports in which the inflation of a MAST garment elevated the blood pressure leading to conversion of supraventricular tachycardia. There are many studies using the MAST suit during CPR. Some document increased carotid flow, others increased blood pressure. On the other hand, there is a body of information suggesting that abdominal binding may be harmful. The role of the MAST suit in CPR is uncertain. There is an unwritten rule in many locations that a MAST garment is automatically applied and inflated on any cardiac arrest victim. Many experts are uncomfortable universally recommending this based on the current literature.

All in all, the MAST garment is controversial, to say the least. True evidence of human efficacy is present, but only to a small degree. Many experts feel that this device helps save lives. More definitive indications will hopefully be forthcoming as further research studies, animal and human, emerge.

Bibliography

Abbot J., et al, *Protocols for Prehospital Emergency Medical Care.* Williams & Wilkins, Baltimore: 1980.

Allen, J. C., and Beam, T. R., *Infectious Disease for the House Officer.* Williams & Wilkins, Baltimore: 1982.

Baldwin, L., and Pierce, R. *Mobile Intensive Care, A Problem-Oriented Approach.* C.V. Mosby Company, St. Louis: 1978.

Barber, J. M., and Budassi, S. A. *Manual of Emergency Care, Practices & Procedures.* C.V. Mosby Company, St. Louis: 1979.

Beary, J. E., et. al, ed. *Manual of Rheumatology and Outpatient Orthopedic Disorders.* Little, Brown & Company, Boston: 1981.

Braker, Wm., et al., *Effects of Exposure to Toxic Gases—First Aid and Medical Treatment,* 2nd edition. Matheson, Lyndhyrst: 1972.

Buttarvoli, P. M., and Stair, T. O., *Common Simple Emergencies.* Brady Communications Company, Inc., Bowie: 1985.

Campbell, J. W., and Frisse, M., ed. *Manual of Medical Therapeutics,* 24th edition. Little, Brown & Company, Boston: 1983.

Cane, R. D., and Shapiro, B. A., *Case Studies in Critical Care Medicine.* Year Book Medical Publishers, Inc., Chicago: 1985.

Committee on Trauma, American College of Surgeons, *Advanced Trauma Life Support Student Manual,* Chicago: 1981.

Cowley, R. A., and Dunham, C. M. *Shock Trauma/Critical Care Manual,* University Park Press, Baltimore: 1982.

Hanson, Wm., Jr., ed. *Clinics in Emergency Medicine* (Volume 5—Toxic Emergencies). Churchill-Livingston, New York: 1984.

Jacobs, L. M., Jr., and Bennett, B. R. *Emergency Patient Care—Prehospital Ground and Air Procedures.* Macmillan Publishing Company, New York: 1983.

Kizer, K. W., ed. *Emergency Medicine Clinics of North America* (Volume 2—Environmental Emergencies). W.B. Saunders Company, Philadelphia: 1984.

Kwaan, H. C., and Rosen, S. T. *Modern Concepts of Cardiovascular Disease.* Year Book Medical Publishers, Inc., Chicago: September 1984.

McIntyre, K. M., and Lewis, A. J., ed. *Textbook of Advanced Cardiac Life Support,* American Heart Association, Dallas: 1983.

Montana Emergency Services Bureau. *Montana Basic Life Support Field Protocols.* State of Montana: 1982.

National Diving Accident Network, *Diving Accident Manual,* 1981.

Nowak, R. M., and Tomlanovich, M. C., ed. *Emergency Medicine Clinics of North America* (Volume 1—Adult Respiratory Emergencies). W. B. Saunders Company, Philadelphia: 1983.

O'Dorisio, T. M., and Cataland, S. "Symptomatic Hypercalcemia." In *Emergency Medicine Survey,* Williams & Wilkins, Baltimore: 1984.

Rippe, J. M., and Csete, M. E., ed. *Manual of Intensive Care Medicine.* Little, Brown & Company, Boston: 1983.

Rosen, P., et al., ed. *Emergency Medicine—Concepts and Clinical Practice,* C. V. Mosby Company, St. Louis: 1983.

Samuels, M. A., ed. *Manual of Neurologic Therapeutics.* Little, Brown & Company, Boston: 1978.

Schwatz, G. R., et al., ed. *Principles and Practices of Emergency Medicine.* W. B. Saunders Company, Philadelphia: 1978.

Shoemaker, W. C., et al., ed. *Textbook of Critical Care.* W. B. Saunders Company, Philadelphia: 1984.

Shoemaker, W. C., and Thompson, W. L., ed. *Critical Care—State of the Art* (Volume 3). Society of Critical Care Medicine, Fullerton: 1982.

Schrier, R. W., ed. *Manual of Nephrology.* Little, Brown & Company, Boston: 1981.

Schrier, R. W., ed. *Renal & Electrolyte Disorders.* Little, Brown & Company, Boston: 1976.

Tintinalli, J. E., ed. *Emergency Medicine Clinics of North America* (Volume 1—Resuscitation). W.B. Saunders Company, Philadelphia: 1983.

Waterbury, L. *Hematology for the House Officer.* Williams & Wilkins, Baltimore: 1981.

Wyngaarden and Smith, *Cecil Textbook of Medicine,* 17th edition. W.B. Saunders Company, Philadelphia: 1985.

Yates, A. P., et al., *Emergency—A Practical Manual.* Synapse, Pittsburgh: 1978.

Index